T0091834

High-Risk IV Medications
in Special Patient Populations

Sandra L. Kane-Gill • Joseph Dasta

(Editors)

High-Risk IV Medications in Special Patient Populations

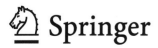

Springer

Editors
Sandra L. Kane-Gill, Pharm.D., M.Sc.,
FCCP, FCCM
Associate Professor of Pharmacy
and Therapeutics
University of Pittsburgh
School of Pharmacy
Center for Pharmacoinformatics
and Outcomes Research
Pittsburgh, PA
USA

Prof. Joseph Dasta, M.Sc., FCCM, FCCP
The Ohio State University, Ohio
USA

ISBN 978-0-85729-605-4   e-ISBN 978-0-85729-606-1
DOI 10.1007/978-0-85729-606-1
Springer London Dordrecht Heidelberg New York

British Library Cataloguing in Publication Data
A catalogue record for this book is available from the British Library

Library of Congress Control Number: 2011932318

Cover design: eStudioCalamar, Figueres/Berlin

Printed on acid-free paper

Springer is part of Springer Science+Business Media (www.springer.com)

Sandy: I dedicate this book to my husband, Michael and my parents, Bob and Lucille. Their love and support is greatly appreciated.
Joe: I dedicate this book to my loving and supportive wife Desma and our daughter Dana.

Preface

Critically ill patients are at risk for a higher frequency and severity of adverse drug events (ADEs) compared to non-critically ill patients. A contributing factor to this risk is the use of high-risk medications in the treatment of critically ill patients, often in combination. High-risk medications as defined by the Institute for Safe Medication Practices are drugs when used in error increases the risk for injury to the patient. The Joint Commission defines high-risk medications as "medications involved in a high percentage of medication errors or sentinel events and medications that carry a high risk for abuse, error, or other adverse outcomes". According to the Institute for Safe Medication Practice's list, many high-risk medications are those administered intravenously (IV), which is a more common route of administration in critically ill patients. Also, the therapeutic categories for high-risk medications are drugs more frequently administered to patients in the intensive care unit. Examples of high-risk medications include anticoagulants, opioids, sedatives, anti-hypertensives, anti-infectives, and electrolytes. Regulatory bodies are requiring active institutional surveillance of high-risk medications. Hypervigilant monitoring of high-risk medications is necessary to prevent patient harm, especially in populations that have dosing challenges.

Special patient populations typically refer to individuals that deviate from the norm. When prescribing medications, there are subsets of individuals that require specific dosing considerations. Special patient populations for purposes of this book are considered individuals that require atypical dosing considerations of drugs due to non-average weight (overweight and underweight), hepatic or renal dysfunction, extracorporeal circulation devices, advanced age, pharmacogenetic alterations, are hemodynamically unstable, or require therapeutic hypothermia. In general, critically ill patients constitute a majority of this special patient population. Dosing challenges are a safety concern in these special patient populations since there is a risk of unwanted ADEs from overdosing and therapeutic inefficacy from underdosing. Often, the lack of data on dosing in special patient populations requires clinicians to extrapolate pharmacokinetic drug characteristics based in either volunteers or non-ICU patients to estimate appropriate doses in the critically ill.

Dosing challenges of high-risk medications in special patient populations further compounds the risk of injury to the patient. This book will review high-risk IV medication dosage considerations for special patient populations. Also, safety concerns of high-risk medications are discussed to aid the clinician in cautious monitoring. The goal of this book is to provide clinicians with tools to minimize adverse drug events with IV high-risk medications while proving maximal beneficial clinical effects of these drugs to the critically ill.

Contents

Contributors

Mitchell S. Buckley, Pharm.D.
Department of Pharmacy
Banner Good Samaritan Medical Center
Phoenix, AZ, USA

**James C. Coons, Pharm.D., BCPS
(AQ Cardiology)**
Department of Pharmacy
Allegheny General Hospital
Pittsburgh, PA, USA

Sandeep Devabhakthuni, Pharm.D.
Department of Pharmacy
University of Pittsburgh Medical Center
Pittsburgh, PA, USA

**John W. Devlin, Pharm.D., BCPS
FCCM, FCCP**
Pharmacy Practice
Northeastern University
Boston, MA, USA

**Sandra L. Kane-Gill, Pharm.D.,
M.Sc., FCCP, FCCM**
Associate Professor of Pharmacy and
Therapeutics, University of Pittsburgh,
School of Pharmacy, Center for
Pharmacoinformatics and Outcomes
Research, Pittsburgh, PA, USA

Jaclyn M. LeBlanc, Pharm.D., BCPS
Department of Pharmacy
Saint John Regional Hospital
(Horizon Health Network)
Saint John, NB, Canada

Robert MacLaren, B.Sc., Pharm.D.
Department of Clinical Pharmacy
University of Colorado Denver School
of Pharmacy, Aurora, CO, USA

Dorothy McCoy, Pharm.D., BCPS-ID
Department of Pharmacy Practice and
Administration, Ernest Mario School
of Pharmacy, Piscataway, NJ, USA

Scott W. Mueller, Pharm.D.
Department of Clinical Pharmacy
University of Colorado Denver School
of Pharmacy, Aurora, CO, USA

**Marilee D. Obritsch, Pharm.D.,
BCPS**
Department of Pharmacy
Hillcrest Medical Center, Tulsa
OK, USA

Christopher A. Paciullo, Pharm.D.
Department of Pharmaceutical Services
Emory University Hospital, Atlanta
GA, USA

**Pamela L. Smithburger, Pharm.D.
BCPS**
Department of Pharmacy and
Therapeutics, University of Pittsburgh,
Pittsburgh, PA, USA

Zachariah Thomas, Pharm.D.
Department of Pharmacy Practice and
Administration, Ernest Mario School
of Pharmacy, Piscataway, NJ, USA

Abbreviations

α	alpha
ABW	actual body weight
ACC	American College of Cardiology
ACCP	American College of Chest Physicians
ACE	angiotensin converting enzyme
ACS	acute coronary syndrome
ACT	activated clotting time
ADE	adverse drug event
A-fib	atrial fibrillation
AHA	American Heart Association
ALT	alanine aminotransferase
aPTT	activated partial thromboplastin time
ARB	Angiotensin receptor blocker
ARDS	acute respiratory distress syndrome
ARF	acute renal failure
AST	aspartate aminotransferase
AT	antithrombin
AUC	area under the curve
AUC24	area under the 0–24 concentration time curve
AV	atrioventricular
β	beta
BMI	body mass index
BP	blood pressure
BUN	blood urea nitrogen
CABG	coronary artery bypass grafting
CAPD	Continuous ambulatory peritoneal dialysis
CAVHF	Continuous arterio-venous hemofiltration
CCPD	Continuous cyclic peritoneal dialysis
C_{max}	maximum concentration
CNS	central nervous system
CO	cardiac output
COMT	catechol-O-methyl transferase

CrCl	creatinine clearance
CRI	chronic renal insufficiency
CRRT	continuous renal replacement therapy
C_{ss}	steady-state drug concentration
CVA	cerebrovascular accident
CVVHD	continuous veno-venous hemodialysis
CVVHDF	Continuous veno-venous hemodiafiltration
CVVHF	Continuous veno-venous hemofiltration
CYP	cytochrome P450
d	day
DA	dopamine
DA-2	dopamine type-2
DFT	defibrillation threshold
DOB	dobutamine
DrotAA	drotrecogin alpha activated
DTI	direct thrombin inhibitors
DVT	deep vein thrombosis
DW	dosing weight
EARLY_ACS	The Early Glycoprotein IIb/IIIa Inhibition in Non-ST-Segment Elevation Acute Coronary Syndrome Trial
EKG	electrocardiogram
EPI	epinephrine
EPIC	Evaluation of c7E3 for the Prevention of Ischemic Complications
EPILOG	Evaluation in PTCA to Improve Long-Term Outcome with Abciximab GP IIb/IIIa Blockade
EPISTENT	Evaluation of Platelet IIb/IIIa Inhibitor for Stenting
ESPRIT	Enhanced Suppression of the Platelet IIb/IIIa Receptor with Integrilin Therapy trial
ESSENCE	Efficacy Safety Subcutaneous Enoxaparin in Non-Q-wave Coronary Events
EXTRACT	The Enoxaparin and Thrombolysis Reperfusion for Acute Myocardial Infarction Treatment
FDA	Food and Drug Administration
GABA	γ-aminobutyric acid
GI	gastrointestinal
GP	glycoprotein
GU	genitourinary
GUSTO	Global Utilization of Streptokinase and Tissue Plasminogen Activator for Occluded Arteries
HD	hemodialysis
HIT	heparin-induced thrombocytopenia
IBW	ideal body weight
ICD	internal cardiodefibrillator
ICH	intracranial hemorrhage
ICU	intensive care unit

INR	international normalized ratio
ISO	isoproterenol
IU	international units
IV	intravenous
kg	kilogram
L	liter
LMWH	low-molecular-weight heparin
MAO	monoamine oxidase
MAP	mean arterial pressure
mcg	microgram
mg	milligram
MI	myocardial infarction
MIC	minimum inhibitory concentration
MIL	milrinone
min	minute
mL	milliliters
NE	norepinephrine
NNRTIs	non-nucleoside reverse transcriptase inhibitors
NS	normal saline
NSAIDs	non-steroidal anti-inflammatory drugs
NSTEMI	non-ST-segment elevation myocardial infarction
OR	odds ratio
PAI	plasminogen activator inhibitor
PCI	percutaneous coronary intervention
PE	pulmonary embolism
PK	pharmacokinetic
PRISM-PLUS	Platelet Receptor Inhibition in Ischemic Syndrome Management in Patients Limited by Unstable Signs and Symptoms trial
PROWESS	Protein C Worldwide Evaluation in Severe Sepsis
PT	prothrombin time
PVC	polyvinyl chloride
q	day once daily
RF	renal failure
RR	relative risk
SBECD	sulfobutylether-beta-cyclodextrin
SC	subcutaneously
SCCM	Society of Critical Care Medicine
SCr	serum creatinine
SLE	systemic lupus erythematosus
SOFA	Sequential Organ Failure Assessment
STEMI	ST-segment-elevation myocardial infarction
SVR	systemic vascular resistance
SYNERGY	The Superior Yield of the New Strategy of Enoxaparin, Revascularization and Glycoprotein IIb/IIa Inhibitors
T3/T4	thyroid hormones 3 and 4

TARGET	Do Tirofiban and Abciximab Give Similar Efficacy Trial
TdP	Torsades de Pointes
TIMI	thrombolysis in myocardial infarction
T_{max}	time to reach Cmax
tPA	tissue plasminogen activator
TRH	thyrotropin-releasing hormone
TSH	thyroid-stimulating hormone
U	units
UA	unstable angina
UFH	unfractionated heparin
VASO	vasopressin
V_d	volume of distribution
VT	ventricular tachycardia
VTE	venous thromboembolism
WHO	World Health Organization

Chapter 1
Thrombolytics/Anticoagulants

James C. Coons and Sandeep Devabhakthuni

Introduction

Critically ill patients are at an increased risk of venous thromboembolism, which is a common complication that is associated with significant mortality and requires appropriate anticoagulation.[1,2] Recently, anticoagulants have been identified as high-alert medications by the Institute for Healthcare Improvement and the Institute for Safe Medication Practices because of their risk for significant patient harm if misused.[2] A study by Fanikos and colleagues demonstrates that 1.67 medication errors occur for every 1,000 patients receiving anticoagulation therapy, and unfractionated heparin (UFH) accounts for a majority (66.2%) of medication errors. Furthermore, approximately 6.2% of patients affected by anticoagulant errors require some type of medical intervention, and 1.5% of patients experience prolonged hospitalization due to anticoagulant effects.[3] The most common types of medication errors regarding anticoagulant use are omission (29%), improper dose/quantity (27.9%), and prescribing (14.5%) errors.[4]

Improper anticoagulant dosing and prescribing errors occur because of various factors in critically ill patients including significant changes in pharmacokinetics and pharmacodynamics, both of which require dose adjustments or heightened awareness for increased susceptibility to adverse events such as bleeding.[5] Another concern is that most anticoagulants require weight-based dosing. Many anticoagulants are dosed according to actual (not ideal) body weight in the intensive care setting, which can lead to underestimation and overestimation, resulting in lack of effectiveness and adverse drug events, respectively.

J.C. Coons (✉)
Department of Pharmacy, Allegheny General Hospital,
Pittsburgh, PA, USA
e-mail: jcoons@wpahs.org

S.L. Kane-Gill and J. Dasta (eds.),
High-Risk IV Medications in Special Patient Populations,
DOI: 10.1007/978-0-85729-606-1_1, © Springer-Verlag London Limited 2011

This chapter will review dosing considerations based on these factors as well as safety concerns for each anticoagulant commonly used in critically ill patients.

Direct Thrombin Inhibitors (Argatroban, Bivalirudin, Lepirudin)

Dosing Considerations

Obesity: Pharmacodynamic and pharmacokinetic properties of direct thrombin inhibitors are summarized in Table 1.1.[6-10] Much of the limited data regarding dosing for obese patients are derived from clinical experience with argatroban.[12,13] Based on available evidence for argatroban, dose adjustment is not required in obese patients up to a body mass index (BMI) of 51 kg/m². In 83 patients (32 obese patients) with suspected heparin-induced thrombocytopenia (HIT) and actual body weights of 40.9–130 kg (BMI 15.5–50.8 kg/m²), argatroban dosing requirements, activated partial thromboplastin time (aPTT) responses, and clinical outcomes were similar between obese (BMI ≥ 30 kg/m²) and nonobese patients.[12] Also, similar therapeutic levels of anticoagulation were achieved with infusion rates of 1 mcg/kg/min in obese patients compared to nonobese patients, and the thrombotic risk in HIT was not shown to be affected by BMI.

In the interventional setting such as a percutaneous coronary intervention (PCI), higher doses of argatroban are recommended.[6] The effect of this higher dosing regimen for argatroban in the setting of PCI was studied in 225 patients (85 obese patients) with BMI of 16.3–50.9 kg/m². The authors concluded that there was no association between BMI and the first activated clotting time (ACT) after bolus

Table 1.1 Comparison of clinical properties of direct thrombin inhibitors[6-10]

Property	Argatroban	Bivalirudin (Angiomax®)	Lepirudin (Refludan®)
Binding to thrombin[a]	Reversible	Partially reversible	Irreversible
Elimination half-life	40–50 min	25 min	1.3–2 h
Primary route of elimination	Hepatic	Renal (20%) Enzymatic (80%)	Renal
Effect on INR	Increase	Slight increase	Slight increase
Dialyzability	Yes (20%)	Yes (25%)	Yes[b]
Anti-hirudin antibody development	No	May cross-react with anti-hirudin antibodies	Yes (up to 60% of patients)[c]

INR international normalized ratio
[a]No antidote exists for any of the direct thrombin inhibitors
[b]High-flux dialyzers with polysulfone membranes are the most effective means of removal[11]
[c]Development of antibodies can lead to lepirudin-antihirudin complexes, which can lead to decreased renal clearance, resulting in potential increased anticoagulant effect

administration, mean infusion dose, need for additional boluses, or time to ACT ≤ 160 s after argatroban cessation. Also, clinical outcomes did not differ between obese and nonobese patients in experiencing ischemic or hemorrhagic complications. Thus, dose adjustment for obesity in both non-interventional and interventional setting is not needed for argatroban.

No formal evaluations of dosing considerations in obesity have been conducted for bivalirudin or lepirudin. Experience with dosing these agents is from large clinical trials that included obese patients. The highest reported weight for patients who were enrolled in bivalirudin clinical trials was 199 kg.[14-16] However, no formal post-hoc analyses were performed examining weight as an influence on clinical and bleeding outcomes for any of these clinical trials. For lepirudin, the manufacturer recommends that in patients who weight ≥110 kg, the maximum weight of 110 kg should be used when determining the appropriate dose.[8]

Thinness/emaciation: There are very limited data on dosing considerations in underweight or nutritionally deficient patients. In the clinical trials assessing safety and efficacy, the lowest reported weights among patients receiving argatroban and bivalirudin were 40.9 kg[13] and 35 kg[14], respectively. In a large, randomized trial, 10,141 patients diagnosed with a non-ST-segment elevation acute coronary syndrome were randomized to receive a 72-h treatment with lepirudin (bolus: 0.4 mg/kg, infusion: 0.15 mg/kg/h) or standard unfractionated heparin (bolus: 5,000 Us, infusion: 15 U/kg/h).[17] The patients in the lepirudin group received the same regimen, regardless of body weight. Hemorrhagic adverse events were stratified based on body weight for analysis (98 patients weighed < 50 kg, 4,720 patients weighed 50–100 kg, and 228 patients weighed > 100 kg). Patients who received lepirudin and weighed < 50 kg had a two-fold higher incidence of hemorrhage (16.33% vs. 8.64% vs. 9.65%, respectively) whereas patients receiving heparin had similar incidence, regardless of body weight. Because lepirudin dosage was not adjusted for patients < 50 kg, this probably led to overdosage in this subgroup. Therefore, it would be reasonable to lower the initial lepirudin loading dose and initial maintenance infusion by 25–50% in patients with very low body weight.[8,17]

Kidney Injury: Pharmacokinetic considerations (Table 1.1) demonstrate that both lepirudin and bivalirudin are affected by renal impairment, whereas argatroban is primarily affected by hepatic dysfunction.[6-8] Table 1.2 provides an overview of dosing recommendations based on clinical studies that were recently conducted for evaluation of renal or hepatic impairment. Table 1.3 summarizes the available data on dosing considerations in renal impairment for all three direct thrombin inhibitors. The retrospective nature of these trials limits the dosing recommendations; however, no prospective, controlled trials have been conducted.

No initial dose adjustment is necessary for argatroban in renal impairment.[25,26] One study demonstrated by regression analysis that each 30 mL/min decrease in creatinine clearance corresponded to a decrease in the therapeutic dose of ~0.1–0.6 mcg/kg/min.[26] Thus, it is imperative to monitor aPTT closely and readjust argatroban therapy appropriately. Pharmacokinetic data have not been reported in patients with renal impairment in the setting of a PCI.

Table 1.2 Dosing recommendations for direct thrombin inhibitors in renal or hepatic impairment[6-8,18-24]

Agent	Dose adjustment in renal impairment	Dose adjustment in hepatic impairment
Argatroban	Not necessary Exception: concomitant hepatic impairment or medical conditions affecting hepatic perfusion (e.g., heart failure, anasarca, or multiple organ damage)[a]	Infusion: initiate at 0.5 mcg/kg/min then titrate to aPTT 1.5–3.0 × baseline
Bivalirudin (Angiomax®)	Bolus: no adjustment necessary Management of ACS involving PCI: Infusion: CrCl < 30 mL/min: 1 mg/kg/h HD: 0.25 mg/kg/h Management of HIT: Infusion: CrCl > 60 mL/min: 0.15 mg/kg/h CrCl 30–60 mL/min: 0.08–1 mg/kg/h CrCl < 30 mL/min or CRRT: 0.03–0.05 mg/kg/h	Not necessary
Lepirudin (Refludan®)	Bolus: 0.2–0.4 mg/kg (should be avoided in patients with renal impairment) Infusion: CrCl > 60 mL/min: 0.075 mg/kg/h CrCl 30–60 mL/min: 0.045 mg/kg/h CrCl < 30 mL/min: 0.0225 mg/kg/h HD: initial dose of 0.05–0.1 mg/kg and repeat intravenous bolus doses of 0.1 mg/kg if aPTT ratio is below 1.5 CRRT: initial dose of 0.1–0.2 mg/kg then repeat intravenous bolus doses of 0.05–0.1 mg/kg if aPTT ratio is below 1.5 **OR** Continuous infusion: 0.005–0.01 mg/kg/h	Not necessary

CrCl creatinine clearance calculated by using the Cockcroft-Gault equation, *HD* hemodialysis, *aPTT* activated partial thromboplastin time, *ACS* acute coronary syndrome, *PCI* percutaneous coronary intervention, *HIT* heparin-induced thrombocytopenia, *CRRT* continuous renal replacement therapy

[a]Dose adjustments similar to those recommended for hepatic impairment only

Table 1.3 Selected clinical trials on use of direct thrombin inhibitors in renal impairment

Reference	Agent	Study design	Study n/N[a]	Dosing	Outcomes	Renal function[b]			p Value
						Normal (CrCl >60 mL/min)	Moderate (CrCl = 30–60 mL/min)	Severe (CrCl <30 mL/min)	
Hursting et al.[25]	Argatroban	Retrospective study in non-HIT patients undergoing PCI	26/152	Load: 250–300 mcg/kg Maintenance: 15 mcg/kg/min	Death	0/126 (0%)		0/26 (0%)	1.0
					MI	2/126 (1.6%)		0/26 (0%)	1.0
					Major bleeding	2/126 (1.6%)		0/26 (0%)	1.0
Guzzi et al.[26]	Argatroban	Retrospective	116/260	2 mcg/kg/min	Death (any cause)	24/144 (16.7%)	9/80 (11.2%)	13/36 (36.1%)	p<0.017[b]
					New thrombosis	21/144 (14.6%)	6/80 (7.5%)	3/36 (8.3%)	
					Major bleeding	9/144 (6.2%)	3/80 (3.8%)	1/36 (2.8%)	
Kiser et al.[18]	Bivalirudin	Retrospective	25/37	Normal: 0.14 ± 0.04 mg/kg/h Moderate: 0.1 ± 0.07 mg/kg/h Severe or RRT: 0.05 ± 0.05 mg/kg/h	Thrombosis during therapy	0/12 (0%)	0/11 (0%)	1/14 (7%)	NR
					Significant bleeding	0/12 (0%)	1/11 (9%)	1/14 (7%)	NR
					Mortality	1/12 (8%)	2/11 (18%)	5/14 (36%)	NR

(continued)

Table 1.3 (continued)

Reference	Agent	Study design	Study n/N[a]	Dosing	Outcomes	Renal function[b]			
						Normal (CrCl>60 mL/min)	Moderate (CrCl= 30–60 mL/min)	Severe (CrCl<30 mL/min)	p Value
Tschudi et al.[19]	Lepirudin	Prospective	15	Normal:0.08 mg/kg/h Moderate: 0.04 mg/ kg/h	Life-threatening bleeding	0/5	0/5	0/5	NR
				Severe:0.01–0.02 mg/ kg/h	Thrombotic complications	0/5	0/5	0/5	NR

MI myocardial infarction, *HIT* heparin-induced thrombocytopenia, *PCI* percutaneous coronary intervention, *NR* not reported
[a]n/N number of renally impaired patients/total study population, unless total study population includes only renally impaired patients (one number provided)
[b]Reported for comparison of death between moderate and severe renal impairment groups; rest of p values not provided but authors reported no significant differences in the other outcomes
[b]CrCl creatinine clearance based on Cockroft-Gault equation

For bivalirudin, several pharmacokinetic studies have demonstrated that dosage should be reduced by 20–90% in renal impairment due to increased risk of bleeding.[27-30] Plasma clearance in patients with moderate or severe renal impairment is reduced by 21% and 24%, respectively.[30] In the setting of PCI, no formal evaluations have been conducted to investigate appropriate dosing regimen in patients with significant renal impairment. The manufacturer provides suggested dose adjustments in this patient population (Table 1.3).[7] For the management of HIT, one recent clinical trial in 37 HIT patients treated with bivalirudin (Table 1.4) determined a feasible dosing adjustment protocol based on renal function that resulted in 51% of the patients achieving target aPTT without increasing risk of clinically significant bleeding.[18]

Similar to bivalirudin, the pharmacokinetics of lepirudin are altered in patients with renal insufficiency with a decline of renal lepirudin clearance that is associated with an increase of lepirudin half-life and area-under-the-curve.[19] Recent publications have demonstrated that lower lepirudin doses than those officially recommended by the manufacturer may be sufficient in achieving target aPTT and reducing the risk of overanticoagulation.[20,31,32] One recent clinical trial determined an experimental dosing regimen based on a retrospective study of 31 HIT patients who received lepirudin.[19] The efficacy of the doses used was demonstrated by increasing platelets and decreasing D-dimer concentration, resulting in rare thrombotic complications (four patients) and decreased major bleeding complications (four patients).[19] Based on this experience, the same investigators derived a lepirudin dosing regimen with an omission of a initial loading bolus, which was then prospectively evaluated in 15 HIT patients (Table 1.4).[19] The investigators demonstrated efficacy and safety of lepirudin by increasing platelet counts and decreasing D-dimer concentrations, resulting in no thrombotic or life-threatening bleeding complications. Based on these results, lepirudin is a feasible option for the management of HIT in patients with renal impairment, provided that appropriate dosage adjustments are made.

Hemodialysis/Continuous Renal Replacement Therapy: The pharmacokinetic responses in patients with end-stage renal disease requiring hemodialysis (HD) or continuous renal replacement therapy (CRRT) have been investigated for all three direct thrombin inhibitors. Comparable argatroban elimination parameters were reported in 13 non-HIT patients[21] undergoing HD while receiving argatroban 2 mcg/kg/min with or without a loading dose of 250 mcg/kg as well as in five HIT patients[33] receiving renal replacement therapy and argatroban 0.5–2 mcg/kg/min. Two case reports have identified a subset of patients with end-stage renal disease and concomitant hepatic impairment or conditions such as anasarca affecting hepatic function, who may require reduced dosage such as those recommended for patients with chronic hepatic impairment only.[34,35] Both case reports demonstrated a significant overshooting of aPTT. Therefore, dosage reduction is recommended for patients with end-stage renal disease with either concomitant hepatic impairment or medical conditions decreasing hepatic perfusion (Table 1.3). Argatroban is a preferred agent in patients with renal impairment compared to the other direct thrombin inhibitors.

Table 1.4 Fondaparinux for treatment of VTE in obese patients[56]

	Fondaparinux (n = 2,201)				Heparins (n = 2,217)			
	Evaluated by ABW		Evaluated by BMI		Evaluated by ABW		Evaluated by BMI	
	ABW ≤ 100 kg	ABW > 100 kg	BMI < 30 kg/m²	BMI ≥ 30 kg/m²	ABW ≤ 100 kg	ABW > 100 kg	BMI < 30 kg/m²	BMI ≥ 30 kg/m²
N (%)	1946 (88)	251 (11)	1560 (71)	594 (27)	1971 (89)	245 (11)	1551 (70)	622 (28)
Median (range)	76 (33–100)	110 (100–176)	26 (13–30)	33 (30–80)	76 (33–100)	111 (100–217)	26 (13–30)	33 (30–78)
VTE N (%)	75 (3.9)	10 (4)	61 (3.9)	22 (3.7)	87 (4.4)	14 (5.7)	70 (4.5)	30 (4.8)
Major bleeding N (%)	25 (1.3)	1 (0.4)	23 (1.5)	2 (0.3)	23 (1.2)	2 (0.8)	18 (1.2)	7 (1.1)

Adapted from Davidson et al.[56]

ABW total body weight, *BMI* body mass index, *VTE* venous thromboembolism recurrent at 3 months

Recent clinical trials have suggested that both bivalirudin and lepirudin require dosage adjustment in patients with dialysis requirements. Limited data for use of bivalirudin in dialysis-dependent patients demonstrate that reductions up to 90% in dosage may be necessary.[28] A retrospective analysis of 396 dialysis-dependent patients undergoing PCI and receiving either bivalirudin or heparin demonstrated a similar rate of major bleeding (3.4% vs. 3.1%, p=0.9) and composite endpoint of death, myocardial infarction, urgent target vessel revascularization (1.8% vs. 0.8%, p=0.7) when compared to heparin.[36] The investigators used the manufacturer recommended dosing regimen in the setting of PCI for bivalirudin, which is provided in Table 1.3. Another retrospective study of 18 critically ill patients with hepatic and/or renal dysfunction who received bivalirudin due to the diagnosis of HIT demonstrated that bivalirudin is primarily influenced by renal dysfunction only.[27] In this study, ten patients that required CRRT received a mean infusion rate of 0.04±0.03 mg/kg/h. For all patients in that study, no clinically significant bleeding occurred and only one patient (6%) experienced thrombosis. Although bivalirudin is partially cleared by hemodialysis, this study demonstrated that dosage requirements for patients requiring CRRT (0.04±0.3 mg/kg/h) were similar to those in patients not receiving CRRT (0.08±0.21 mg/kg/h).

Like bivalirudin, dosage requirements for lepirudin in patients requiring dialysis should be reduced. Evidence indicate that the manufacturer's recommendation for hemodialysis patients (initial bolus of 0.2 mg/kg followed by 0.01 mg/kg every other day if aPTT ratio<1.5)[8] results in significant and prolonged overanticoagulation.[37] Based on the available evidence in patients requiring HD, intravenous doses should be limited to 0.05–0.1 mg/kg and frequency of dosing should be guided by aPTT results. Repeat intravenous boluses are necessary, and the expected interval between doses may be as long as 6–12 days.[37-39] There are no uniform dosing guidelines in patients receiving CRRT in the literature. Only case reports on the management of HIT in this patient population have been published.[22-24] All of the case reports demonstrated that lepirudin can be administered safely without significant overanticoagulation. For dosing lepirudin in the setting of CRRT, the investigators experimented with either giving intermittent intravenous boluses or continuous infusion (with or without an initial loading bolus) at a significantly reduced rate. The dosing regimens used are summarized in Table 1.3. The common finding was that patients receiving continuous infusions were more likely to have higher aPTT responses, potentially increasing the risk of bleeding. Thus, intermittent bolus therapy with lepirudin as guided by aPTT ratio may be more appropriate.[22]

Liver Dysfunction: Formal evaluations in the setting of liver dysfunction have not been conducted for bivalirudin or lepirudin. Per manufacturers' recommendations, both of these agents do not need to be dose adjusted for moderate or severe hepatic dysfunction.[7,8] In contrast, argatroban has been shown to have a four-fold decrease in clearance and three-fold increase in elimination half-life in adults with moderate hepatic impairment when compared to healthy subjects.[40] Table 1.3 summarizes the recommended reduction in argatroban dose in hepatic impairment (assessed as Child-Pugh score>6 or total serum bilirubin>1.5 mg/dL).[41] More recently, many clinical studies have suggested that reduced argatroban doses may be necessary in HIT patients with medical conditions that decrease hepatic perfusion or increase congestion such as heart failure, multiple organ damage, anasarca, and postcardiac surgery.[41-43] In one retrospective study, therapeutic responses were achieved at lower maintenance infusion rates in patients with heart failure compared to those without heart failure (0.6 mcg/kg/h vs. 1.0 mcg/kg/h).[44] However, these findings have not been confirmed by pharmacokinetic studies. Based on these findings, dosage reduction should be considered similar to the recommendations defined for hepatic impairment (e.g., initial infusion rate of 0.5 mcg/kg/h).[6] In the setting of PCI, the use of argatroban in patients with significant hepatic impairment has not been investigated; thus, argatroban should be avoided in this situation.

Hypothermia: Formal pharmacokinetic evaluations on direct thrombin inhibitors are currently not available.

Safety Concerns

Safety concern	Rationale	Comments/recommendations
Risk of hemorrhage	While on anticoagulant therapy, patients are at a higher risk of bleeding.[6-8] Thus, direct thrombin inhibitors should be used with caution in certain disease states and other circumstances that can increase risk of hemorrhage	Avoid in patients with active major bleeding (e.g., intracranial or gastrointestinal hemorrhage).[6-8] Caution in patients with increased risk of bleeding including:[6-8] Severe uncontrolled hypertension Spinal anesthesia Recent lumbar puncture; Recent major bleeding (e.g., intracranial, gastrointestinal, or intraocular bleeding) Major surgery such as those involving the brain or spinal cord Hematologic conditions with increased bleeding tendencies (e.g., congenital or acquired coagulopathy) Advanced renal impairment Recent cerebrovascular accident or stroke Gastric ulcerations

Safety concern	Rationale	Comments/recommendations
Development of anti-hirudin antibodies	Formation of anti-hirudin antibodies has been observed in up to 60% of HIT patients treated with lepirudin. Prolonged therapy for 10 days or more will increase likelihood of antibody development. This may increase the anticoagulant effect of lepirudin potentially due to delayed renal elimination of lepirudin-anti-hirudin complexes[45]	Strict monitoring of aPTT is warranted if prolonged therapy of lepirudin is anticipated
Drug-drug interactions	Pharmacodynamic interactions could be a concern if used concurrently with other medications known to increase risk of bleeding	An example of a pharmacodynamic interaction is the concurrent administration of a direct thrombin inhibitor (argatroban, bivalirudin, and lepirudin) with an antiplatelet agent (aspirin, warfarin, or thienopyridines). Monitoring of complete blood count with platelets and aPTT is warranted
	No significant pharmacokinetic interactions through the CYP450 system exist for any of the direct thrombin inhibitors. While there are no pharmacokinetic interactions between argatroban and warfarin, both agents can prolong INR	Argatroban and warfarin co-therapy can prolong INR more than with warfarin monotherapy.[45,46] INRs > 5 commonly occur while on co-therapy and typically do not cause bleeding. In this situation, it is recommended to hold argatroban when INR > 4 and check INR in 4–6 h after stopping. If INR > 2, then argatroban can be discontinued. Argatroban and warfarin should be co-administered for at least 5 days and until warfarin has a therapeutic effect for at least 2 days[47]

INR international normalized ratio

Fondaparinux

Dosing Considerations

Obesity: The reports of fondaparinux use in obese patients are limited to subgroup and post-hoc analyses of patients that that received prophylaxis or treatment for venous thromboembolism (VTE). The volume of distribution (Vd) of fondaparinux is mainly limited to the plasma compartment (Vd of 7–11 L). Distribution to extravascular fluid therefore is expected to be minimal.[48] The plasma clearance increases by 9% for each 10-kg increase in body weight. A prospective crossover study evaluated pharmacokinetic (PK) parameters in morbidly obese volunteers (n = 10). The mean BMI was 51.5 kg/m^2 (35.1–76.6) and actual body weight (ABW) was 145.1 kg (93.2–248.3). A dose of 5 mg led to proportional increases for maximum concentration (Cmax), time to reach Cmax (Tmax) and the area under the 0–24 concentration time curve (AUC24). The 2.5 mg dose did not achieve target levels of Cmax and AUC24, but did for Tmax.[49]

Dosing for Venous Thromboembolism (VTE) Prophylaxis in Obesity

Fondaparinux has been evaluated for prophylaxis of VTE following major orthopedic surgery of the lower limbs. The highest weight enrolled in these trials was 169 kg.[50] Overall, efficacy among patients with a BMI < 30 and ≥ 30 kg/m^2 was similar. Subgroup analyses in abdominal surgery also showed similar efficacy and risk of major bleeding compared to dalteparin and intermittent pneumatic compression alone. The highest weight in these trials was 215 kg (BMI 82.2 kg/m^2).[51,52] While there appears to be no need for dosing adjustment of fondaparinux for prophylaxis of VTE among obese patients based on clinical trial experience, the number of morbidly obese included was relatively low. The single aforementioned PK study by Raftopoulos et al. suggests use of a 5 mg dose, rather than 2.5 mg, for prophylaxis of VTE in morbidly obese patients.[49]

Dosing for VTE Treatment in Obesity

The Matisse trials for treatment of deep vein thrombosis (DVT) or pulmonary embolism (PE) defined obesity as a BMI ≥ 30 kg/m^2. There were no weight restrictions for entry into these clinical trials. Patients with obesity comprised 26.3% and 28.7% of the overall population in the DVT and PE trials, respectively.[53,54] A subgroup of analysis of the Matisse trials showed no significant differences in recurrent VTE or major bleeding among patients with and without obesity that received fondaparinux compared to either twice-daily subcutaneous enoxaparin (1 mg/kg) or adjusted-dose intravenous unfractionated heparin (UFH).[55] Davidson et al. performed a combined analysis of outcomes from the Matisse trials using obesity definitions based on both BMI and ABW.[56] Results from this analysis are shown in

Table 1.4. Limitations of these data include the post-hoc design as well as a limited number of patients with a BMI > 50 kg/m^2. Nonetheless, these data support the observation that dosing adjustment of fondaparinux for treatment of VTE in obese patients appears unnecessary.

Thinness/emaciation: The total clearance of fondaparinux is reduced by 30% in patients that weigh less than 50 kg and there is a concomitant increase in bleeding risk for such patients.[48] Therefore, the use of fondaparinux for VTE prophylaxis in these patients is contraindicated. Compared to patients that weighed > 50 kg, patients under this weight threshold had higher rates of major bleeding in all settings of VTE prophylaxis (hip fracture surgery, hip replacement, knee replacement, abdominal surgery).[48] Fondaparinux, however, may be used cautiously for the treatment of VTE among patients under 50 kg. The maximum recommended dose for these patients is 5 mg.[48]

Kidney Injury: The primary route of elimination of fondaparinux is renal clearance of unchanged drug (77%). Consequently, patients with impaired renal function are at greater risk for bleeding events. The total clearance of fondaparinux is reduced by 25% in patients with mild renal impairment (CrCl 50–80 mL/min), 40% in moderate renal impairment (CrCl 30–50 mL/min), and 55% in severe renal impairment (CrCl < 30 mL/min) compared to those with normal renal function. Rates of major bleeding among patients that underwent orthopedic surgery ranged from 1.6% for normal renal function to 4.8% among patients with severe renal impairment. A similar range was seen for abdominal surgery (2.1–7.1%) for normal renal function and severe renal impairment, respectively. Major bleeding rates in the setting of VTE treatment in patients with normal renal function and severe renal impairment were 0.4% and 7.3%, respectively.[48] Consequently, fondaparinux is contraindicated in severe renal impairment for both prophylaxis and treatment of VTE. No specific recommendations have been provided for patients with less severe renal impairment although caution should be exercised.[48] Pharmacokinetic data suggest that a dose of 1.5 mg daily provides similar Cmax and AUC24 for patients with moderate renal insufficiency (CrCl 20–50 mL/min) as those with normal renal function that received 2.5 mg daily, although this dose is not currently recommended by the manufacturer.[48,57] Renal function should be monitored periodically while patients receive fondaparinux. If there is any evidence of acute renal failure or severe renal impairment, then fondaparinux should be discontinued immediately. The half-life in patients with normal renal function is approximately 17–21 h. Upon discontinuation, the effects of fondaparinux may persist for 2–4 days (approximates 3–5 half-lives) in patients with normal renal function. The effects would be expected to be longer in patients with renal impairment.[48]

Hemodialysis/Continuous Renal Replacement Therapy: The experience with fondaparinux in patients receiving HD or CRRT is very limited. A prospective, open-label comparison of fondaparinux and UFH was conducted in 12 patients receiving HD. The goal of anticoagulation was to prevent clotting of the dialysis circuit. Although the clearance of fondaparinux was increased by about ten-fold during HD, the total clearance remained low and resulted in accumulation of anti-Xa concentrations during HD. Furthermore, anti-Xa concentrations remained elevated for up to 48 h after HD. The half-life off HD was estimated to be about 60 h.

Both the efficacy and safety profile of UFH was superior to fondaparinux in this trial. Bleeding with fondaparinux was most notable during the interdialytic interval.[58] Case reports describe fondaparinux in patients with both renal failure requiring HD and HIT type II. Both reports described doses of 2.5 mg every other day without bleeding or thrombotic complications. However, dosing was given subcutaneously on non-dialysis days in one report whereas the other report described installation into the dialysis circuit on dialysis days.[59,60] The efficacy and safety of fondaparinux for HIT are not well-established and is addressed below in the *"Safety Concerns"* section.

Liver Dysfunction: Fondaparinux does not undergo hepatic metabolism. Data from single-dose pharmacokinetic studies in patients with moderate hepatic impairment (Child-Pugh Category B) showed a decrease in Cmax and AUC24 by 22% and 39%, respectively. No significant changes in laboratory parameters of coagulopathy (e.g., aPTT, prothrombin time [PT]/INR, antithrombin III) were observed compared to patients with normal hepatic function. In these same patients there was a higher rate of minor bleeding (mild hematomas at blood sampling or injection site). No data exist for patients with severe hepatic impairment.[48] No specific dosage adjustments are recommended for patient with hepatic dysfunction.

Hypothermia: The pharmacokinetics of fondaparinux have not been investigated.

Safety Concerns

Safety concern	Rationale	Comments/recommendations
Risk of hemorrhage	Fondaparinux is a selective factor Xa inhibitor. Therefore, it should be used with caution in certain disease states and other circumstances that can increase risk of hemorrhage.[48]	Avoid in patients with: Severe renal impairment (CrCl<30 mL/min) Active, major bleeding Bacterial endocarditis Thrombocytopenia associated with a positive *in vitro* test for anti-platelet antibody in the presence of fondaparinux Body weight<50 kg (VTE prophylaxis only)[48] Weigh the benefits of fondaparinux use in the context of known risk factors for fondaparinux-associated bleeding: earlier (≤6 h) administration of the first post-operative injection, revascularization for coronary artery disease, and patients≥65 years.[61] A 2.5 mg/day fondaparinux dose has a similar bleeding risk as UFH and prophylactic dose low-molecular-weight heparin (LMWH), but a lower risk than therapeutic dose LMWH. A 7.5 mg/day fondaparinux dose has a similar bleeding risk as therapeutic doses of UFH or LMWH.[61]

Safety concern	Rationale	Comments/recommendations
Risk of spinal/ epidural hematomas	Patients with neuraxial anesthesia or that undergo spinal puncture may develop hematomas if fondaparinux is given. Hematomas may result in long-term or permanent paralysis	Consider benefit vs. risk before neuraxial intervention in patients anticoagulated with fondaparinux
	Use of post-operative indwelling epidural catheters increases risk.[48]	Monitor frequently for signs and symptoms of neurologic impairment.[48]
Patients ≥ 65 years	Age-related decline in glomerular filtration rate and correlation between fondaparinux clearance and creatinine clearance. Significant prolonga-tion of half-life and decrease in clearance with fondaparinux was observed.[62]	Assess renal function prior to initiating therapy. Use fondaparinux cautiously and monitor serum creatinine periodically
	The incidence of major bleeding is increased in the setting of prophylaxis for orthopedic and abdominal surgery as well as DVT/PE treatment among patients ≥ 65 years compared to those < 65 years.[48] In the setting of acute coronary syndromes, there was a non-significant increase in major bleeding for patients ≥65 years (2.7% vs. 1.4%).[63]	
Heparin-induced thrombocytope-nia (HIT) type II	Although there is no cross-reactivity with heparin and an inability for fonda-parinux to bind to platelet factor 4, rare reports of thrombocy-topenia associated with a positive in vitro test for anti-platelet antibody have been described.[64-66]	Fondaparinux is a potential alternative for the treatment of HIT, although there is a paucity of evidence and ambiguity surrounding appropriate dosing.[67,68]

(continued)

Safety concern	Rationale	Comments/recommendations
Drug-drug interactions	Pharmacokinetic-based drug-drug interactions such as Cytochrome P450 inhibition is not a concern with fondaparinux.[48] Pharmacodynamic interactions could be a concern with compounded or additive effects with the administration of drugs known to increase the risk of hemorrhage	An example of a pharmacodynamic interaction is the concomitant administration of fondaparinux and oral antiplatelets such as aspirin and/or thienopyridines (e.g., clopidogrel)

Glycoprotein IIB/IIIA Inhibitors (Abciximab, Eptifibatide, Tirofiban)

Dosing Considerations

Obesity: Pharmacodynamic and pharmacokinetic properties of glycoprotein (GP) IIb/IIIa inhibitors are shown in Table 1.5 below.[69-73] Accompanying data for obese patients are limited and prospective evaluations of clinical outcomes are also lacking. Experience with dosing these agents in obesity is largely derived from post-hoc analyses and maximum doses which were used in the original clinical trials. There is very limited experience with abciximab in patients weighing more than 160 kg (maximum weight included in clinical trials was 164 kg).[74,75] In total, over 1,400 patients that weighed more than 90 kg were included in three landmark trials of abciximab.[75-77] The incidence of death, MI, revascularization, and non-coronary artery bypass grafting (CABG) major bleeding in these patients were consistent with the overall study results.[74] In addition, a post-hoc analysis of abciximab use in the setting of acute myocardial infarction stratified patients by BMI (<25 vs. ≥25 to<30 vs. ≥30 kg/m^2). Overall, obese patients (BMI≥30 kg/m^2) were less likely to develop moderate bleeding, need for transfusions, and thrombocytopenia compared to patients with normal weight (BMI<25 kg/m^2). Severe bleeding rates were similar across categories. Mortality rates were lower in obese patients at 30-days and 1-year.[78] Table 1.6 below provides a summary of dosing recommendations for the use of the three currently available GP IIb/IIIa inhibitors (abciximab, eptifibatide, tirofiban) in obesity. Despite the paucity of data evaluating GP IIb/IIIa inhibitors in obesity, numerous reports have cited obesity as being associated with diminished platelet inhibition.[79] Reasons for this are unclear but may relate to underdosing of

Table 1.5 Comparison of pharmacokinetic and pharmacodynamic properties of glycoprotein IIb/IIIa inhibitors[69-73]

Property	Abciximab (Reopro®)	Eptifibatide (Integrilin®)	Tirofiban (Aggrastat®)
Platelet receptor binding	Non-competitive	Competitive	Competitive
Elimination half-life	30 min	2.5 h	2 h
Normalization of platelet function	Days	4–8 h	4–8 h
Reversibility[a]	No	Yes	Yes
Primary route of elimination	Reticuloendothelial system	Renal (50%)	Renal (39–69%)
Dialyzability	No	Yes	Yes

[a]Reversibility achieved with administration of platelets for abciximab; eptifibatide and tirofiban effects can be reversed with discontinuation due to competitive binding

Table 1.6 Overview of GP IIb/IIIa inhibitor dosing in obesity[69-71,75-77]

Agent	Bolus dose	Maximum actual body weight for bolus	Continuous infusion dose	Maximum actual body weight for continuous infusion
Abciximab (Reopro®)	0.25 mg/kg (maximum 40 mg)[a]	160 kg[a]	0.125 mcg/kg/min (maximum 10 mcg/min)[b]	80 kg[b]
Eptifibatide (Integrilin®)	180 mcg/kg (single or double-bolus)	121 kg	2 mcg/kg/min (normal renal function)	121 kg or 267 lb
Tirofiban (Aggrastat®)	0.4 mcg/kg/min as an infusion for 30 min	153 kg	0.1 mcg/kg/min (normal renal function)	153 kg

[a]The maximum bolus dose used in the EPILOG study[75]
[b]The maximum continuous infusion dose in the EPIC, EPILOG, and EPISTENT studies[75-77]

antiplatelet medications including GP IIb/IIIa inhibitors or the heightened inflammatory state that accompanies obesity.[80]

Thinness/emaciation: There have been no formal evaluations of dosing for underweight or nutritionally deficient patients. The clinical trial experience is limited with all agents. The lowest reported weight among patients enrolled in the abciximab trials was 39 kg.[76] The lowest reported weights for eptifibatide and tirofiban were 37 kg and 30 kg, respectively.[70,71] Unlike obese patients where there may be an excess risk for thrombosis, underweight patients are known to be at increased risk for bleeding complications to antiplatelet medications.[80,81] This may be the result of relative overdosing of these medications, including GP IIb/IIIa inhibitors, or to a lower level of platelet activation.[82]

Kidney Injury: Renal failure is known to increase the risk for both mortality and bleeding in patients with acute coronary syndromes.[83] Reasons for this are likely multifactorial and may reflect underusage of agents such as GP IIb/IIIa inhibitors and the higher incidence of uremic bleeding from platelet dysfunction.[73,83] Observational data suggest that GP IIb/IIIa inhibitor use decreases mortality in ACS patients with renal impairment but at the expense of increased bleeding.[83] Formal evaluations of GP IIb/IIIa inhibitors in these patients are limited as renal dysfunction was an exclusion criterion for most studies. As an example, only 18 patients with a serum creatinine (SrCr) between 2 and 4 mg/dL were included in the eptifibatide clinical trial experience and patients with a SrCr > 4 mg/dL were excluded.[70,84] Tirofiban trials excluded patients with a SrCr > 2 mg/dL or 2.5 mg/dL.[71,85-87] Pooled data from several landmark trials of abciximab showed that only 63 out of 7,562 patients had a SrCr > 2 mg/dL.[73] Pharmacokinetic considerations (Table 1.5) demonstrate that abciximab dosing is not affected by renal impairment.[69] Conversely, the small molecules eptifibatide and tirofiban are renally eliminated and therefore have recommendations for dose adjustment or avoidance. Table 1.7 provides an overview of dosing recommendations in renal impairment per the manufacturer. Table 1.8 summarizes the available data on studies of GP IIb/IIIa inhibitors in such patients. These trials are limited by their retrospective and/or observational designs. The cumulative observations are that renal insufficiency increases the risk for bleeding and that GP IIb/IIIa inhibitor use further compounds this risk. However, variability was seen in the interaction between GP IIb/IIIa inhibitor use, renal insufficiency, and bleeding. In summary, abciximab is the preferred agent in the setting of severe renal impairment, whereas eptifibatide and tirofiban are best avoided. For mild to moderate renal impairment eptifibatide and tirofiban should be dose-adjusted according to the manufacturers recommendations. These recommendations should be strictly adhered to as a recent observational analysis found that excess dosing of eptifibatide and tirofiban occurred in 27% of patients and was associated with a significant increase in major bleeding.[82]

Hemodialysis/Continuous Renal Replacement Therapy: Data for the use of GP IIb/IIIa inhibitors in patients with end-stage renal disease that receive HD or CRRT are limited. The molecular weights of the GP IIb/IIIa inhibitors are as follows: abciximab (47,615), eptifibatide (832), tirofiban (495).[73] The molecular size coupled with the non-competitive binding of abciximab renders it not dialyzable. Whereas the small size and competitive binding of eptifibatide and tirofiban suggest that they are dialyzable. Despite these considerations, patients with end-stage renal disease that were dialysis-dependent were excluded from studies of eptifibatide and tirofiban. Dialysis is a contraindication to eptifibatide use and tirofiban should be used with caution.[70,71] An analysis of the National Cardiovascular Data Registry Cath PCI registry found that approximately 14% of dialysis-dependent patients received eptifibatide during PCI and these patients were at significantly greater risk for in-hospital bleeding.[96] A case report of eptifibatide (Table 1.8) showed that acute HD reversed the inhibitory effect on platelet aggregation in two patients.[92] Abciximab has been used in patients that were HD-dependent (Table 1.8), although the data

Table 1.7 Overview of GP IIb/IIIa inhibitor dosing recommendations in renal impairment[69-71]

Agent	Recommendations for dose adjustment in renal impairment
Abciximab (Reopro®)	Not applicable
Eptifibatide (Integrilin®)	Decrease continuous infusion dose by 50% (e.g., from 2 to 1 mcg/kg/min) for estimated creatinine clearance [CrCl] <50 mL/min[a]
	Contraindicated if dialysis-dependent
Tirofiban (Aggrastat®)	Decrease continuous infusion dose by 50% (e.g., from 0.1 to 0.05 mcg/kg/min) for estimated CrCl <30 mL/min
	Use with caution in chronic hemodialysis (HD)

CrCl estimated creatinine clearance as calculated by the Cockcroft-Gault equation

[a]Note that for eptifibatide dosing the manufacturer advises that ABW be used for estimation of CrCl since studies used the original Cockcroft-Gault equation based on this weight

Table 1.8 Studies of GP IIb/IIIa inhibitors in renal impairment[84,88-93]

Agent	Study design	Number of patients	Definition of renal failure (RF)	Safety outcomes
Abciximab	Retrospective chart review[88]	182	Baseline SrCr ≥ 2 mg/dL	Major bleeding 21% (abciximab) vs. 15% (control); p=0.39
		(n=87 abciximab; n=95 control) n=21/87 received HD		Bleeding definition: cerebrovascular, retroperitoneal, gastrointestinal, or any transfusion
	Retrospective evaluation of registry[89]	1040	SrCr ≥ 1.3 mg/dL	Major bleeding 4.5% (RF) vs. 0.6% (no RF); p=0.003; OR 5.1; 95% CI 1.9–13.8) for bleeding with renal insufficiency and abciximab
		(n=44 with RF; n=996 without RF)		
		n=5/44 received HD		Bleeding definition: any bleed requiring transfusion
	Retrospective evaluation of registry[90]	4158	Stratification as follows: CrCl ≥ 70, 50–69, or <50 mL/min	RR 2.14 (95% CI, 1.12–4.10; p=0.022) for major bleeding with abciximab; RR 2.49 (95% CI, 1.12–5.55; p=0.025) for minor bleeding; interaction between abciximab and CrCl non-significant
		(n=1,248 abciximab; n=2,910 control)		
				Bleeding definition: TIMI criteria

(continued)

Table 1.8 (continued)

Agent	Study design	Number of patients	Definition of renal failure (RF)	Safety outcomes
Eptifibatide	Prospective, observational[91]	175	CrCl<35 mL/min (not required for study inclusion)	OR 9.12 (95% CI, 1.58–52.52; p=0.01) for TIMI major bleeding with renal dysfunction and eptifibatide; OR 6.10 (95% CI, 1.24–30.02; p=0.03) for GUSTO bleeding Bleeding definition: TIMI and GUSTO criteria
	Subgroup analysis of ESPRIT trial[84]	2044 (n=289 with RF; n=1,755 without RF)	CrCl<60 mL/min	TIMI/GUSTO major bleeding 1.1% (eptifibatide) vs. 0.4% (control); p value not reported: interaction between eptifibatide and CrCl non-significant Bleeding definition: TIMI and GUSTO criteria
	Case report[92]	3 n=2/3 required HD	ARF (n=1); CRI (n=1); end-stage renal disease (n=1)	Prolonged inhibition of platelet aggregation in each case; platelet function restored to normal with HD in 2 cases; 1 case developed ICH before HD
Tirofiban	Subgroup analysis of PRISM-PLUS[93]	1537	Stratification as follows: CrCl≥75, 60–75, 30–60, or <30 mL/min	Neither renal insufficiency nor addition of tirofiban significantly increased major bleeding; composite of TIMI major/minor bleeding was increased with worsening renal function (p=0.004) and tirofiban (p=0.04) Bleeding definition: TIMI criteria

RF renal failure, TIMI thrombolysis in myocardial infarction[94], TIMI major bleed intracranial hemorrhage or a decrease in hematocrit ≥15% or hemoglobin (Hb) ≥5 g/dL, TIMI minor bleed observed blood loss and a drop of ≥10% in Hct or ≥3 g/dL in Hb or if no bleeding was observed a drop of ≥12% in Hct or ≥4 g/dL in Hb, GUSTO Global Utilization of Streptokinase and Tissue Plasminogen Activator for Occluded Arteries[95], GUSTO severe or life-threatening bleed intracranial hemorrhage or bleeding that caused hemodynamic compromise and required intervention, GUSTO moderate bleed bleeding that required transfusion without hemodynamic compromise, GUSTO minor bleed bleeding that does not meet criteria for severe or moderate bleeding, SrCr serum creatinine, HD hemodialysis, CrCl creatinine clearance, OR odds ratio, RR relative risk, ESPRIT Enhanced Suppression of the Platelet IIb/IIIa Receptor with Integrilin Therapy trial, ARF acute renal failure, CRI chronic renal insufficiency, ICH intracranial hemorrhage, PRISM-PLUS Platelet Receptor Inhibition in Ischemic Syndrome Management in Patients Limited by Unstable Signs and Symptoms trial are limited. Consequently, abciximab is the preferred agent for patients that are dialysis-dependent.

Liver Dysfunction: Studies of GP IIb/IIIa inhibitors in the setting of liver dysfunction are lacking. According to the product information, the plasma clearance of tirofiban is not significantly different between patients with mild to moderate hepatic insufficiency and healthy patients.[71] No mention of hepatic impairment is provided in the product information for either eptifibatide or abciximab.

Hypothermia: The use of therapeutic hypothermia as part of the management of post-cardiac arrest syndrome is known to impair coagulation and inhibit platelet function which may predispose to bleeding.[97] The pharmacokinetics of GP IIb/IIIa inhibitors have been investigated in an in vitro study of mild hypothermia (32–34°C). Blood samples from six healthy volunteers were used to analyze the effects of all three commercially available GP IIb/IIIa inhibitors. The principle finding was that mild hypothermia enhanced the platelet inhibitory effects of submaximal doses of eptifibatide and tirofiban, but not abciximab.[98] The authors suggest that doses of eptifibatide and tirofiban may need to be modified but do not provide specific recommendations. However, other authors noted that doses of these agents are not adjusted for patients that receive therapeutic hypothermia at their institution.[97] Nonetheless, it would be prudent to monitor for signs and symptoms of bleeding in patients that receive GP IIb/IIIa inhibitors during therapeutic hypothermia, particularly eptifibatide and tirofiban.

Safety Concerns

Safety concern	Rationale	Comments/recommendations
Risk of hemorrhage	GP IIb/IIIa inhibitors inhibit platelet aggregation and have the potential to increase the risk of bleeding particularly at the arterial access site for cardiac catheterization or from the gastrointestinal (GI) or genitourinary (GU) tract and pulmonary and retroperitoneal sites. Use of concomitant medications which affect hemostasis (e.g., anticoagulation, thrombolytics, nonsteroidal anti-inflammatory drugs) further increase this risk[69-71]	Strategies to minimize bleeding risk should include: Use of low-dose, weight-adjusted UFH Discontinuation of anticoagulation after catheterization (unless indications exist beyond ACS/PCI)

(continued)

Safety concern	Rationale	Comments/recommendations
		Careful vascular access site management
		Early femoral arterial sheath removal
		Dose adjust eptifibatide for CrCl < 50 mL/min and tirofiban for CrCl < 30 mL/min
		Consider abciximab for patients receiving dialysis
		Avoid in patients with:
		Active internal bleeding
		GI or GU bleeding within 6 weeks
		Recent cerebrovascular accident (within 30 days) or any history of hemorrhagic cerebrovascular accident (CVA)
		Bleeding diathesis
		Thrombocytopenia
		Major surgery or trauma within 6 weeks
		Intracranial neoplasm, arterio-venous malformation, or aneurysm
		Severe, uncontrolled hypertension (e.g., systolic blood pressure (BP) > 200 mmHg or diastolic BP > 110 mmHg)
		Dependency on dialysis (eptifibatide)
		Hypersensitivity to the GP IIb/IIIa inhibitor[69-71]
Acute, profound thrombocytopenia	Decline in platelet count to less than 20,000 platelets/mm³ within 24 h of administration has been reported. The incidence is approximately 0.7% of abciximab patients. Case reports of this reaction with eptifibatide and tirofiban have also been documented	Monitor platelet count at baseline, within 4 h, and 24 h after initiation of any GP IIb/IIIa inhibitor
	The mechanism is unclear but thought to be immune-mediated[99]	Discontinue GP IIb/IIIa inhibitor and anticoagulant (e.g., heparin) and give platelet transfusions as needed[99]

Safety concern	Rationale	Comments/recommendations
Readministration	Potential for antigenicity exists with abciximab, but not eptifibatide or tirofiban	Same recommendations with regard to platelet count monitoring apply as with initial administration. Monitor for signs and symptoms of hypersensitivity
	Human anti-chimeric IgG antibodies may develop in 6–7% of patients with abciximab	
	Theoretical potential for hypersensitivity reactions including anaphylaxis, augmented thrombocytopenia, and/or decreased efficacy[99]	
Initial invasive vs. initial conservative strategy	The GUSTO-IV ACS study of abciximab found no benefit among patients not planned for early revascularization[100]	Abciximab is indicated upstream only if there is no appreciable delay to angiography and PCI is likely to be performed; otherwise, eptifibatide or tirofiban is preferred
	Benefits of eptifibatide and tirofiban have been shown in patients not planned for routine PCI[101]	If an initial conservative strategy is selected and a GP IIb/IIIa inhibitor is used, then eptifibatide or tirofiban should be used[101]
GP IIb/IIIa inhibitor selection for PCI	The TARGET study reported a significantly lower event rate for the composite of death/nonfatal MI/urgent target vessel revascularization with abciximab compared to tirofiban[102]	While any GP IIb/IIIa inhibitor may be used for PCI, abciximab may be considered over tirofiban based on the TARGET study[102]
	No large, randomized, prospective trials have directly compared abciximab and eptifibatide or tirofiban and eptifibatide	
Routine early vs. delayed, provisional use	The EARLY-ACS study of eptifibatide found no difference in ischemic events between these strategies despite an increase in bleeding with routine, early use[103]	It is reasonable to start a GP IIb/IIIa inhibitor at the time of primary PCI for ST-segment-elevation MI (STEMI). The usefulness of GP IIb/IIIa inhibitors for STEMI prior to arrival in the catheterization laboratory is uncertain[104]
Admixture	Abciximab is the Fab fragment of the chimeric human-murine monoclonal antibody 7E3. Consequently, filtration is needed for particle or aggregate removal from the protein solution[69]	Abciximab must be filtered using a sterile, non-pyrogenic, low protein-binding 0.2 or 0.5 μm syringe filter prior to administration of the bolus and upon admixture or during administration of the continuous infusion[69]

(continued)

Safety concern	Rationale	Comments/recommendations
Drug-drug Interactions	Pharmacokinetic-based drug-drug interactions such as Cytochrome P450 inhibition is not a concern with GP IIb/IIIa inhibitors. Pharmacodynamic interactions could be a concern with compounded or additive effects with the administration of drugs known to affect the risk of bleeding	An example of a pharmacodynamic interaction is the concomitant administration of a GP IIb/IIIa inhibitor and oral antiplatelet agents such as aspirin and/or thienopyridines and anticoagulants. Monitoring of complete blood count with platelets and aPTT or anti-factor-Xa concentrations should occur

Low-Molecular Weight Heparins (Enoxaparin, Dalteparin, Tinzaparin)

Dosing Considerations

Obesity: Pharmacodynamic data with LMWH exist for patients weighing as much as 190 kg.[105] Clinical trials of LMWH in the setting of ACS, however have enrolled patients with a maximum weight of 196 kg.[106] There is an inverse correlation between ABW and anti-Xa concentrations in obese patients.[107,108] The association between ABW and thrombosis is less certain than BMI.[109] While BMI is the benchmark used by the World Health Organization (WHO) for the definition of obesity, the majority of studies evaluating LMWH used ABW.[110] Table 1.9 provides a summary of dosing recommendations for the use of the three currently available LMWHs (enoxaparin, dalteparin, tinzaparin) across FDA-approved indications. Guidance with respect to dosing in obesity is provided where appropriate.

Dosing for VTE Prophylaxis in Obesity

Numerous clinical studies have suggested that higher fixed doses of enoxaparin and dalteparin may be justified over standard doses for VTE prophylaxis.[115] Studies evaluating the use of LMWH for patients that are morbidly obese are primarily limited to the bariatric surgery population. Table 1.10 provides a summary of pharmacodynamic and clinical studies of LMWH for VTE prophylaxis in patients with obesity.[114] The largest prospective study conducted to date in this setting suggested a lower rate of DVT complications with use of a higher dose of enoxaparin (40 mg SC q 12 h) compared to standard dosing (30 mg SC q 12 h) although overall results were inconclusive.[116] Based on this and other published data, it may be reasonable to increase the dose of LMWH by 30% in patients that are morbidly obese (BMI > 40 kg/m^2).[114-116]

Table 1.9 Overview of LMWH dosing in obesity[111-115]

Indication	Enoxaparin	Dalteparin	Tinzaparin
VTE prophylaxis	30 mg q 12 h (knee arthroplasty, hip arthroplasty)	2,500–5,000 international units (IU) q day (abdominal surgery)[a]	Not indicated
	40 mg q day (hip arthroplasty, abdominal surgery, medical patients)	5,000 IU q day (hip arthroplasty, medical patients)[b]	
	Increase dose in patients with morbid obesity (BMI > 40 kg/m²)[114,115]	Increase dose in patients with morbid obesity[114,115]	
VTE treatment	1 mg/kg q 12 h or 1.5 mg/kg q day (inpatient treatment of deep vein thrombosis [DVT] with or without pulmonary embolism [PE])	200 IU/kg q day (month 1); 150 IU/kg q day (months 2–6) (extended treatment of VTE in patients with cancer)	175 IU/kg q day (inpatient treatment of DVT with or without PE)
	1 mg/kg q 12 h (outpatient treatment of DVT)	Total daily dose should not exceed 18,000 IU[112,114]	Weight-based dosing is appropriate for heavy/obese patients[114]
	Weight-based dosing without dose capping[114]		
	Twice daily dosing preferred[114]		
UA/NSTEMI	1 mg/kg q 12 h	120 IU/kg q 12 h with dose capping at 10,000 IU q 12 h[112]	Not indicated
STEMI	30 mg intravenous (IV) bolus plus a 1 mg/kg SC dose, followed by 1 mg/kg q 12 h with dose capping of the first two doses at 100 mg[111] for patients greater than or equal to 75 years, no initial IV bolus, then 0.75 mg/kg SC q 12 h with dose capping of the first two doses at 75 mg	Not indicated	Not indicated

Adapted from references[111-115]

Note: All doses given subcutaneously (SC), except where noted

LMWH low-molecular-weight heparins, *VTE* venous thromboembolism, *q day* once daily, *BMI* body mass index, *DVT* deep vein thrombosis, *PE* pulmonary embolism, *UA* unstable angina, *NSTEMI* non-ST-segment-elevation myocardial infarction, *STEMI* ST-segment-elevation myocardial infarction

[a]DVT prophylaxis in abdominal surgery with dalteparin: May also give 2,500 IU followed by 2,500 IU 12 h later then 5,000 IU q day

[b]DVT prophylaxis in hip replacement with dalteparin: Administer 2,500 IU 2 h before surgery followed by 2,500 IU 4–8 h after surgery, then 5,000 IU q day or 5,000 IU evening before surgery followed by 2,500 IU 4–8 h after surgery; If begun postoperatively, administer 2,500 IU 4–8 h after surgery then 5,000 IU q day

Table 1.10 Pharmacodynamic and clinical studies of LMWH for VTE prophylaxis in obese patients

Study	Pts.	LMWH	n/N[a]	Dosing	Study design	Definition of obese	Outcome	Nonobese	Obese
Pharmacodynamic outcomes							*Anti-Xa concentrations*		
Frederiksen et al.[107]	Surgical	Enoxaparin	NA/19	40 mg (single)	Prospective cohort		Correlation with body weight	Negative correlation	
Simone (2008)	Bariatric surgery	Enoxaparin	40 mg q12h vs. 60 mg q12h, 3 doses	Prospective cohort			Mean	0.21 U/mL vs. 0.43 U/mL	
							Subtherapeutic (<0.18 U/mL)	$p < 0.001$ 44% vs. 0%	
							Supratherapeutic (>0.44 U/mL)	$p = 0.02$ 0% vs. 57%	
Borkgren-Okonek (2008)	Bariatric surgery	Enoxaparin	223	40 mg bid if BMI ≤50 kg/m^2 vs. 60 mg bid if BMI >50 kg/m^2	Prospective open-label		4 h after 3rd dose	0.32 IU/mL vs. 0.26 IU/mL	
Clinical outcomes							*VTE or major bleeding*		
Kucher (2005)	Medically ill	Dalteparin	558/3706	5,000 U/day	RCT retrospective subgroup	Men: BMI ≥30 kg/m^2	VTE	2.8%	2.8%
							Major bleeding	1.6%	0%
		Placebo	560/3706			Women: BMI ≥28.6 kg/m^2	VTE	5.2%	4.3%
							Major bleeding	0.3%	0.7%

Study	Surgery	Drug	n/N	Dose	Study type	BMI	VTE bleeding[b]		
Samama et al.[109]	Orthopedic surgery	Enoxaparin	NA/817	40 mg/day	Retrospective analysis	BMI >32 kg/m²	VTE bleeding[b]	16.7% no relationship with body weight	31.8% (p < 0.001 vs. non-obese)
Scholten et al.[116]	Bariatric surgery	Enoxaparin	481	30 mg q12h 40 mg q12h	Prospective cohort	Mean BMI 50–51 kg/m²	VTE Major bleeding VTE Major bleeding		5.4%c 1.1% 0.6%c 0.3%
Escalante-Tattersfield (2008)	Bariatric surgery	Enoxaparin	618	40 mg q12h	Retrospective	BMI > 35 kg/m²	VTE Postoperative bleeding		0.16% 1.6%
Kardys (2008)	Bariatric surgery	Enoxaparin	31	40 mg q12h	Retrospective chart review	Mean BMI 71 kg/m² (38–107)	VTE		9.5%

From Nutescu et al.[114] Reprinted with permission

BMI body mass index, *LMWH* low-molecular-weight heparin, *NA* not available, *RCT* randomized clinical trial, *VTE* venous thromboembolism

[a]n/N = obese patients/total study population. If the total study population included only obese patients, just 1 number is given

[b]Bleeding not defined as major or minor

[c]Significant difference in VTE rate with 30-mg dose vs. 40-mg dose; p < 0.01

Because data for LMWH dosing in morbidly obese patients has been generated in the bariatric surgery setting, it is unclear if the same recommendations apply to other patients. Finally, peak anti-Xa monitoring can be used to guide therapy for morbidly obese patients. Peak concentrations should be drawn 4 h following subcutaneous injection. While there is no clear consensus on the exact therapeutic range for anti-factor Xa concentrations, some authors have advocated a range of 0.2–0.4 IU/mL for prophylaxis (peak plasma concentration drawn 3–5 h post-dose).[114]

Dosing for VTE Treatment in Obesity

LMWHs reside mainly in the intravascular compartment (volumes of distribution approximately 5–7 L).[117] Subsequently, recommendations for weight-based dosing for the treatment of VTE have been met with concerns about increased bleeding risk and subsequent suggestions for dose-capping.[114] Similar to UFH though, LMWHs also seem to follow a saturable non-renal route of elimination.[118] Pharmacodynamic studies further support this view and reinforce the use of ABW as the preferred method of dosing.[114] Enoxaparin demonstrated a similar volume of distribution and clearance between obese and nonobese volunteers and an appropriate increase in anti-factor-Xa activity with weight adjusted dosing as high as 144 kg (1.5 mg/kg once daily).[119] A follow-up study of enoxaparin showed a consistent trend with patient weights up to 159 kg.[120] Similar results have also been seen for dalteparin at weights up to 190 kg and with tinzaparin up to 165 kg.[121-123] Table 1.11 provides a summary of pharmacodynamic and clinical studies of LMWH for VTE treatment and ACS in patients with obesity.[114] An additional consideration with enoxaparin is that twice-daily dosing may be preferred to once-daily dosing for acute VTE in obese patients.[56,124] Anti-Xa concentration monitoring is generally not needed for patients weighing ≤ 190 kg based on pharmacodynamic data. However, monitoring of these concentrations is reasonable in patients with morbid obesity.[114] Similar to prophylaxis there is no established therapeutic anti-factor Xa range for treatment. General ranges though have been proposed for VTE treatment (0.5–1 IU/mL for twice-daily dosing and 1–2 IU/mL for once-daily dosing [peak plasma concentration drawn 3–5 h post-dose]).[114]

Dosing for ACS in Obesity

Only enoxaparin and dalteparin have been studied for patients with NSTEMI and accordingly are Food and Drug Administration (FDA)-approved for these patients. However, enoxaparin is the only LMWH specifically recommended for the management of ACS by the American College of Cardiology/American Heart Association (ACC/AHA) treatment guidelines.[126,127] While weight-based dosing has been recommended, questions about the appropriateness of a dose cap for LMWH have been debated.[128,129] A retrospective analysis of the combined database of the TIMI 11B and Efficacy Safety Subcutaneous Enoxaparin in Non-Q-wave Coronary

Table 1.11 Pharmacodynamic and clinical studies of LMWH for VTE treatment and ACS in obese patients

Study	LMWH (or comparator)	n/N[a]	Dosing	Study design	Definition of obese	Outcome	Nonobese	Obese
Pharmacodynamic outcomes								
							Anti-Xa concentrations	
Smith and Canton[121]	Dalteparin	21	196.5 U/kg once daily	Retrospective open-label	>90 kg	Mean		0.9 SD ± 1.1
			126.2 U/kg q12h					1.1 SD ± 0.23
Yee (2000)	Dalteparin	10/20	200 IU/kg/day or 120 IU/kg q12h	Pharmacodynamic	BMI ≥30 kg/m^2	Volume of distribution	8.36 (n = 10)	12.36 (n = 10; p = 0.11 vs. nonobese)
Wilson (2001)	Dalteparin	37	200 IU/kg once daily	Prospective cohort	100–120% ideal body weight	Mean		1.01 (95% CI 0.89–1.13) (n = 13)
					120–140% ideal body weight			0.97 (95% CI 0.85–1.09) (n = 14)
					>140% ideal body weight			1.12 (95% CI 0.96–1.28) (n = 10)
Sanderink (2002)	Enoxaparin	24/48	1.5 mg/kg sc once daily	Pharmacodynamic	BMI 30–40 kg/m^2		(n = 24)	14–19% higher vs. nonobese (n = 24; p < 0.05)

(continued)

Table 1.11 (continued)

Study	LMWH (or comparator)	n/N[a]	Dosing	Study design	Definition of obese	Outcome	Nonobese	Obese
Bazinet et al.[120]	Enoxaparin	81/233	1.5 mg/kg once daily	Prospective open-label	BMI > 30 kg/m^2	Mean	1.13 (95% CI 1.04–1.22)	1.15 (95% CI 1.02–1.28)
			1 mg/kg bid				1.12 (95% CI 1.03–1.20)	1.17 (95% CI 1.08–1.25)
Hainer (2002)	Tinzaparin	35	175 IU/kg	Pharmacodynamaic	100–160 kg	Mean	0.87 (95% CI 0.78–0.96)	0.81 (95% CI 0.76–0.86)
		37	75 IU/kg				0.30 (95% CI 0.28–0.32)	0.34 (95% CI 0.303–0.375)
Barrett (2001)	Tinzaparin	NA/425	175 IU/kg once daily	Data analysis of 2 RCTs	BMI > 30 kg/m^2	LMWH clearance		22% decrease
Clinical outcomes								
VTE treatment						*VTE or major bleeding*		
Al-Yaseen dalteparin (2005)		193	200 IU/kg once daily	Retrospective chart review	>90 kg kg/m^2	Recurrent VTE		1.6% (95% CI 0.2–5.8)
			100 IU/kg q 12h			Major bleeding		0.8 (95% CI 0.02–4.5)
						Recurrent VTE		1.4% (95% CI 0.03–7.6)
						Major bleeding		1.4% (95% CI 0.03–7.6)

Study	Drug	N	Dose	Design	Criteria	Outcome		
Merli et al.[124]	Enoxaparin	900	1 mg/kg once daily	RCT	Men: BMI >26.9 kg/m², women: BMI >27.2 kg/m²	Recurrent VTE	4.4%	7.3%
			1.5 mg/kg q 12h				2.9%	3.4%
	UFH		Adjusted				4.1%	2.5%
RIETE registry Barba (2005)	NA	294/8845	Different doses	Registry analysis	>100 kg	Recurrent VTE	10%	0.7% (OR 0.7; 95% CI 0.2–2.7 vs. nonobese)
						Major bleeding	1.3%	1.0% (OR 0.8; 95% CI 0.2–2.5 vs. nonobese)
ACS						*Ischemic events or major bleeding*		
Klein (1997)	Dalteparin placebo	NA/1482	Days 1–6: 120 IU/kg q12h days 7–45: 7,500 IU once daily	RCT subgroup analysis	BMI > 26	Death, MI, UR	15.7%	8.4%
							13.3%	11.4%
FRISC FRISC Investigators (1996)	Dalteparin Placebo	731/1497	120 IU/kg q12 (10,000 IU cap)	RCT subgroup analysis	BMI > 26	Death, MI	0.8%	2.5%
							5.5%	4.0%

(continued)

Table 1.11 (continued)

Study	LMWH (or comparator)	n/N[a]	Dosing	Study design	Definition of obese	Outcome	Nonobese	Obese
Spinler et al.[125]	Enoxaparin	921/3516	1 mg/kg q12h	RCT subgroup analysis	BMI ≥ 30	Death, MI, UR	1.6%	14.3%
						Major bleeding	1.6%	0.4%
	UFH	918/3481	Adjusted doses			Death, MI, UR	19.2%	18.0%
						Major bleeding	1.0%	1.2%
	Enoxaparin/UFH					Death, MI, UR	16.2%	17.6% (p = 0.39 vs. nonobese)
						Major bleeding	0.8%	1.3% (p = 0.12 vs. nonobese)

From Nutescu[114] Reprinted with permission

ACS acute coronary syndromes, *BMI* body mass index, *LMWH* low-molecular-weight heparin, *MI* myocardial infarction, *NA* not available, *OR* odds ratio, *RCT* randomized clinical trial, *UFH* unfractionated heparin, *UR* urgent revascularization, *VTE* venous thromboembolism

[a]n/N obese patients/total study population. If the total study population included only obese patients, just 1 number is given

Events (ESSENCE) trials showed that approximately 26% of the population was obese (defined as BMI ≥ 30 kg/m^2) and 540 patients weighed more than 100 kg.[125] The maximum patient weight observed in these studies was 158.6 kg. Ultimately, obesity did not affect clinical outcomes in this combined analysis.[125] The Superior Yield of the New strategy of Enoxaparin, Revascularization and Glycoprotein IIb/IIIa inhibitors (SYNERGY) trial enrolled patients with a weight as high as 196 kg (SYNERGY). This represents the highest patient weight included in the context of enoxaparin dosing for ACS.[106] However, a recent retrospective analysis of enoxaparin found a higher risk of bleeding in patients weighing more than 150 kg that received 1 mg/kg dosing compared to those of normal body weight. There were only 35 patients in this subgroup with a weight of >150 kg.[130] Nonetheless, it is currently recommended that enoxaparin dosing for ACS be based on ABW with dose adjustment based on anti-factor Xa concentrations for patients >190 kg or on evidence of bleeding if anti-Xa concentrations are unavailable.[114] A proposed general target range for anti-factor Xa concentrations for ACS is 0.5–1.5 IU/mL (peak plasma concentration drawn 3–5 h post-dose).[114]

Thinness/emaciation: The lowest reported total body weight among LMWH treatment trials for ACS or VTE was 26 kg.[131] However, formal evaluations of LMWH dosing in patients with low body weight and/or emaciation have not been conducted. A prospective registry described clinical characteristics and outcomes in patients with extreme body weight that were treated for acute VTE. Approximately 2% (n = 169) of the registry weighed <50 kg and 161 of these patients received LMWH. Patients were predominantly female and had more severe underlying disease (e.g., malignancy). Patients that weighed less than 50 kg had an increased risk of bleeding complications, and 3 of 5 patients that developed major bleeding had received >200 IU/kg/day of LMWH.[132] Consequently, it would seem prudent to consider lower doses of LMWH in patients at lower extremes of body weight.

Kidney Injury: LMWHs are primarily eliminated renally. Consequently, their biologic half-lives are prolonged in patients with renal failure and these patients are at increased risk of bleeding.[108] Pharmacokinetic studies have demonstrated a linear correlation between the anti-Xa concentration of LMWHs and CrCl. Anti-Xa concentrations were most notably increased when the CrCl was <30 mL/min.[108] Consequently, most clinical trials of LMWHs have excluded patients with severe renal impairment, defined as an estimated CrCl (Cockcroft-Gault) ≤30 mL/min.[114] The published experience with LMWHs in the setting of renal impairment has generally been limited to enoxaparin. No explicit dosage adjustments have been made with either dalteparin or tinzaparin. Tinzaparin has the highest molecular weight among the currently available agents, which may result in a higher hepatic clearance.[108] However, tinzaparin was associated with a higher risk of death compared to UFH when used in elderly patients with renal insufficiency (70 years or older with CrCl ≤30 mL/min or 75 years or older with CrCl ≤60 mL/min) for the treatment of VTE. Therefore, tinzaparin use in this setting should be avoided.[113] Table 1.12 below provides a summary of dosing recommendations for LMWH in severe renal impairment.

Table 1.12 Overview of LMWH dosing in severe renal impairment (CrCl < 30 mL/min)[111-114]

Indication	Enoxaparin	Dalteparin	Tinzaparin
VTE prophylaxis	30 mg q day	Use with caution	Not indicated
VTE treatment	1 mg/kg q day	Dose adjust to anti-Xa target range of 0.5–1.5 IU/mL for long-term treatment of pts with cancer[a]	Dose with caution in pts with severe renal impairment
UA/NSTEMI	1 mg/kg q day	Use with caution	Not indicated
STEMI	30 mg intravenous (IV) bolus plus a 1 mg/kg SC dose, followed by 1 mg/kg SC q day. For patients ≥ 75 years, no initial IV bolus, then 0.75 mg/kg SC q day	Not indicated	Not indicated

Adapted from references[111-114]

Note: All doses given subcutaneously (SC), except where noted

LMWH low-molecular-weight heparins, *CrCl* creatinine clearance, *VTE* venous thromboembolism, *q day* once daily, *UA* unstable angina, *NSTEMI* non-ST-segment-elevation myocardial infarction, *STEMI* ST-segment-elevation myocardial infarction, *SC* subcutaneously, *IV* intravenously

[a]Measure anti-Xa concentrations 4–6 h after dalteparin dose and only after a patient has received 3–4 doses[112]

Dosing for VTE Prophylaxis in Kidney Injury

Pharmacodynamic data with enoxaparin show a significant increase in anti-Xa concentrations in patients with CrCl < 30 mL/min compared to patients with a CrCl ≥ 30 mL/min.[133] Data with dalteparin and tinzaparin are much more limited, but suggest no evidence of anti-Xa accumulation in patients with severe renal impairment. A summary of published literature describing LMWHs for prophylaxis in the setting of renal impairment is shown in Table 1.13.[114] None of the studies suggest an increase in bleeding complications, although it is recommended to reduce the dose of enoxaparin to 50% of the usual dose (e.g., 30 mg once daily if dosing 30 mg twice daily) or to 30 mg once daily if dosing 40 mg once daily for CrCl < 30 mL/min.[111] No dosage adjustments are recommended for dalteparin or tinzaparin. Patients with mild-to-moderate renal impairment (CrCl 30–90 mL/min) do not require dosing adjustment of LMWHs.[114] Because these studies have generally been conducted with shorter durations of LMWH use (4–10 days), it may be necessary to monitor anti-Xa concentrations in patients receiving extended prophylaxis.[114]

Table 1.13 Pharmacodynamic and clinical studies of LMWH for VTE prophylaxis in renal impairment

Reference	LMWH	Study n/N[a]	Design	Dosing	Mild outcome	CrCl, mL/min			
						Moderate (50–80)	Severe (30–50)	(<30)	
Pharmacodynamic outcomes					*Anti-Xa levels*				
Sanderink (2002)	Enoxaparin	36/48	Prospective cohort	40 mg/day, 4 doses	Exposure vs. healthy volunteers	20% higher (n = 12; p = 0.10)	21% higher (n = 12; p = 0.10)	65% higher (n = 12; p = 0.0001)	
Mahé (2007)	Enoxaparin	125	Prospective cohort	40 mg/day, <10 days	Maximum (mean)	0.60 (n = 28)	0.61 (n = 58)	0.72 (n = 39; p > 0.05 vs. all others)	
Mahé (2007)	Enoxaprin	28	Prospective open-label	40 mg/day, ≥8 days	Accumulation day 1–8 correlation with CrCl		1.22 (n = 28; p < 0.0001) no correlation (n = 28)		
	Tinzaparin	27		4,500 IU/day, ≥8 days	Accumulation day 1–8 correlation with CrCl		1.05 (n = 27; p = 0.29) no correlation (n = 27)		
Tincani (2006)	Dalteparin	115	Prospective cohort	5,000 IU/day or 2,500 IU/day, ≥6 days	Mean ± SD	0.030 ± 0.086 (n = 12)	0.030 ± 0.075 (n = 73)	0.048 ± 0.084 (n = 24; p = 0.72)	
Rabbat (2005)	Dalteparin	19	Prospective observational cohort	5,000 IU/day	Correlation with CrCl	No correlation (n = 8)			
Schmid (2007)	Dalteparin	38	Prospective observational cohort	Not specified, mean 7.5 days	Mean (95%)	0.46 (0.21–0.57) (n = 8)	0.40 (0.19–0.87) (n = 13)	0.48 (0.33–0.63) (n = 8)	
Douketis (2008)	Dalteparin	156	Prospective open-label cohort	5,000 IU/day, until discharge up to 30 days	Pts. (n) with trough anti-Xa > 0.40 IU/mL			0 (n = 120)	

(continued)

Table 1.13 (continued)

Reference	LMWH	Study n/N[a]	Design	Dosing	Mild outcome	CrCl, mL/min Moderate (50–80)	Severe (30–50)	(<30)
Clinical outcomes					VTE or major bleeding			
Mahé (2007)	Enoxaparin	28	Prospective open-label	40 mg/day, ≥8 days	Symptomatic VTE			None (n = 28)
					Major bleeding		1 (n = 28)	
	Tinzaparin	27		4,500 IU/day, ≥8 days	Symptomatic VTE			None (n = 27)
					Major bleeding		2 (n = 27)	
Mahé (2007)	Enoxaparin	125		40 mg/day, <10 days	Serious bleeding	Anti-Xa levels similar between pts. with and without bleeding (n = 125; p = 0.77)		
Tincani (2006)	Dalteparin	115	Prospective cohort	5,000 IU/day or 2,500 IU/day, ≥6 days	Major bleeding or VTE	None (n = 115)		
Rabbat (2005)	Dalteparin	19	Prospective observational cohort	5,000 IU/day	VTE	1 (n = 19)		
					Major bleeding	1 (n = 19)		
Douketis (2008)	Dalteparin	156	Prospective open-label cohort	5,000 IU/day, until discharge up to 30 days	DVT (95% CI)			5.1 (2.5–10.2) (n = 156)
					Major bleeding (95% CI)			7.2 (4.0–12.8) (n = 156)

From Nutescu et al.[114] Reprinted with permission

CrCl creatinine clearance, *DVT* deep-vein thrombosis, *LMWH* low-molecular-weight heparin, *VTE* venous thromboembolism

[a]n/N renally impaired patients/total study population. If the total study population included only renally impaired patients, just one number is given

Dosing for VTE Treatment and ACS in Kidney Injury

Therapeutic dosing of LMWH in the setting of severe renal impairment leads to consistently higher anti-Xa concentrations.[108-114] An inverse correlation between CrCl and anti-Xa concentrations has been noted with enoxaparin, although this relationship is less certain with dalteparin and tinzaparin.[114,134,135] A summary of published literature describing therapeutic dosing of LMWHs in the setting of renal impairment is shown in Table 1.14.[114] Increased bleeding complications as a result of decreased LMWH clearance are well-documented.[108,114] An analysis of the ESSENCE and TIMI 11B data showed an increased risk of major bleeding with therapeutic doses of enoxaparin in patients with CrCl $\leq$ 30 mL/min.[125] A meta-analysis also showed a significantly increased risk of major bleeding in patients with a CrCl $\leq$ 30 mL/min and use of therapeutic-dose enoxaparin. However, this observation was not found when an empiric dose reduction was applied to enoxaparin.[136] Consequently, the dose of enoxaparin should be reduced by 50% (1 mg/kg twice daily to 1 mg/kg once daily) for patients with CrCl < 30 mL/min.[111] Some authors have advocated this dose adjustment to include patients with a CrCl between 20 and 30 mL/min as data for the use of LMWH with CrCl < 20 mL/min are very limited.[114] UFH is preferred in patients with a CrCl < 20 mL/min due to ease of monitoring with aPTT and full reversal with protamine.

Hemodialysis/Continuous Renal Replacement Therapy: Data for the use of LMWH in patients with end-stage renal disease that receive HD or CRRT are limited. While the experience with therapeutic dosing is limited due to ambiguity about optimal dosing and bleeding risk, LMWHs have been used to prevent thrombosis of the extracorporeal dialysis circuit.[138] LMHWs have a mean molecular weight of about 5,000 Da (range, 2,000–9,000).[108] However, LMWHs are not generally removed by HD or CRRT including continuous veno-venous hemofiltration (CVVHF).[139,140] A pharmacokinetic study of reduced doses of dalteparin (single 2,500 IU IV bolus; mean dose 39 U/kg) and enoxaparin (40 mg IV bolus; mean dose 0.7 mg/kg) in patients on HD found no evidence of accumulation with reduced dosing over 4 weeks of treatment, but anti-Xa concentrations decreased more rapidly with dalteparin. This finding provides further support that enoxaparin is more dependent on renal elimination than dalteparin.[141] While tinzaparin was not evaluated in this study, other data did not demonstrate accumulation in patients on HD.[142] A meta-analysis of LMWHs used for preventing thrombosis of the extracorporeal dialysis circuit showed comparable safety and effectiveness to UFH.[138] Enoxaparin was variably removed by the CRRT circuit in one study that included critically ill patients undergoing CVVHF and continuous veno-venous hemodialysis (CVVHD), but the need for dosing adjustments remains unclear.[143]

Because the risk of bleeding complications is higher among patients with severe renal insufficiency that receive therapeutic doses of LMWH, UFH is considered preferred in the setting of dialysis.[108] An analysis of the National Cardiovascular Data Registry Cath PCI registry found that approximately 10% of dialysis-dependent patients received enoxaparin during percutaneous coronary intervention and these patients were at significantly greater risk for in-hospital bleeding.[96]

Table 1.14 Pharmacodynamic and clinical studies of LMWH for VTE treatment and ACS in renal impairment

Reference	LMWH (or comparator)	n/N[a]	Dosing	Study design	Outcome	CrCl, mL/min			
						Normal (>80)	Mild (50–50)	Moderate (30–50)	Severe (<30)
Pharmacodynamic outcomes									
Anti-Xa concentrations									
Bazinet et al.[120]	Enoxaparin	233	1.5 mg/kg once daily	Prospective, open-label	Mean (95% CI) supra-target (>2.0 IU)	1.10 (1.00–1.20) (n = 38) 0%		1.21 (1.09–1.33) (n = 27) 4%	1.18 (0.92–1.44) (n = 14) 0%
			1 mg/kg q12h		Mean (95% CI) supra-target (>1.1 IU)	1.06 (0.99–1.14) (n = 68) 40%		1.25 (1.12 to 1.39) (n = 27) 63%	1.27 (1.15 to 1.40) (n = 22) 77%
Becker et al.[134]	Enoxaparin	445	Initial 30-mg iv bolus, 1 or 1.25 mg/kg sc q12h	RCT subgroup	Peak level ± SD (3rd dose)	1.25 ± 0.37 (n = 273)	1.41 ± 0.44[b] (n = 149)		1.58 ± 0.58[c] (n = 11)
					Trough level ± SD (3rd dose)	0.58 ± 0.35	0.71 ± 0.42[b]		0.83 ± 0.49[c]
Bruno (2003)	Enoxaparin		Initial 30-mg iv bolus, 1 or 1.25 mg/kg sc q12h	Modeling study	LMWH clearance vs. normal			17% decrease	27% decrease
Hulot (2005)	Enoxaparin	350/532	Mean 0.83 ± 0.19 mg/kg q12h	Retrospective analysis	LMWH clearance vs. normal	(n = 182)	17% decrease (n = 192)	31% decrease (n = 103)	44% decrease (n = 55)

Study	Drug	N	Dose	Design	Measure/Outcome		
Chow et al.[135]	Enoxaparin	18	1 mg/kg q12h	Prospective cohort	Mean	0.91 (n = 13)	1.34 (n = 5) (p < 0.05)
					Correlation with CrCl	Yes	
Pautas (2002)	Tinzaparin	200	175 IU/kg once daily	Prospective cohort	Correlation with CrCl	No	
Shprecher (2005)	Dalteparin	11/22	100 IU/kg q12h	Prospective open-label cohort	Anti-X	0.55 ± 0.20 (n = 11)	0.47 ± 0.25[b] (n = 11)
Siguret (2000)	Tinzaparin	30	175 IU/kg	Prospective cohort	Correlation anti-Xa and CrCl?	No	
Barrett (2001)	Tinzaparin	131/187	175 IU/kg once daily		LMWH clearance		24% decrease
Clinical outcomes VTE/ACS treatment							
Lim et al.[136] Enoxaparin			Therapeutic dose adjusted meta-analysis to CrCl or anti-Xa	Meta-analysis	*Ischemic events or major bleeding*		
					Major bleeding	2.4%	8.3%
					Major bleeding	1.9%	0.9%
ACS							
Spinler et al.[125]	Enoxaparin	69/3,501	1 mg/kg q12h	RCT retrospective subgroup	Death, MI, urgent revascularization	15.7%	18.8%

(continued)

J.C. Coons and S. Devabhakthuni

Table 1.14 (continued)

Reference	LMWH (or comparator)	n/N[a]	Dosing	Study design	Outcome	CrCl, mL/min			
						Normal (>80)	Mild (50–50)	Moderate (30–50)	Severe (<30)
	UFH	74/3,468	Iv, dose adjusted		Major bleeding	1.2%			7.5%
					Death, MI, urgent revascularization	18.4%			32.4%
	Enoxaparin/ UFH	143/6,969			Major bleeding	1.0%			5.8%
					Death, MI, urgent revascularization	17.0%			25.9%
					Major bleeding	1.1%			6.6%
Thorevska (2004)	Enoxaparin	620	1 mg/kg sc q12h	Retrospective cohort	Major bleeding		12.4%[d]		36.6%[f]
	UFH		iv, dose adjusted				16.9%[d]		30.7%[f]
Collet (2003)	Enoxaparin	174/515	1 mg/kg q12h (65% of dose for CrCl ≤ 30 mL/ min, adjusted to anti-Xa levels)	Prospective cohort	Death, MI	5.6%			25.0%
					Major or minor bleeding	2.4%			4.7%

Study	Drug	n/N	Study type	Dosing	Outcome				
Collect (2005)	Enoxaparin UFH	4,687/11,881	NA, registry data Prospective cohort		Death	1.75%[g]		4.30%[h]	15.35%
					Major bleeding	1.24%[g]		2.03%[h]	5.9%
					Death	2.74%[g]		7.8%[h]	18.58%
					Major bleeding	2.18%[g]		4.36%[h]	9.29%
					Major bleeding			OR 2.4	OR 3.8
Bruno (2003)	Enoxaparin	448	NA, registry data Modeling study	Initial 30 mg iv bolus, 1 or 1.25 mg/kg sc q12h					
Fox et al.[137]	Enoxaparin	initial 30 mg iv bolus, 1 mg/kg sc q12h[i]			Death, MI	5.1%[j]	9.6%[k]	19.4%[h]	33.0%
					Major bleeding	1.2%[j]	2.3%[k]	3.5%[h]	5.7%
	UFH	mg/kg sc q12h[i]			Death, MI	7.3%[j]	12.1%[k]	19.4%[h]	37.7%
					Major bleeding	0.8%[j]	1.6%[k]	1.9%[h]	2.8%
	Enoxaparin/ UFH				Death, MI	6.2%[j]	10.9%[k]	19.4%[h]	35.4%
					Major bleeding	1.0%[j]	1.9%[k]	2.7%[h]	4.2%

From Nutescu[114] Reprinted with permission

ACS acute coronary syndromes, CrCl creatinine clearance, GFR glomerular filtration rate, LMWH low-molecular-weight heparin, MI myocardial infarction, NA not available, OR odds ratio, RCT randomized clinical trial, UFH unfractionated heparin, VTE venous thromboembolism

[a]n/N = renally impaired patients/total study population. If the total study population included only renally impaired patients, just 1 number is given

[b]CrCl 40–80 mL/min

[c]CrCl ≤ 40 mL/min

[d]GFR 41–60 mL/min

[e]GFR 21–40 mL/min

[f]GFR ≤ 20 mL/min

[g]CrCl > 60 mL/min

[h]CrCl 30–60 mL/min

[i]Dose adjustments for CrCl < 30 mL/min and ≥75 years of age

[j]CrCl > 90 mL/min

[k]CrCl 60–90 mL/min

Liver Dysfunction: Formal evaluations of LMWHs in the setting of liver dysfunction are lacking. Tinzaparin has a higher molecular weight than both enoxaparin and dalteparin and consequently may undergo greater hepatic clearance.[108] Based on this observation either enoxaparin or dalteparin may be preferred.

Hypothermia: The use of therapeutic hypothermia as part of the management of post-cardiac arrest syndrome is known to impair coagulation and inhibit platelet function which may predispose to bleeding.[97] However, no official recommendations for dose adjustments of LMWH are available in the setting of hypothermia at this time.

Safety Concerns

Safety concern	Rationale	Comments/recommendations
Risk of hemorrhage	LMWHs inhibit blood coagulation and should be used with caution in certain disease states and other circumstances that can increase risk of hemorrhage[111-113]	Avoid in patients with: Active major bleeding History of HIT Hypersensitivity to LMWH, UFH, pork products, or benzyl alcohol
	The additional risk of major hemorrhage with LMWH is between 0% and 2%, depending on concomitant disease states, medications, and the duration and intensity of treatment[61]	Caution in patients with increased risk of hemorrhage, including: Bleeding diathesis Uncontrolled hypertension History of recent gastrointestinal ulceration Diabetic retinopathy Renal dysfunction Bacterial endocarditis Congenital or acquired bleeding disorders Hemorrhagic stroke Recent brain, spinal, or opthalmological surgery Recent percutaneous coronary intervention (obtain hemostasis at puncture site before sheath removal; administer dose no sooner than 6–8 h after sheath removal) Concomitant platelet inhibitors[111-113]
Risk of spinal/epidural hematomas	Patients with neuraxial anesthesia or that undergo spinal puncture may develop hematomas if LMWH is given. Hematomas may result in long-term or permanent paralysis	Consider benefit vs. risk before neuraxial intervention in patients anticoagulated with LMWH

Safety concern	Rationale	Comments/recommendations
	Use of post-operative indwelling epidural catheters increases risk[111-113]	Monitor frequently for signs and symptoms of neurologic impairment[111-113]
Critically ill patients	Pharmacokinetic variability in critically ill patients that received LMWHs (enoxaparin) has been demonstrated. Reasons are likely multifactorial and may relate to inadequate SC absorption due to vasoconstriction with low cardiac output and/or use of vasopressors as well as the presence of peripheral edema[144,145]	Consider use of alternative anticoagulation where possible, such as IV unfractionated heparin, IV direct thrombin inhibitors, or SC fondaparinux
	Anti-Xa concentrations were significantly lower in critically ill vs. non-critically ill patients in one study in which SC 40 mg daily doses of enoxaparin were used.[144] Significant variability in anti-Xa concentrations was also found in multiple trauma patients that received SC 30 mg twice daily doses of enoxaparin[145]	Alternatively, dose adjustments of LMWH based on anti-Xa concentrations, higher empiric SC doses, or the use of a continuous IV infusion (enoxaparin) have been proposed but are not validated and therefore not recommended for routine use[144,146]
	Continuous IV infusion enoxaparin has been studied as a means of providing more predictable anti-Xa activity. In one analysis, a two-fold lower anti-Xa clearance was seen among patients in the ICU compared to the general ward[146,147]	
Heparin-induced thrombocytopenia type II (HIT)	Because of the cross-reactivity between LMWHs and UFH, LMWHs should not be used in patients with or a history of HIT[108,111-113]	LMWHs are contraindicated[108,111-113]
Elderly (age ≥ 75 years)	Age-related decline in renal function. Excess bleeding complications may be minimized by using a dose-reduction strategy for enoxaparin (EXTRACT-TIMI-25 trial)[148]	Use all LMWHs with caution in elderly patients with renal insufficiency. See Table 1.12 for specific dosage adjustments based on CrCl where applicable. Alternatively, UFH should be considered. Tinzaparin, in particular, should be avoided[113]

(continued)

Safety concern	Rationale	Comments/recommendations
	An increased mortality risk was observed among elderly patients with renal insufficiency that received tinzaparin compared to UFH for VTE[113]	Enoxaparin for STEMI: 1) omit initial 30 mg IV bolus; 2) reduce SC dose from 1 to 0.75 mg/kg q 12 h; 3) dose cap first 2 SC doses to 75 mg[111]
Drug-drug Interactions	Pharmacokinetic-based drug-drug interactions such as Cytochrome P450 inhibition is not a concern with UFH. Pharmacodynamic interactions could be a concern with compounded or additive effects with the administration of drugs known to affect the risk of bleeding	An example of a pharmacodynamic interaction is the concomitant administration of UFH and antiplatelet agents such as aspirin and/or thienopyridines. Monitoring of complete blood count with platelets and aPTT or anti-factor-Xa concentrations should occur

Thrombolytics (Alteplase, Anistreplase, Reteplase, Streptokinase, Tenecteplase, Urokinase)

Dosing Considerations

Obesity: Pharmacodynamic and pharmacokinetic properties of the various thrombolytic agents are summarized in Table 1.15.[149-154] Previous evidence suggests an inverse relationship between fibrinolytic activity and the ratio of observed to standard weight.[155-157] In a study of 34 subjects with varying ratio of observed to standard weight, decreased plasma fibrinolytic activity was observed in obese subjects due to decreased production of plasminogen activator.[155] Body mass index has been shown to be an independent predictor of 30-day mortality and in-hospital bleeding, stroke, and cardiogenic shock in patients experiencing an ST-segment elevation ACS.[156,157] However, in patients diagnosed with this type of ACS, significantly higher rate of mortality has been demonstrated among patients with BMI when employing thrombolysis as a reperfusion strategy.[156,157] Based on recommendations made by the manufacturers, all of the thrombolytics have maximum dose limits (Table 1.15), leading to potentially lower thrombolytic dose per body weight in patients with high BMI.[149-153] Having a maximum dose limit could alter the relative effectiveness of thrombolytics when comparing clinical outcomes to those in patients undergoing a PCI, which is less likely to be influenced by BMI.[156]

While many studies have confirmed the influence of BMI on clinical outcomes, very limited data are available on the effectiveness of thrombolytic therapy compared to PCI in patients with varying BMI. One retrospective analysis examined 7,630 patients with STEMI receiving either PCI (46%) or thrombolytic therapy (54%), who were stratified into three groups by BMI: (1) BMI 20–24.9 kg/m^2

Table 1.15 Comparison of clinical properties of thrombolytics[149-154]

Property	Alteplase	Anistreplase[a]	Reteplase	Streptokinase	Tenecteplase	Urokinase
Molecular weight (Da)	70,000	131,000	39,000	47,000	70,000	34,500
Half-life (min)	<5	100	13–16	18–83	20–24	20
Elimination	Hepatic	Hepatic	Renal	Renal	Hepatic	Hepatic
Fibrin selective	Yes	No	Yes	No	Yes	No
Potential allergenicity	<0.2%	Unknown	No	1–4%	<1%	<1%
Systemic fibrinogen depletion	+	+++	++	+++	Minimal	+++
Maximum intravenous dose in ACS	100 mg (body weight ≥67 kg)	30 U	20 U (two 10 U boluses given 30 min apart)	1,50,000 U	50 mg (body weight ≥90 kg)	4,400 IU/kg, followed by 4,400 IU/kg/h for 12 h
Hemodialyzable[b]	Unlikely (no data)	Unlikely (no data)	No data	No data	Unlikely (no data)	No data

ACS acute coronary syndrome, *IU* international units

[a]No longer available in the United States

[b]Although no data were found for any of the thrombolytics, some of them are unlikely to be dialyzable based on pharmacokinetic parameters including molecular weight

(n = 2,277); (2) BMI 25–29.9 kg/m^2 (n = 3,763); and (3) BMI ≥ 30 kg/m^2 (n = 1,590).[158] The investigators demonstrated that BMI was inversely related to death, shock, stroke, and bleeding in patients receiving either reperfusion therapy. However, patients receiving thrombolytic therapy were more likely to experience in-hospital death, regardless of BMI (group I: OR 1.69 [95% CI 1.19–2.44], group II: OR 1.89 [95% CI 1.39–2.56], group III: OR 1.85, [95% CI 1.08–3.22]). There were also trends in decreased rate of stroke and nonfatal bleeding in obese patients. The findings from this study suggested that obese patients may benefit from higher thrombolytic dosing. However, until future studies have investigated the impact of higher thrombolytic dosing on the risk of clinically significant bleeding, the maximum thrombolytic doses recommended by the manufacturers should be used.

Thinness/emaciation: There are no reports on dosing considerations in underweight or nutritionally deficient patients. Because the incidence of bleeding has been demonstrated to be the highest in STEMI patients with low BMI (<20 kg/m^2), it would be reasonable to consider decreasing the fibrinolytic dose; however, this would have the potential to reduce target vessel reperfusion in this patient population.[158] Until formal pharmacokinetic evaluations are performed in patients with low BMI, the recommended dosing regimen by manufacturers should be used.

Kidney Injury: Pharmacokinetic considerations (Table 1.15) demonstrate that both reteplase and streptokinase are affected by renal impairment, whereas the other thrombolytics are primarily affected by hepatic impairment.[149-153] Patients with chronic kidney disease have platelet abnormalities that could increase risk of thromboembolic events when untreated and potentially augment bleeding episodes with concomitant antiplatelet and antithrombotic therapy.[137,159] Much of the limited data in patients with significant renal impairment are derived from alteplase therapy. In a retrospective study of 74 patients who received thrombolytic therapy for acute ischemic stroke, patients with a creatinine clearance (CrCl) <60 mL/min were not found to be associated with increased risk of intracranial hemorrhage, poor functional outcome, or death. This trial demonstrated that alteplase (given at the manufacturer's recommended dose of 0.9 mg/kg up to a maximum of 90 mg) is safe for treatment of stroke in patients with renal impairment.[160] Another study of 196 stroke patients receiving recombinant tissue plasminogen activator (tPA) determined that impaired renal function is an independent predictor of poor outcomes and increased risk of intracranial hemorrhage. However, the study did not investigate the correlation of renal function and clinical outcomes with the use of recombinant tPA.[161]

A retrospective analysis was conducted in 79 patients with myocardial infarction treated with either streptokinase (64 patients) or alteplase (15 patients), to examine whether renal and hepatic function influence elimination and metabolism of thrombolytics and their efficacy in PCI.[162] The authors determined a positive correlation between streptokinase use and high serum creatinine concentrations (p = 0.001). Yet, patients receiving streptokinase and undergoing rescue PCI had similar serum creatinine concentrations compared to patients who did not receive a PCI and experienced similar clinical outcomes. There were no correlations found between alteplase use and serum creatinine concentrations.

Based on the current available data, dosage adjustments in patients with renal impairment are not necessary when administering thrombolytic therapy.

Hemodialysis/Continuous Renal Replacement Therapy: No formal pharmacokinetic evaluations have been conducted in patients with end-stage renal disease requiring either hemodialysis or continuous renal replacement therapy.

Liver Dysfunction: Many of the thrombolytics are metabolized and cleared by the liver, including alteplase (clearance > 80%), tenecteplase (clearance significantly less than alteplase), and urokinase (primarily metabolized in liver with small fractions found in bile and urine).[149,152,153] Patients with liver disease (e.g., alcoholic cirrhosis, primary biliary cirrhosis, and hepatic malignancy) are more likely to have appreciable increases in plasma concentration of tPA and specific plasminogen activator inhibitors (PAI-1, PAI-2).[163] This balance between tPA and the inhibitors may be disrupted in liver disease due to reduced hepatic clearance of tPA and tPA-PAI-1 complex, which may account for increased concentrations of free and complexed tPA.[163] This has pertinent clinical considerations because increased concentrations of tPA may increase the risk of bleeding in patients with hepatic impairment.

In a retrospective analysis of 79 patients with myocardial infarction treated with either streptokinase (64 patients) or alteplase (15 patients), the investigators examined whether renal and hepatic function influence elimination and metabolism of thrombolytics and efficacy of PCI.[162] The authors determined that there was no correlation observed between use of streptokinase and serum alanine transaminase concentrations. Similarly, there were no correlations found between alteplase use and hepatic enzymes. The authors stated that clearance of alteplase was not significantly changed in moderate impairment; however, clearance was significantly influenced by severe hepatic impairment (e.g., fibrosis or cirrhosis).

Based on the very limited date in patients with hepatic impairment, no dosage adjustments are required at this time.

Hypothermia: To date, there are no formal clinical evaluations on the effect of therapeutically-induced hypothermia in patients receiving a thrombolytic. However, some studies have demonstrated *in vitro* temperature dependence changes on fibrinolysis using human clot lysis.[163,164] Using a human clot model demonstrated that lowering the temperature prolonged the lysis time from 111 min at T = 37.5°C to 186 min at T = 30°C.[164] The investigators demonstrated that the conversion from plasminogen to plasmin exhibited a temperature dependence. Clinically, this could potentially increase the risk of bleeding in patients who are undergoing therapeutically-induced hypothermia. Future studies investigating the effect of hypothermia on thrombolytics in patients with either STEMI or acute ischemic stroke are warranted.

Safety Concerns

Safety concern	Rationale	Comments/recommendations
Risk of hemorrhage	Intracranial hemorrhage and major bleeding are the most serious side effects of fibrinolytic agents. The risk of intracranial hemorrhage is highest with fibrin-specific agents (e.g., alteplase and tenecteplase) than with streptokinase. Yet, risk of systemic bleeding other than intracranial hemorrhage is higher with streptokinase.[165]	Closely monitor for signs/ symptoms of bleeding and neurological function Absolute Contraindications: Active internal bleeding Previous intracranial hemorrhage at any time or ischemic stroke within 3 months Known intracranial neoplasm Known structural vascular lesion Suspected aortic dissection significant closed head or facial trauma within 3 months
	Certain risk factors are known to increase incidence of intracranial hemorrhage in patients receiving thrombolytics: patients over 65 years, female sex, and low body weight (<70 kg).[154]	
	Thus, thrombolytics should be used with caution in certain disease states and other circumstances that can increase risk of hemorrhage. Patients with high risk of major hemorrhage, including intracranial hemorrhage, have either absolute or relative contraindications defined by ACC/AHA Guidelines for management of patients with STEMI.[165]	Relative Contraindications (benefit outweighs risk of major hemorrhage): Severe, uncontrolled hypertension (BP > 180/110 mmHg) History of previous ischemic stroke >3 months or dementia Current use of anticoagulants known bleeding diathesis Traumatic or prolonged (>10 min) CPR or major surgery <3 weeks ago Noncompressible vascular puncture Recent internal bleeding within 2–4 weeks ago Pregnancy Active peptic ulcer
UFH dosing	In patients receiving thrombolytics, concomitant therapy with UFH is required in order to prevent possible thrombotic events; however, the addition of UFH can increase risk of intracranial bleeding if high doses are used.[166]	Initiate a lower dose of unfractionated heparin in patients receiving a thrombolytic:[167] Initial dose: 60 U/kg (maximum 4,000 U) Maintenance dose: 12 U/kg/h (maximum 1,000 U/h)

Safety concern	Rationale	Comments/recommendations
Readministration	Due to development of antibodies, streptokinase may be ineffective after 5 days up to 12 months from the first administration due to increased likelihood of resistance.[151] Although sustained antibody development to alteplase has not been documented previously, detectable concentrations have been reported.[149]	Administer with caution
Drug-drug interactions	Pharmacodynamic interactions could be a concern if used concurrently with other medications known to increase risk of bleeding.[149-153]	An example of a pharmacodynamic interaction is the concurrent administration of a thrombolytic (e.g., alteplase, streptokinase, and reteplase) with an anticoagulant (e.g., heparin, bivalirudin, fondaparinux, etc.) or antiplatelet agent (e.g., aspirin, warfarin, or thienopyridines). Monitoring of complete blood count with platelets and aPTT is warranted

BP blood pressure, *ACC* American College of Cardiology, *AHA* American Heart Association, *STEMI* ST-segment Elevation Myocardial Infarction

Unfractionated Heparin

Dosing Considerations

Obesity: The volume of distribution of UFH approximates blood volume (40–70 mL/kg) given its saturable clearance within vascular endothelium. Adipose tissue is less vascularized than lean tissue and therefore heparin does not distribute well into adipose tissue.[168-170] Debate over what type of weight to use when dosing heparin in the setting of obesity is ongoing. The use of ABW for dosing may lead to supratherapeutic heparin concentrations whereas ideal body weight (IBW) may lead to subtherapeutic concentrations by failing to account for the additional vasculature seen in adipose tissue.[170,171] An overview of the issues surrounding heparin dosing for both prophylaxis and treatment in the setting of obesity is described below.

Dosing for VTE Prophylaxis in Obesity

The optimal dosing of UFH for VTE prophylaxis in obesity or morbid obesity is unclear. Studies evaluating the use of UFH for patients that are morbidly obese are limited to the bariatric surgery population. Numerous observational studies have evaluated fixed doses of 5,000–7,500 U given SC every 8–12 h.[172-174] None of these studies, however, included a standardized assessment for DVT and PE. Consequently, the incidence of such events was low. Other small studies have examined IV infusions or SC regimens adjusted based on anti-Xa concentrations. These studies have not been shown to be superior to traditional fixed doses and should be avoided due to the risk for over-anticoagulation.[175-177] The utility of anti-Xa monitoring to predict effectiveness or bleeding events is unclear. The American College of Chest Physicians (ACCP) advocate higher doses of UFH for inpatient bariatric surgery. Specific recommendations are to give UFH three-times daily (Grade 1C) at higher doses than usual for nonobese patients (Grade 2C).[115] Because data for UFH dosing in morbidly obese patients have been generated in the bariatric surgery setting, it is unclear if the same recommendations apply to other patients.

Dosing for VTE Treatment in Obesity

Use of a weight-based dosing nomogram for heparin has long been established as a means of providing more prompt therapeutic anticoagulation without increasing the risk of major bleeding.[178] Various nomograms have been published for treatment of acute VTE, ACS, and stroke. Current ACCP guidelines for management of VTE recommend an initial IV bolus dose of 80 U/kg or 5,000 U with an initial continuous IV infusion of 18 U/kg/h or 1,300 U/h.[179] The landmark study by Raschke et al. established the current dosing regimen for VTE and used ABW for dosing. However, only nine patients in that study weighed more than 100 kg and the highest patient weight included was 131 kg.[178] Consequently, several evaluations have described other dosing schemes based on IBW, dosing weight (DW), a modified DW which averages ABW and IBW, ABW with maximum allowable initial doses ("dose caps"), or even estimates of plasma volume. A summary of published reports describing different evaluations of weight with respect to treatment doses of heparin is shown in Table 1.16.[169-171,180-187] Although ABW still appears to be the preferred means of dosing heparin for patients that are not morbidly obese, comparative data between different types of weight-based strategies and laboratory and clinical outcomes are limited.

Despite the various approaches to determine the most appropriate type of weight to employ for treatment doses of UFH, evidence suggests that the rates of nontherapeutic aPTT by 24–48 h remain around 60% with weight-based dosing in general.[188] Alternative means of dosing heparin have been proposed based on the estimation of blood volume. Equations for estimating blood volume and initial heparin dose which take into account sex, ABW, height, and age have been published.

Table 1.16 Overview of therapeutic heparin dosing in obesity

Dosing method/initial bolus and infusion regimen	Definition of obesity or patient weight	Study design	No. patients	Primary endpoint
Empiric[170] Bolus 10,000 U Infusion 1000 U/h	210 kg	Case report	1	Dose required to maintain therapeutic aPTT (3,800 U/h)
ABW[180] Bolus 80 U/kg (20,400 U) Infusion rate 18 U/kg/h (4,590 U/h)	255 kg	Case report	1	Dose required to maintain therapeutic aPTT (1,280 U/h)
DW = IBW + 0.3 (ABW-IBW) if obese[171] ABW (with maximum) Bolus 80 U/kg (10,000 U) Infusion 15 U/kg/h (1,500 U/h) if non-obese	≥10 kg above IBW	Retro-spective	213	ABW vs. IBW vs. DW; less deviation of infusion rates leading to first therapeutic aPTT with ABW (p<0.001)
ABW[169] Bolus 70 U/kg Infusion 15 U/kg/h	ABW ≥30% above IBW	Retro-spective	40	Obese vs. non-obese; no differences in % change between initial and final infusion rates, time to therapeutic aPTT, or final infusion rates
Total blood volume[181] Bolus 450 U/L of estimated blood volume (L)[a] Infusion = 344.335 + (estimated blood volume × 257.962) − (age in years × 4.951)	Median ABW 77 kg (range, 30–184 kg)	Prospective case series	197	Initial target anti-Xa concentrations (62% at 8 h) improved vs. weight-based protocol

(continued)

Table 1.16 (continued)

Dosing method/initial bolus and infusion regimen	Definition of obesity or patient weight	Study design	No. patients	Primary endpoint
Modified DW[182] = (ABW + IBW)/2	182 kg	Case report	1	Therapeutic aPTT achieved within 10 h (2,160 U/h)
ABW (with maximum)[183] Bolus 80 U/kg (10,000 U) Infusion 15 U/kg/h (2,100 U/h)	ABW >50% above IBW	Retro-spective	53	Obese vs. non-obese; no differences in therapeutic aPTT, time to therapeutic aPTT, or follow-up aPTT
ABW[184] Bolus 80 U/kg Infusion 18 U/kg/h	BMI ≥ 40 kg/m²	Retro-spective	101	Morbidly obese vs. non-morbidly obese; greater aPTT values at 6–12 h and more supratherapeutic aPTTs in morbidly obese group
Bolus 5,000 U[185] (non-weight based) Infusion 15 U/kg/h (maximum 1,500 U/h)	388 kg	Case report	1	Initial therapeutic aPTT achieved at 55 h (3,650 U/h)
ABW[186] Bolus (60–80 U/kg) Infusion (12–18 U/kg/h)	BMI ≥ 40 kg/m²	Prospective, observational, cohort	273	BMI ≥ 40 vs. 25–39.9 vs. <25 kg/m²; mean infusion rate required to achieve first therapeutic aPTT 11.5 vs. 12.5 vs. 13.5 U/kg/h, respectively (p = 0.001)

Men: $(0.3669 \times \text{height in m}^3) + (0.03219 \times \text{weight in kg}) + 0.6041$

Women: $(0.3561 \times \text{height in m}^3) + (0.03308 \times \text{weight in kg}) + 0.1833$

U units, *ABW* actual body weight, *aPTT* activated partial thromboplastin time, *DW* dosing weight, *IBW* ideal body weight, *BMI* body mass index

[a]Estimated blood volume (L) calculated below from Nadler et al.[187]

Evaluation of this protocol has shown improved anti-factor Xa results, but not clinical outcomes.[181]

Dosing for Acute Coronary Syndromes (ACS) in Obesity

The American College of Cardiology/American Heart Association (ACC/AHA) and ACCP guidelines recommend an initial IV bolus dose of 60 U/kg (maximum 4,000 U) and an initial continuous IV infusion of 12 U/kg/h (maximum 1,000 U/h) based on ABW or estimated weights for NSTEMI, unstable angina, and STEMI.[126,127,189] A protocol for subsequent weight-based dose adjustments has not been validated. Despite these recommendations, registry data have indicated that only one-third of heparin doses for NSTEMI were appropriate.[82] Furthermore, a subgroup analysis of the EXTRACT-TIMI 25 trial demonstrated that body weight was an independent predictor of markedly high or low anticoagulation which translated to an increased risk of bleeding and recurrent MI, respectively.[190]

Dosing for Morbidly Obese

The use of ABW or IBW may result in overdosing or underdosing, respectively for morbidly obese patients. Use of ABW with a maximum limit may also delay the time to achievement of a therapeutic aPTT for these patients.[185] Dosing recommendations for morbid obesity, defined as ABW at least 200% of IBW or BMI $\geq$ 40 kg/m^2, are limited but one recent report recommends use of a modified dosing weight (DW = IBW + 0.4 [ABW-IBW] or DW = IBW + 0.3 [ABW-IBW]) for initial heparin dosing requirements.[185] Authors of the largest study of heparin in morbid obesity to date recommend a maximum initial infusion rate of 14 U/kg/h based on ABW for patients meeting the BMI definition ($\geq$40 kg/m^2).[186] While BMI is used by the World Health Organization to define obesity, at this time it is not generally used for medication dosing in the clinical setting. In summary, the use of dose limits for UFH in morbidly obese patients is controversial. Ideally, these patients should be evaluated on an individual basis. However, a review of the available literature in Table 1.16 suggests that a maximum bolus dose of 10,000 U may be reasonable to minimize the risk of overanticoagulation. Maximum infusion rates are less certain, although the highest report dose required to maintain a therapeutic aPTT was 3,800 U/h.[170]

Thinness/emaciation: Formal evaluations of UFH dosing in patients with low body weight and/or emaciation have not been conducted. However, a prospective registry described clinical characteristics and outcomes in patients with extreme body weight that were treated for acute VTE. Approximately 2% (n = 169) of the registry weighed <50 kg, although only eight of the 169 patients received UFH. Patients were predominantly female and had more severe underlying disease (e.g., malignancy). Patients that weighed less than 50 kg had an increased risk of bleeding complications, but only 1 of 5 with major bleeding had received UFH. This may reflect underlying co-morbidities, UFH, or both.[132] Consequently, it seems prudent to consider lower doses of UFH in patients at lower extremes of body weight.

Kidney Injury: At low to therapeutic concentrations, heparin exhibits non-linear and rapid clearance via protein binding and endothelial uptake. In contrast, higher doses of heparin or continued administration saturate endothelial binding and result in renal elimination through a slower dose-independent route.[191] Lower doses (25 U/kg) appear to have a half-life of 30 min whereas higher doses (100 and 400 U/kg) have half-lives of 60–150 min.[191] Specific dosage adjustments for heparin in the setting of renal impairment have not been determined. However, a higher SCr was shown to be an independent predictor of nontherapeutic antico-agulation with heparin in an EXTRACT-TIMI 25 sub-analysis. Specifically, a 0.2 mg/dL increment increase in SCr was associated with a significant 8% increase in the risk of markedly high anticoagulation. Patients with severe renal impair-ment (SCr > 2.5 mg/dL in males or >2 mg/dL in females) were excluded from this analysis.[190] In another analysis, renal insufficiency (defined as SCr > 2 mg/dL, CrCl < 30 mL/min, or need for dialysis) was also shown to be a risk factor for excess dosing of heparin in ACS registry data.[82] No formal studies have evaluated specific dosage adjustments in this setting, however, use should be approached with caution and strict monitoring of the aPTT or anti-Xa concentrations are rec-ommended. Despite the challenges in dosing UFH in patients with renal impair-ment, some authors have advocated its use over newer anticoagulants with extended half-lives and predominant renal clearance (e.g., enoxaparin, fonda-parinux). Specifically, UFH has been recommended for treatment of VTE in patients with an estimated CrCl < 30 mL/min.[192]

Hemodialysis/Continuous Renal Replacement Therapy: The need to provide anticoagulation of the extracorporeal circuit is generally met with the use of UFH (bolus of up to 5,000 IU; continuous infusion rate of 200–1,600 U/h).[138,193] Target anti-Xa concentrations have been proposed at >0.5 IU/mL.[194] However, no formal evaluations of dosing have been conducted in this population. UFH has a mean molecular weight of 15,000 Da (range, 3,000–30,000).[108] Hemodialysis would only be expected to remove negligible amount of larger molecules including UFH. Conversely, hemofiltration (CVVHF) will generally clear solutes up to 20,000 Da.[193] Therefore UFH should be more likely to be removed by CVVHF than hemodialysis.[193] However, a study of critically ill patients that received CVVHF demonstrated no appreciable removal of UFH despite the molecular weight con-siderations. The authors speculated that UFH bound to antithrombin III (AT III) may render the complexes too large or the negative charge of UFH may prevent removal through the filter membrane.[140] No dosing adjustments of UFH have been evaluated in this population. While it might seem intuitive to empirically reduce the dose of UFH during CRRT, critically ill patients may have a deficiency of AT III that could lead to clotting of the hemofilter circuit therefore requiring higher doses of UFH.[140]

Liver Dysfunction: UFH is metabolized mainly through the reticuloendothelial sys-tem via a saturable mechanism.[195] Consequently, no dosage adjustments would be expected in patients with liver dysfunction, although formal evaluations are lacking.

Hypothermia: A small study of patients that underwent cardiopulmonary bypass examined the effect of hypothermia on UFH concentrations. The investigators demonstrated insignificant UFH decay during hypothermia (25 °C) as opposed to a linear decline in concentrations with rewarming (37°C). Therefore, re-dosing of UFH during periods of hypothermia in the setting of cardiopulmonary bypass is likely not needed.[196] The use of therapeutic hypothermia as part of the management of post-cardiac arrest syndrome is known to impair coagulation and inhibit platelet function which may predispose to bleeding. Monitoring of aPTT levels during UFH therapy should be accompanied by a recording of the patient's temperature during hypothermia so that the laboratory may test the sample at that temperature.[97] No official recommendations for dose adjustments of UFH are available in the setting of hypothermia at this time.

Safety Concerns

Safety concern	Rationale	Comments/recommendations

Risk of hemorrhage	UFH inhibits blood coagulation, impairs platelet function, and increases capillary permeability. Bleeding can occur at virtually any site
	
	The additional risk of major bleeding conferred with therapeutic UFH appears to be <3%. The exact risk depends on intensity and duration of treatment as well as concurrent medications and disease states[61]
		Avoid in patients with:
		  Severe thrombocytopenia
		  When blood coagulation tests (e.g., aPTT) cannot be performed at appropriate intervals to monitor therapeutic doses of UFH

	Certain conditions are known to have an increased risk of hemorrhage (e.g., severe hypertension, subacute bacterial endocarditis, major surgery, need for lumbar puncture or spinal anesthesia, hemophilia, thrombocytopenia, certain vascular purpuras, ulcerative lesions, continuous drainage of the stomach or small intestine, and liver disease with impaired hemostasis)[195]	Uncontrollable active bleeding except when due to disseminated intravascular coagulation) Weigh the benefits of UFH use in the context of known risk factors for UFH-associated bleeding: recent surgery, trauma, age>70 years, and renal failure. Additionally, intermittent IV UFH has been related to higher bleeding compared to continuous IV and SC UFH infusions. While the bleeding risk is anticipated to be increased with higher intensity UFH, this relationship has not been consistently documented[61]

(continued)

Safety concern	Rationale	Comments/recommendations
Heparin-induced thrombocytopenia type II (HIT)	Antibody-mediated reaction in response to heparin bound to platelet factor 4 (PF4) that results in platelet activation and thrombin generation	Platelet count monitoring is suggested
	Clinicopathologic syndrome diagnosed with presence of "HIT antibodies" along with one of the following: unexplained platelet count fall (30–50% from baseline), presence of thrombosis, skin lesions at heparin injection sites, or acute systemic reactions after IV bolus administration of heparin	Investigate HIT if patient meets clinical criteria as defined under clinicopathologic syndrome. Additionally, platelet count fall generally occurs between days 5–14 unless the patient has been exposed to heparin within the preceding 100 days (can occur within 24 h)
	Serologic testing is more effective in ruling out HIT than confirming the diagnosis (lower specificity than sensitivity). However, a strong positive result is associated with a higher risk for HIT[67]	Discontinue heparin by all routes and change to alternative anticoagulant (e.g., direct thrombin inhibitor) if HIT is strongly suspected or confirmed. Withhold warfarin therapy until the platelet count has recovered substantially (e.g., >150 × 10^9/L)[67]
Drug-drug Interactions	Pharmacokinetic-based drug-drug interactions such as Cytochrome P450 inhibition is not a concern with UFH. Pharmacodynamic interactions could be a concern with compounded or additive effects with the administration of drugs known to affect the risk of bleeding	An example of a pharmacodynamic interaction is the concomitant administration of UFH and antiplatelet agents such as aspirin and/or thienopyridines. Monitoring of complete blood count with platelets and aPTT or anti-factor-Xa concentrations should occur

References

1. Attia J, Ray JG, Cook DJ, et al. Deep vein thrombosis and its prevention in critically ill adults. *Arch Intern Med.* 2001;161:1268-1279.
2. Geerts WH, Heit JA, Clagett GP, et al. Prevention of venous thromboembolism. *Chest.* 2001;119:132S-175S.
3. Fanikos J, Stapinski C, Koo S, et al. Medication errors associated with anticoagulant therapy in a hospital. *Am J Cardiol.* 2004;94(4):532-535.
4. Hicks RW, Becker SC, Cousins DD, eds. MEDMARX data report: a report on the relationship of drug names and medication errors in response to the institute of medicine's call to action (2003–2006 findings and trends 2002–2006). Rockville, MD: Center for the Advancement of Patient Safety, US Pharmacopeia; 2008.

5. Michaels AD, Spinler SA, Leeper B, et al. Medication errors in acute cardiovascular and stroke patients: a scientific statement from the American Heart Association Acute Cardiac Care Committee of the Council on Clinical Cardiology. *Circulation*. 2010;121:1644-1682.

6. Product information. Argatroban. Research Triangle Park, NC: GlaxoSmithKline; March 2009.

7. Product information. Angiomax® (bivalirudin). Parsippany, NJ: The Medicines Company; December 2005.

8. Product information. Refludan® (lepirudin). Montville, NJ: Berlex Laboratories; October 2004.

9. Nutescu EA, Shapiro NL, Chevalier A. New anticoagulant agents: direct thrombin inhibitors. *Clin Geriatr Med*. 2006;22(viii):33-56.

10. Nutescu EA, Wittkowsky AK. Direct thrombin inhibitors for anticoagulation. *Ann Pharmacother*. 2004;38:99-109.

11. Institute for Safe Medication Practices. ISMP's list of high-alert medications. 2008. Available at: http://www.ismp.org/Tools/highalertmedications.pdf. Accessed November 23, 2010.

12. Hursting MJ, Jang IK. Effect of body mass index on argatroban therapy during percutaneous coronary intervention. *J Thromb Thrombolysis*. 2008;25:273-279.

13. Rice L, Hursting MJ, Baillie GM, et al. Argatroban anticoagulation in obese versus nonobese patients: implications for treating heparin-induced thrombocytopenia. *J Clin Pharmacol*. 2007;47(8):1028-1034.

14. Lincoff AM, Bittl JA, Harrington RA, et al. Bivalirudin and provisional glycoprotein IIb/IIIa blockade compared with heparin and planned glycoprotein IIb/IIIa blockade during percutaneous coronary intervention: REPLACE-2 randomized trial. *JAMA*. 2003;289:853-863.

15. Bittl JA, Chaitman BR, Feit F, et al. Bivalirudin versus heparin during coronary angioplasty for unstable or postinfarction angina: final report reanalysis of the bivalirudin angioplasty study. *Am Heart J*. 2001;142:952-959.

16. Mahaffey KW, Lewis BE, Wildermann NM, for the ATBAT Investigators, et al. The anticoagulant therapy with bivalirudin to assist in the performance of percutaneous coronary intervention in patients with heparin-induced thrombocytopenia (ATBAT) study: main results. *J Invasive Cardiol*. 2003;15:611-616.

17. Yusuf S, Pogue J, Anand S, et al. Effects of recombinant hirudin (lepirudin) compared with heparin on death, myocardial infarction, refractory angina, and revascularization procedures in patients with acute myocardial ischemia without ST elevation: a randomized trial. *Lancet*. 1999;353:429-438.

18. Kiser TH, Burch JC, Klem PM, et al. Safety, efficacy, and dosing requirements of bivalirudin in patients with heparin-induced thrombocytopenia. *Pharmacotherapy*. 2008;28:1115-1124.

19. Tschudi M, Lammle B, Alberio L. Dosing lepirudin in patients with heparin-induced thrombocytopenia and normal or impaired renal function: a single-center experience with 68 patients. *Blood*. 2009;113:2402-2409.

20. Tardy B, Lecompte T, Boelhen F, et al. Predictive factors for thrombosis and major bleeding in an observational study in 181 patients with heparin-induced thrombocytopenia treated with lepirudin. *Blood*. 2006;108:1492-1496.

21. Murray PT, Reddy BV, Grossman EF, et al. A prospective comparison of three argatroban treatment regimens during hemodialysis in end-stage renal disease. *Kidney Int*. 2004;66: 2446-2453.

22. Gajra A, Vajpayee N, Smith A, et al. Lepirudin for anticoagulation in patients with heparin-induced thrombocytopenia treated with continuous renal replacement therapy. *Am J Hematol*. 2007;82:391-393.

23. Fischer KG, van de Loo A, Bohler J. Recombinant hirudin (lepirudin) as anticoagulant in intensive care patients treated with continuous hemodialysis. *Kidney Int*. 1999;56:S46-S50.

24. Saner F, Hertl M, Broelsch CE. Anticoagulation with hirudin for continuous veno-venous hemodialysis in liver transplantation. *Acta Anaesthesiol Scand*. 2001;45:914-918.

25. Hursting MJ, Jang IK. Impact of renal function on argatroban therapy during percutaneous coronary intervention. *J Thromb Thrombolysis*. 2010;29:1-7.

26. Guzzi LM, McCollum DA, Hursting MJ. Effect of renal function on argatroban therapy in heparin-induced thrombocytopenia. *J Thromb Thrombolysis*. 2006;22:169-176.
27. Kiser TH, Fish DN. Evaluation of bivalirudin treatment for heparin-induced thrombocytopenia in critical ill patients with hepatic and/or renal dysfunction. *Pharmacotherapy*. 2006;26: 452-460.
28. Seybert AL, Coons JC, Zerumsky K. Treatment of heparin-induced thrombocytopenia: is there a role for bivalirudin? *Pharmacotherapy*. 2006;26:229-241.
29. Robson R. The use of bivalirudin in patients with renal impairment. *J Invasive Cardiol*. 2000;12:F33-F36.
30. Robson R, White H, Aylward P, et al. Bivalirudin pharmacokinetics and pharmacodynamics: effect of renal function, dose, and gender. *Clin Pharmacol Ther*. 2002;71:433-439.
31. Lubenow N, Eichler P, Lietz T, et al. Lepirudin in patients with heparin-induced thrombocytopenia: results of the third prospective study (HAT-3) and a combined analysis of HAT-1, HAT-2, and HAT-3. *J Thromb Haemost*. 2005;3:2428-2436.
32. Hacquard M, de Maistre E, Lecompte T. Lepirudin: is the approved dosing schedule too high? *J Thromb Haemost*. 2005;3:2593-2596.
33. Tang IY, Cox DS, Patel K, et al. Argatroban and renal replacement therapy in patients with heparin-induced thrombocytopenia. *Ann Pharmacother*. 2005;39:231-236.
34. Williamson DR, Boulanger I, Tardif M, et al. Argatroban dosing in intensive care patients with acute renal failure and liver dysfunction. *Pharmacotherapy*. 2004;24(3):409-414.
35. de Denus S, Spinler SA. Decreased argatroban clearance unaffected by hemodialysis in anasarca. *Ann Pharmacother*. 2003;37:1237-1240.
36. Delhaye C, Maluenda G, Wakabayashi K, et al. Safety and in-hospital outcomes of bivalirudin use in dialysis patients undergoing percutaneous coronary intervention. *Am J Cardiol*. 2010;105:297-301.
37. Wittkowsky AK, Kondo LM. Lepirudin dosing in dialysis-dependent renal failure. *Pharmacotherapy*. 2000;20(9):1123-1128.
38. Bucha E, Nowak G, Czerwinski R, et al. R-hirudin as anticoagulant in regular hemodialysis therapy: finding of therapeutic r-hirudin blood/plasma concentrations and respective dosages. *Clin Appl Thromb Hemost*. 1999;5:164-170.
39. Vanholder RC, Camez AA, Veys NM, et al. Recombinant hirudin: a specific thrombin inhibiting anticoagulant for hemodialysis. *Kidney Int*. 1994;45:1754-1759.
40. Swan SK, Hursting MJ. The pharmacokinetics and pharmacodynamics of argatroban: effects of age, gender, and hepatic or renal dysfunction. *Pharmacotherapy*. 2000;20:318-329.
41. Levine RL, Hursting MJ, McCollum D. Argatroban therapy in heparin-induced thrombocytopenia with hepatic dysfunction. *Chest*. 2006;129:1167-1175.
42. Hoffman WD, Czyz Y, McCollum D, et al. Reduced argatroban doses after coronary artery bypass graf surgery. *Ann Pharmacother*. 2008;42:309-316.
43. Begelman SM, Baghdasarian SB, Singh IM, et al. Argatroban anticoagulation in intensive care patients: effects of heart failure and multiple organ system failure. *J Intensive Care Med*. 2008;23:313-320.
44. Nutescu EA, Shapiro NL, Chevalier A, et al. New anticoagulant agents: direct thrombin inhibitors. *Clin Geriatr Med*. 2006;22:33-56.
45. Sheth SB, DiCicco RA, Hursting MJ, et al. Interpreting the International Normalized Ratio (INR) in individuals receiving argatroban and warfarin. *Thromb Haemost*. 2001;85:435-440.
46. Hursting MJ, Zehnder JL, Joffrion JL, et al. The International Normalized Ratio during concurrent warfarin and argatroban anticoagulation: differential contributions of each agent and effects of the choice of thromboplastin used. *Clin Chem*. 1999;45:409-412.
47. Warkentin TE, Greinacher A, Koster A, et al. Treatment and prevention of heparin-induced thrombocytopenia: American College of Chest Physicians evidence-based clinical practice guidelines. 8th ed. *Chest*. 2008;133:340S-380S.
48. Product information. Arixtra (fondaparinux). Research Triangle Park, NC: GlaxoSmithKline; October 2010.

49. Raftopoulos I, Cortese-Hassett A, Gourash W, et al. Pharmacokinetic properties of fonda-parinux sodium in morbidly obese volunteers indicate that a single, weight-independent daily dose for thromboprophylaxis is feasible. In: Society of American Gastrointestinal and Endoscopic Surgeons (SAGES). Philadelphia, PA, April 8–12, 2008. Abstract # ETP079.

50. Turpie AGG. Use of selective factor Xa inhibitors in special populations. *Am J Orthop.* 2002;31(suppl 11):11-15.

51. Agnelli G, Bergqvist D, Cohen AT, et al. Randomized clinical trial of postoperative fonda-parinux versus perioperative dalteparin for prevention of venous thromboembolism in high-risk abdominal surgery. *Br J Surg.* 2005;92:1212-1220.

52. Turpie AGG, Bauer KA, Caprini JA, et al. Fondaparinux combined with intermittent pneu-matic compression vs. intermittent pneumatic compression alone for prevention of venous thromboembolism after abdominal surgery: a randomized, double-blind comparison. *J Thromb Haemost.* 2007;5:1854-1861.

53. Buller HR, Davidson BL, Decousus H, et al. Subcutaneous fondaparinux versus intravenous unfractionated heparin in the initial treatment of pulmonary embolism. *N Engl J Med.* 2003;349(18):1695-1702.

54. Buller HR, Davidson BL, Decousus H, et al. Fondaparinux or enoxaparin for the initial treat-ment of symptomatic deep venous thrombosis: a randomized trial. *Ann Intern Med.* 2004; 140:867-873.

55. Buller HR for the MATISSE Investigators. Efficacy and safety of fondaparinux (Arixtra®) in the initial treatment of venous thromboembolism in obese patients [abstract]. *Blood* 2004; Abstract No. 706.

56. Davidson BL, Buller HR, Decousus H, et al. Effect of obesity on outcomes after fondaparinux, enoxaparin, or heparin treatment for acute venous thromboembolism in the Matisse trials. *J Thromb Haemost.* 2007;5:1191-1194.

57. Turpie AGG, Lensing AWA, Fuji T, Boyle DA. Pharmacokinetic and clinical data supporting the use of fondaparinux 1.5 mg once daily in the prevention of venous thromboembolism in renally impaired patients. *Blood Coagul Fibrinolysis.* 2009;20:114-121.

58. Kalicki RM, Aregger F, Alberio L, et al. Use of the pentasaccharide fondaparinux as an anti-coagulant during haemodialysis. *Thromb Haemost.* 2007;98:1200-1207.

59. Wellborn-Kim JJ, Mitchel GA, Terneus WF Jr, et al. Fondaparinux therapy in a hemodialysis patient with heparin-induced thrombocytopenia type II. *Am J Health Syst Pharm.* 2010;67: 1075-1079.

60. Haase M, Bellomo R, Rocktaeschel J, et al. Use of fondaparinux (Arixtra®) in a dialysis patient with symptomatic heparin-induced thrombocytopaenia type II. *Nephrol Dial Transplant.* 2005;20:444-446.

61. Schulman S, Beyth RJ, Kearon C, et al. Hemorrhagic complications of anticoagulant and thrombolytic treatment. *Chest.* 2008;133:257S-298S.

62. Boneu B, Necciari J, Cariou R, et al. Pharmacokinetics and tolerance of the natural pentasac-charide (SR90107/Org31540) with high affinity to antithrombin III in man. *Thromb Haemost.* 1995;74:1468-1473.

63. Yusuf S, Mehta SR, Chrolavicius S, et al. Comparison of fondaparinux and enoxaparin in acute coronary syndromes. *N Engl J Med.* 2006;354:1464-1476.

64. Warkentin TE, Maurer BT, Aster RH. Heparin-induced thrombocytopenia associated with fondaparinux. *N Engl J Med.* 2007;356:2653-2655.

65. Rota E, Bazzan M, Fantino G. Fondaparinux-related thrombocytopenia in a previous low-molecular-weight (LMWH)-induced heparin-induced thrombocytopenia (HIT). *Thromb Haemost.* 2008;99:779-781.

66. Alsaleh KA, Al-Nasser SM, Bates SM, et al. Delayed-onset HIT caused by low-molecular-weight heparin manifesting during fondaparinux prophylaxis. *Am J Hematol.* 2008;83:876-878.

67. Warkentin TE, Greinacher A, Koster A, Lincoff AM. Treatment and prevention of heparin-induced thrombocytopenia: American College of Chest Physicians Evidence-Based Clinical Practice Guidelines (8th ed). *Chest.* 2008;133(suppl 6):340S-380S.

68. Blackmer AB, Oertel MD, Valgus JM. Fondaparinux and the management of heparin-induced thrombocytopenia: the journey continues. *Ann Pharmacother*. 2009;43:1636-1646.
69. Product information. Reopro (abciximab). Leiden, NL: Centocor B.V.; and Indianapolis, IN: Eli Lilly and Company; November 2005.
70. Product information. Integrilin (eptifibatide). Kenilworth, NJ: Schering-Plough; January 2009.
71. Product information. Aggrastat (tirofiban). Deerfield, IL: Baxter Healthcare Corporation; and Somerset, NJ: Medicure Pharma, Inc.; July 2008.
72. Crouch MA, Nappi JM, Cheang KI. Glycoprotein IIb/IIIa receptor inhibitors in percutaneous coronary intervention and acute coronary syndrome. *Ann Pharmacother*. 2003;37:860-875.
73. Smith BS, Gandhi PJ. Pharmacokinetics and pharmacodynamics of low-molecular-weight heparins and glycoprotein IIb/IIIa receptor antagonists in renal failure. *J Thromb Thrombolysis*. 2001;11:39-48.
74. Data on file, Eli Lilly and Company and/or one of its subsidiaries.
75. EPILOG Investigators. Platelet glycoprotein IIb/IIIa receptor blockade and low-dose heparin during percutaneous coronary revascularization. *N Engl J Med*. 1997;336:1689-1696.
76. Investigators EPIC. Use of a monoclonal antibody directed against the platelet glycoprotein IIb/IIIa receptor in high-risk coronary angioplasty. *N Engl J Med*. 1994;330:956-961.
77. EPISTENT Investigators. Randomized-placebo and balloon-angioplasty-controlled trial to assess safety of coronary stenting with use of platelet glycoprotein IIb/IIIa blockade. *Lancet*. 1998;352:7-92.
78. Nikolsky E, Stone GW, Grines CL, et al. Impact of body mass index on outcomes after primary angioplasty in acute myocardial infarction. *Am Heart J*. 2006;151(1):168-175.
79. Ang L, Palakodeti V, Khalid A, et al. Elevated plasma fibrinogen and diabetes mellitus are associated with lower inhibition of platelet reactivity with clopidogrel. *J Am Coll Cardiol*. 2008;52:1052-1059.
80. Bhatt DL. What makes platelet angry. *J Am Coll Cardiol*. 2008;52(13):1060-1061.
81. Wiviott SD, Braunwald E, McCabe CH, et al. Prasugrel versus clopidogrel in patients with acute coronary syndromes. *N Engl J Med*. 2007;357:2001-2015.
82. Alexander KP, Chen AY, Roe MT, et al. Excess dosing of antiplatelet and antithrombin agents in the treatment of non-ST-segment elevation acute coronary syndromes. *JAMA*. 2005;294: 3108-3116.
83. Freeman RV, Mehta RH, Al Badr W, et al. Influence of concurrent renal dysfunction on outcomes of patients with acute coronary syndromes and implications of the use of glycoprotein IIb/IIIa inhibitors. *J Am Coll Cardiol*. 2003;41(5):718-724.
84. Reddan DN, O'Shea JC, Sarembock IJ, et al. Treatment effects of eptifibatide in planned coronary stent implantation in patients with chronic kidney disease (ESPRIT Trial). *Am J Cardiol*. 2003;91:17-21.
85. Platelet Receptor Inhibition in Ischemic Syndrome Management in Patients Limited by Unstable Signs and Symptoms (PRISM-PLUS) Study Investigators. Inhibition of the platelet glycoprotein IIb/IIIa receptor with tirofiban in unstable angina and non-Q-wave myocardial infarction. *N Engl J Med*. 1998;338:1488-1497.
86. Platelet Receptor Inhibition in Ischemic Syndrome Management (PRISM) Study Investigators. A comparison of aspirin plus tirofiban with aspirin plus heparin for unstable angina. *N Engl J Med*. 1998;338:1498-1505.
87. The Randomized Efficacy Study of Tirofiban for Outcomes and Restenosis (RESTORE) Study Investigators. Effects of platelet glycoprotein IIb/IIIa blockade with tirofiban on adverse cardiac events in patients with unstable angina or acute myocardial infarction undergoing coronary angioplasty. *Circulation*. 1997;96:1445-1453.
88. Jeremias A, Bhatt DL, Chew DP, et al. Safety of abciximab during percutaneous coronary intervention in patients with chronic renal insufficiency. *Am J Cardiol*. 2002;89:1209-1211.
89. Frilling B, Zahn R, Fraiture B, et al. Comparison of efficacy and complication rates after percutaneous coronary interventions in patients treated with and without renal insufficiency treated with abciximab. *Am J Cardiol*. 2002;89:450-452.

90. Best PJM, Lennon R, Gersh BJ, et al. Safety of abciximab in patients with chronic renal insufficiency who are undergoing percutaneous coronary interventions. *Am Heart J.* 2003;146:345-350.

91. Rasty S, Borzak S, Tisdale JE. Bleeding associated with eptifibatide targeting higher risk patients with acute coronary syndromes: incidence and multivariate risk factors. *J Clin Pharmacol.* 2002;42:1366-1373.

92. Sperling RT, Pinto DS, Ho KKL, Carrozza JP Jr. Platelet glycoprotein IIb/IIIa inhibition with eptifibatide: prolongation of inhibition of aggregation in acute renal failure and reversal with hemodialysis. *Catheter Cardiovasc Inter.* 2003;59:459-462.

93. Januzzi JL, Snapinn SM, DiBattiste PM, et al. Benefits and safety of tirofiban among acute coronary syndrome patients with mild to moderate renal insufficiency. *Circulation.* 2002;105:2361-2366.

94. Chesebro JH, Knatterud G, Roberts R, et al. Thrombolysis in Myocardial Infarction (TIMI) Trial, phase I: a comparison between intravenous tissue plasminogen activator and intravenous streptokinase: clinical findings through hospital discharge. *Circulation.* 1987;76:142-154.

95. The GUSTO Investigators. An international randomized trial comparing four thrombolytic strategies for acute myocardial infarction. *N Engl J Med.* 1999;329:673-682.

96. Tsai TT, Maddox TM, Roe MT, et al. Contraindicated medication use in dialysis patients undergoing percutaneous coronary intervention. *JAMA.* 2009;302(22):2458-2464.

97. Arpino PA, Greer DM. Practice pharmacologic aspects of therapeutic hypothermia after cardiac arrest. *Pharmacotherapy.* 2008;28(1):102-111.

98. Frelinger AL III, Furman MI, Barnard MR, et al. Combined effects of mild hypothermia and glycoprotein IIb/IIIa antagonists on platelet-platelet and leukocyte-platelet aggregation. *Am J Cardiol.* 2003;92:1099-1101.

99. Tcheng JE. Clinical challenges of platelet glycoprotein IIb/IIIa receptor inhibitor therapy: bleeding, reversal, thrombocytopenia, and retreatment. *Am Heart J.* 2000;139:S38-S45.

100. Simoons ML. Effect of glycoprotein IIb/IIIa receptor blocker abciximab on outcome in patients with acute coronary syndromes without early coronary revascularization: the GUSTO-IV ACS randomized trial. *Lancet.* 2001;357:1915-1924.

101. Anderson JL, Adams CD, Antman EM, et al. ACC/AHA 2007 guidelines for the management of patients with unstable angina/non-ST-elevation myocardial infarction: a report of the American College of Cardiology/American Heart Association Task Force on Practice Guidelines (Writing Committee to Revise the 2002 Guidelines for the Management of Patients with Unstable Angina/Non-ST-Elevation Myocardial Infarction): developed in collaboration with the American College of Emergency Physicians, American College of Physicians, Society for Academic Emergency Medicine, Society for Cardiovascular Angiography and Interventions, and Society of Thoracic Surgeons. *J Am Coll Cardiol.* 2007;50:e1-e157.

102. Topol EJ, Moliterno DJ, Herrmann HC, et al. Comparison of two platelet glycoprotein IIb/IIIa inhibitors, tirofiban and abciximab, for the prevention of ischemic events with percutaneous coronary revascularization. *N Engl J Med.* 2001;344:1888-1894.

103. Giugliano RP, White JA, Bode C, for the EARLY ACS Investigators, et al. Early versus delayed, provisional eptifibatide in acute coronary syndromes. *N Engl J Med.* 2009;360:2176-2190.

104. Kushner FG, Hand M, Smith SC Jr, et al. 2009 focused updates: ACC/AHA guidelines for the management of patients with ST-elevation myocardial infarction (updating the 2004 guideline and 2007 focused update) and ACC/AHA/SCAI guidelines on percutaneous coronary intervention (updating the 2005 guideline and 2007 focused update): a report of the American College of Cardiology Foundation/American Heart Association Task Force on Practice Guidelines. *J Am Coll Cardiol.* 2009;54:2205-2241.

105. Wilson SJ, Wilbur K, Burton E, Anderson DR. Effect of patient weight on the anticoagulant response to adjusted therapeutic dosage of low-molecular-weight heparin for the treatment of venous thromboembolism. *Haemostasis.* 2001;31:42-48.

106. The SYNERGY Trial Investigators. Enoxaparin vs unfractionated heparin in high-risk patients with non-ST-segment elevation acute coronary syndromes managed with an intended early invasive strategy. *JAMA*. 2004;292:45-54.
107. Frederiksen SG, Hedenbro JL, Norgren L. Enoxaparin effect depends on body-weight and current doses may be inadequate in obese patients. *Br J Surg*. 2003;90:547-548.
108. Hirsh J, Bauer KA, Donati MB, et al. Parenteral anticoagulants. *Chest*. 2008;133: 141S-159S.
109. Samama MM, Verhille C, Carchy L. Relation between weight, obesity and frequency of deep vein thrombosis after enoxaparin in orthopedic surgery (abstract 300). *Thromb Haemost*. 1995;73:977.
110. WHO. Physical status: the use and interpretation of anthropometry. Report of a WHO Expert Committee. WHO Technical Report Series 854. Geneva: World Health Organization; 1995.
111. Lovenox (enoxaparin sodium injection) prescribing information. Bridgewater, NJ: Sanofi-Aventis; 2009.
112. Fragmin (dalteparin sodium injection) prescribing information. New York, NY: Pfizer; March 2010.
113. Innohep (tinzaparin sodium injection) prescribing information. Parsippany, NJ: LEO Pharm Inc; May 2010.
114. Nutescu EA, Spinler SA, Wittkowsky A, Dager WE. Low-molecular-weight heparins in renal impairment and obesity: available evidence and clinical practice recommendations across medical and surgical settings. *Ann Pharmacother*. 2009;43:1064-1083.
115. Geerts WH, Bergqvist D, Pineo GF, et al. Prevention of venous thromboembolism. *Chest*. 2008;133:381S-453S.
116. Scholten DJ, Hoedema RM, Scholten SE. A comparison of two different prophylactic dose regimens of low molecular weight heparin in bariatric surgery. *Obes Surg*. 2002;12:19-24.
117. Frydman A. Low-molecular weight heparins: an overview of their pharmacodynamics, pharmacokinetics and metabolism in humans. *Haemostasis*. 1996;26(suppl 2):24-38.
118. Troy S, Fruncillo R, Ozawa T, et al. The dose proportionality of the pharmacokinetics of ardeparin, a low molecular weight heparin, in healthy volunteers. *J Clin Pharmacol*. 1995;3:1194-1199.
119. Sanderink G, Liboux AL, Jariwala N, et al. The pharmacokinetics and pharmacodynamics of enoxaparin in obese volunteers. *Clin Pharmacol Ther*. 2002;72:308-318.
120. Bazinet A, Almanrie K, Brunet C, et al. Dosage of enoxaparin among obese and renal impairment patients. *Thromb Res*. 2005;116:41-50.
121. Smith J, Canton E. Weight-based administration of dalteparin in obese patients. *Am J Health Syst Pharm*. 2003;60:683-687.
122. Wilson S, Wilbur K, Burton E, et al. Effect of patient weight on the anticoagulant response to adjusted therapeutic dosage of low-molecular-weight heparin for the treatment of venous thromboembolism. *Haemostasis*. 2001;31:42-48.
123. Hainer J, Barrett J, Assaid C, et al. Dosing in heavy-weight/obese patients with the LMWH tinzaparin: a pharmacodynamic study. *Thromb Haemost*. 2002;87:817-823.
124. Merli G, Spiro TE, Olsson CG, et al. Subcutaneous enoxaparin once or twice daily compared with intravenous unfractionated heparin for treatment of venous thromboembolic disease. *Ann Intern Med*. 2001;134:191-202.
125. Spinler SA, Inverso SM, Cohen M, et al. Safety and efficacy of unfractionated heparin versus enoxaparin in patients who are obese and patients with severe renal impairment: analysis from the ESSENCE and TIMI 11B studies. *Am Heart J*. 2003;146:33-41.
126. Anderson JL, Adams CD, Antman EM, et al. ACC/AHA 2007 guidelines for the management of patients with unstable angina/non-ST-elevation myocardial infarction: a report of the American College of Cardiology/American Heart Association Task Force on Practice Guidelines. *Circulation*. 2007;116:e148-e304.
127. Kushner FG, Hand M, Smith SC Jr, et al. 2009 Focused updates: ACC/AHA guidelines for the management of patients with ST-elevation myocardial infarction and ACC/AHA/SCAI guidelines on percutaneous coronary intervention: a report of the American College of

Cardiology Foundation/American Heart Association Task Force on Practice Guidelines. *Circulation.* 2009;120:2271-2306.

128. Macie C, Forbes L, Foster GA, et al. Dosing practices and risk factors for bleeding in patients receiving enoxaparin for the treatment of an acute coronary syndrome. *Chest.* 2004;125: 1616-1621.

129. Spinler SA, Dobesh P. Dose capping enoxaparin is unjustified and denies patients with acute coronary syndromes a potentially effective treatment. *Chest.* 2005;127(6):2288-2289.

130. Spinler SA, Ou F, Roe MT, et al. Weight-based dosing of enoxaparin in obese patients with non-ST-segment elevation acute coronary syndromes: results from the CRUSADE initiative. *Pharmacotherapy.* 2009;29(6):631-638.

131. Meyer G, Brenot F, Pacouret G, et al. Subcutaneous low-molecular-weight heparin Fragmin versus intravenous unfractionated heparin in the treatment of acute non massive pulmonary embolism: an open randomized pilot study. *Thromb Haemost.* 1995;74:1432-1435.

132. Barba R, Marco J, Martin-Alvarez H, et al. The influence of extreme body weight on clinical outcome of patients with venous thromboembolism: findings from a prospective registry (RIETE). *J Thromb Haemost.* 2005;3:703-709.

133. Sanderink G, Guimart C, Ozoux M-L, et al. Pharmacokinetics and pharmacodynamics of the prophylactic dose of enoxaparin once daily over 4 days in patients with renal impairment. *Thromb Res.* 2002;105:225-231.

134. Becker RC, Spencer FA, Gibson M, et al. Influence of patient characteristics and renal function on factor Xa inhibition pharmacokinetics and pharmacodynamics after enoxaparin administration in non-ST-segment elevation acute coronary syndromes. *Am Heart J.* 2002;143:753-759.

135. Chow SL, Zammit K, West K, Dannenhoffer M, Lopez-Candales A. Correlation of antifactor Xa concentrations with renal function in patients on enoxaparin. *J Clin Pharmacol.* 2003;43:586-590.

136. Lim W, Dentali F, Eikelboom JW, Crowther MA. Meta-analysis: low-molecular-weight heparin and bleeding in patients with severe renal insufficiency. *Ann Intern Med.* 2006;144: 673-684.

137. Fox KA, Antman EM, Montalescot G, et al. The impact of renal dysfunction on outcomes in the EXTRACT-TIMI 25 trial. *J Am Coll Cardiol.* 2007;49:2249-2255.

138. Lim W, Cook DJ, Crowther MA. Safety and efficacy of low molecular weight heparins for hemodialysis in patients with end-stage renal failure: a meta-analysis of randomized trials. *J Am Soc Nephrol.* 2004;15:3192-3206.

139. Ljunberg B, Jacobson SH, Lins LE, Pejler G. Effective anticoagulation by a low molecular weight heparin (Fragmin) in haemodialysis with a highly permeable polysulfone membrane. *Clin Nephrol.* 1992;38:97-100.

140. Singer M, McNally T, Screaton G, et al. Heparin clearance during continuous veno-venous haemofiltration. *Intensive Care Med.* 1994;20:212-215.

141. Pokinghorne KR, McMahon LP, Becker GJ. Pharmacokinetic studies of dalteparin (Fragmin), enoxaparin (Clexane), and danaparoid sodium (Orgaran) in stable chronic hemodialysis patients. *Am J Kidney Dis.* 2002;40:990-995.

142. Hainer JW, Sherrard DJ, Swan SK, et al. Intravenous and subcutaneous weight-based dosing of the low molecular weight heparin tinzaparin (Innohep) in end-stage renal patients undergoing chronic hemodialysis. *Am J Kidney Dis.* 2002;40:531-538.

143. Isla A, Gascon AR, Maynar J, et al. In vitro and in vivo evaluation of enoxaparin removal by continuous renal replacement therapies with acrylonitrile and polysulfone membranes. *Clin Ther.* 2005;27:1444-1451.

144. Priglinger U, Karth GD, Geppert A, et al. Prophylactic anticoagulation with enoxaparin: is the subcutaneous route appropriate in the critically ill? *Crit Care Med.* 2003;31: 1405-1409.

145. Haas CE, Nelsen JL, Raghavendran K, et al. Pharmacokinetics and pharmacodynamics of enoxaparin in multiple trauma patients. *J Trauma.* 2005;59:1336-1344.

146. Feng Y, Green B, Duffull SB, et al. Development of a dosage strategy in patients receiving enoxaparin by continuous intravenous infusion using modeling and simulation. *Br J Pharmacol*. 2006;62(2):165-176.
147. Kane-Gill SL, Feng Y, Bobek MB, et al. Administration of enoxaparin by continuous infusion in a naturalistic setting: analysis of renal function and safety. *J Clin Pharm Ther*. 2005;30:207-213.
148. Antman EM, Morrow DA, McCabe CH, et al. for the EXTRACT-TIMI 25 Investigators. Enoxaparin versus unfractionated heparin with fibrinolysis for ST-elevation myocardial infarction. *N Engl J Med*. 2006;354:1477-1488.
149. Product information. Activase® (alteplase). South San Francisco, CA: Genentech, Inc.; December 2005.
150. Product information. Retevase® (reteplase). Fremont: BioPharma, Inc.; November 2006. Product information.® (streptokinase). Fremont, CA: BioPharma, Inc.; November 2006.
151. Product information. Streptase (Streptokinase®). Ottawa, Ontario: CSL Behring, Canada, Inc.; 2007.
152. Product information. TNKase® (tenecteplase). South San Francisco, CA: Genentech, Inc.; January 2008.
153. Product information. Kinlytic® (urokinase). Tucson, AZ: ImaRx Therapeutics, Inc.; June 2007.
154. Khan IA, Gowda RM. Clinical perspectives and therapeutics of thrombolysis. *Int J Cardiol*. 2003;91:115-127.
155. Bennett MB, Ogston CM, McAndrew GM, et al. Studies on the fibrinolytic enzyme system in obesity. *J Clin Pathol*. 1966;19:241-243.
156. Lee KL, Woodlief LH, Topol EJ, et al. Predictors of 30-day mortality in the era of reperfusion for acute myocardial infarction. Results from an international trial of 41,021 patients. *Circulation*. 1995;91:1659-1668.
157. Mehta RH, Califf RM, Garg J, et al. The impact of anthropomorphic indices on clinical outcomes in patients with acute ST elevation myocardial infarction. *Eur Heart J*. 2007;28:415-424.
158. Mehta RH, Gitt AK, Junger C, et al. Body mass index and effectiveness of reperfusion strategies: implications for the management of patients with ST-elevation myocardial infarction. *J Interv Cardiol*. 2008;21:8-14.
159. Kirtane AJ, Piazza G, Murphy SA, et al. Correlates of bleeding events among moderate- to high-risk patients undergoing percutaneous coronary intervention and treated with eptifibatide: observations from the protect-timi-30 trial. *J Am Coll Cardiol*. 2006;47:2374-2379.
160. Agrwal V, Rai B, Fellows J, et al. In-hospital outcomes with thrombolytic therapy in patients with renal dysfunction presenting with acute ischemic stroke. *Nephrol Dial Transplant*. 2010;25:1150-1157.
161. Lyrer PA, Fluri F, Gisler D, et al. Renal function and outcome among stroke patients treated with IV thrombolysis. *Neurology*. 2008;71:1548-1550.
162. Vincze Z, Brugos B. Does impairment of renal and hepatic function influence the metabolism of thrombolytics in patients with myocardial infarction? *Pharmazie*. 2008;63:245-246.
163. Yenari MA, Palmer JT, Bracci PM, et al. Thrombolysis with tissue plasminogen activator (tPA) is temperature dependent. *Thromb Res*. 1995;77:475-481.
164. Shaw GJ, Dhamija A, Bavani N, et al. Arrhenius temperature dependence of *in vitro* tissue plasminogen activator thrombolysis. *Phys Med Biol*. 2007;52:2953-2967.
165. Antman EM, Anbe DT, Armstrong PW, et al. ACC/AHA guidelines for the management of patients with ST-elevation myocardial infarction: executive summary. A report of the American College of Cardiology/American Heart Association Task Force on Practice Guidelines (Committee to revise the 1999 Guidelines for the Management of Patients with Acute Myocardial Infarction). *Circulation*. 2004;110:588-636.
166. Cannon C. Exploring the issues of appropriate dosing in the treatment of acute myocardial infarction: potential benefits of bolus fibrinolytic agents. *Am Heart J*. 2000;140: S154-S160.

167. Hochman JS, Wali AU, Gavrila D, et al. A new heparin regimen for heparin use in acute coronary syndromes. *Am Heart J.* 1999;137:786-791.
168. Schaefer DC, Hufnagle J, Williams L. Rapid heparin anticoagulation: use of a weight-based nomogram. *Clin Pharm.* 1996;54(8):2517-2521.
169. Spruill WJ, Wade WE, Huckaby G, et al. Achievement of anticoagulation by using a weight-based heparin dosing protocol for obese and nonobese patients. *Am J Health Syst Pharm.* 2001;58:2143-2146.
170. Ellison MJ, Sawyer WT, Mills TC. Calculation of heparin dosage in a morbidly obese woman. *Clin Pharm.* 1989;8:65-68.
171. Yee WP, Norton LL. Optimal weight base for a weight-based heparin dosing protocol. *Am J Health Syst Pharm.* 1998;55:159-162.
172. Miller MT, Rovito PF. An approach to venous thromboembolism prophylaxis in laparoscopic roux-en-Y gastric bypass surgery. *Obes Surg.* 2004;14:731-737.
173. Cotter SA, Cantrell W, Fisher B, Shopnick R. Efficacy of venous thromboembolism prophylaxis in morbidly obese patients undergoing gastric bypass surgery. *Obes Surg.* 2005;15: 1316-1320.
174. Kothari SN, Lambert PJ, Mathiason MA. A comparison of thromboembolic and bleeding events following laparoscopic gastric bypass in patients treated with prophylactic regimens of unfractionated heparin or enoxaparin. *Am J Surg.* 2007;194:709-711.
175. Quebbemann B, Akhondzadeh M, Dallal R. Continuous intravenous heparin infusion prevents peri-operative thromboembolic events in bariatric surgery patients. *Obes Surg.* 2005;15: 1221-1224.
176. Shepherd MF, Rosborough TK, Schwartz ML. Heparin thromboprophylaxis in gastric bypass surgery. *Obes Surg.* 2003;13:249-253.
177. Shepherd MF, Rosborough TK, Schwartz ML. Unfractionated heparin infusion for thromboprophylaxis in highest risk gastric bypass surgery. *Obes Surg.* 2004;14:601-605.
178. Raschke RA, Reilly BM, Guidry JR, et al. The weight-based heparin dosing nomogram compared with a "standard care" nomogram: a randomized controlled trial. *Ann Intern Med.* 1993;119:874-881.
179. Kearon C, Kahn SR, Agnelli G, et al. American College of Chest Physicians. Antithrombotic therapy for venous thromboembolic disease: American College of Chest Physicians Evidence-Based Clinical Practice Guidelines (8th edition). *Chest.* 2008;133(suppl):454S-545S [published correction appears in Chest 2008;134:892].
180. Holliday DM, Watling SM, Yanos J. Heparin dosing in the morbidly obese patient. *Ann Pharmacother.* 1994;28:1110-1111.
181. Rosborough TK, Shepherd MF. Achieving target antifactor Xa activity with a heparin protocol based on sex, age, height, and weight. *Pharmacotherapy.* 2004;24(6):713-719.
182. Schwiesow SJ, Wessell AM, Steyer TE. Use of a modified dosing weight for hepain therapy in a morbidly obese patient. *Ann Pharmacother.* 2005;39:753-756.
183. Dee BM, Thomas ML. Safety and efficacy of a high-intensity, weight-based, intravenous heparin protocol revision in patients who are obese. *Hosp Pharm.* 2008;43:895-902.
184. Barletta JF, DeYoung JL, McAllen K, et al. Limitations of a standardized weight-based nomogram for heparin dosing in patients with morbid obesity. *Surg Obes Relat Dis.* 2008;4:748-753.
185. Myzienski AE, Lutz MF, Smythe MA. Unfractionated heparin dosing for venous thromboembolism in morbidly obese patients: case report and review of the literature. *Pharmacotherapy.* 2010;30(3):105e-112e.
186. Riney JN, Hollands JM, Smith JR, Deal EN. Identifying optimal initial infusion rates for unfractionated heparin in morbidly obese patients. *Ann Pharmacother.* 2010;44:1141-1151.
187. Nadler SB, Hidalgo JU, Bloch T. Prediction of blood volume in normal human adults. *Surgery.* 1962;51:224-232.
188. Dobesh PP and the Heparin Consensus Group. Unfractionated heparin dosing nomograms: road maps to where? *Pharmacotherapy.* 2004;24(8 Pt 2):142S-145S.

189. Goodman SG, Menon V, Cannon CP, et al. Acute ST-segment elevation myocardial infarction. *Chest.* 2008;133:708S-775S.
190. Cheng S, Morrow DA, Sloan S, et al. Predictors of initial nontherapeutic anticoagulation with unfractionated heparin in ST-segment elevation myocardial infarction. *Circulation.* 2009;119: 1195-1202.
191. Bussey H, Francis JL, and the Heparin Consensus Group. Heparin overview and issues. *Pharmacotherapy.* 2004;24(8 Pt 2):103S-107S.
192. Rondina MT, Pendleton RC, Wheeler M, Rodgers GM. The treatment of venous thromboembolism in special populations. *Thromb Res.* 2007;119:391-402.
193. Forni LG, Hilton PJ. Continuous hemofiltration in the treatment of acute renal failure. *N Engl J Med.* 1997;336(18):1303-1309.
194. Ireland H, Lane DA, Curtis JR. Objective assessment of heparin requirements for hemodialysis in humans. *J Lab Clin Med.* 1984;103:643-652.
195. Product information. Heparin sodium. Lake Forest, IL: Hospira, Inc.; March 2008.
196. Cohen JA, Frederickson EL, Kaplan JA. *Anesth Analg.* 1977;56(4):564-569.
197. Simone EP, Madan AK, Tichansky DS, et al. Comparison of two low-molecular-weight heparin dosing regimens for patients undergoing laparoscopic bariatric surgery. *Surg Endosc.* 2008;22:2392-2395.
198. Borkgren-Okonek MJ, Hart RW, Pantano JE, et al. Enoxaparin thromboprophylaxis in gastric bypass patients: extended duration, dose stratification, and antifactor Xa activity. *Surg Obes Relat Dis.* 2008;4:625-631.
199. Kucher N, Leizorovicz A, Vaitkus PT, et al. Efficacy and safety of fixed low-dose dalteparin in preventing venous thromboembolism among obese or elderly hospitalized patients: a subgroup analysis of the PREVENT trial. *Arch Intern Med.* 2005;165:341-345.
200. Escalante-Tattersfield T, Tucker O, Fajnwaks P, et al. Incidence of deep vein thrombosis in morbidly obese patients undergoing laparoscopic Roux-en-Y gastric bypass. *Surg Obes Relat Dis.* 2008;4:126-130.
201. Kardys CM, Stoner MC, Manwaring ML, et al. Safety and efficacy of intravascular ultrasound-guided inferior vena cava filter in super obese bariatric patients. *Surg Obes Relat Dis.* 2008;4:50-54.
202. Yee JY, Duffull SB. The effect of body weight on dalteparin pharmacokinetics: a preliminary study. *Eur J Clin Pharmacol.* 2000;56:293-297.
203. Wilson SJ, Wilbur K, Burton E, et al. Effect of patient weight on the anticoagulant response to adjusted therapeutic dosage of low-molecular-weight heparin for the treatment of venous thromboembolism. *Haemostasis.* 2001;31:42-48.
204. Sanderink GJ, Liboux AL, Jariwala N, et al. The pharmacokinetics and pharmacodynamics of enoxaparin in obese volunteers. *Clin Pharmacol Ther.* 2002;72:308-318.
205. Hainer JW, Barrett JS, Assaid CA, et al. Dosing in heavy-weight/obese patients with the LMWH tinzaparin: a pharmacodynamic study. *Thromb Haemost.* 2002;87:817-823.
206. Barrett JS, Gibiansky E, Hull RD, et al. Population pharmacodynamics in patients receiving tinzaparin for the prevention and treatment of deep vein thrombosis. *Int J Clin Pharmacol Ther.* 2001;39:431-446.
207. Al-Yaseen E, Wells PS, Anderson J, et al. The safety of dosing dalteparin based on actual body weight for the treatment of acute venous thromboembolism in obese patients. *J Thromb Haemost.* 2005;3:100-102.
208. Barba R, Marco J, Martin-Alvarez H, et al. The influence of extreme body weight on clinical outcome of patients with venous thromboembolism: findings from a prospective registry (RIETE). *J Thromb Haemost.* 2005;3:856-862.
209. Klein W, Buchwald A, Hillis SE, et al. Comparison of low-molecular-weight heparin with unfractionated heparin acutely and with placebo for 6 weeks in the management of unstable coronary artery disease. Fragmin in unstable coronary artery disease study (FRIC). *Circulation.* 1997;96:61-68.
210. Low-molecular-weight heparin during instability in coronary artery disease, Fragmin during Instability in Coronary Artery Disease (FRISC) study group. *Lancet.* 1996;347:561-568.

211. Mahe I, Gouin-Thibault I, Drouet L, et al. Elderly medical patients treated with prophylactic dosages of enoxaparin: influence of renal function on anti-Xa activity level. *Drugs Aging.* 2007;24:63-71.

212. Mahe I, Aghassarian M, Drouet L, et al. Tinzaparin and enoxaparin given at prophylactic dose for eight days in medical elderly patients with impaired renal function: a comparative pharmacokinetic study. *Thromb Haemost.* 2007;97:581-586.

213. Tincani E, Mannucci C, Casolari B, et al. Safety of dalteparin for the prophylaxis of venous thromboembolism in elderly medical patients with renal insufficiency: a pilot study. *Haematologica.* 2006;91:976-979.

214. Rabbat CG, Cook DJ, Crowther MA, et al. Dalteparin thromboprophylaxis for critically ill medical-surgical patients with renal insufficiency. *J Crit Care.* 2005;20:357-363.

215. Schmid P, Brodmann D, Fischer AG, et al. Pharmacokinetics of dalteparin in prophylactic dosage in patient with impaired renal function (abstract). *J Thromb Haemost.* 2007;5(suppl 2):-P-T-674.

216. Douketis J, Cook D, Meade M, et al. Canadian Critical Care Trials Group. Prophylaxis against deep vein thrombosis in critically ill patients with severe renal insufficiency with the low-molecular-weight heparin dalteparin: an assessment of safety and pharmacodynamics: the DIRECT study. *Arch Intern Med.* 2008;168:1805-1812.

217. Bruno R, Baille P, Retout S, et al. Population pharmacokinetics and pharmacodynamics of enoxaparin in unstable angina and non-ST-segment elevation myocardial infarction. *Br J Clin Pharmacol.* 2003;56:407-414.

218. Hulot JS, Montalescot G, Lechat P, et al. Dosing strategy in patients with renal failure receiving enoxaparin for the treatment of non-ST-segment elevation acute coronary syndrome. *Clin Pharmacol Ther.* 2005;77:542-552.

219. Pautas E, Gouin I, Bellot O, et al. Safety profile of tinzaparin administered once daily at a standard curative dose in two hundred very elderly patients. *Drug Saf.* 2002;25:725-733.

220. Shprecher AR, Cheng-Lai A, Madsen EM, et al. Peak antifactor Xa activity produced by dalteparin treatment in patients with renal impairment compared with controls. *Pharmacotherapy.* 2005;25:817-822.

221. Siguret V, Pautas E, Fevrier M, et al. Elderly patients treated with tinzaparin (Innohep) administered once daily (175 anti-Xa IU/kg): anti-Xa and anti-IIa activities over 10 days. *Thromb Haemost.* 2000;84:800-804.

222. Thorevska N, Amoateng-Adjepong Y, Sabahi R, et al. Anticoagulation in hospitalized patients with renal insufficiency. *Chest.* 2004;125:856-863.

223. Collet JP, Montalescot G, Fine E, et al. Enoxaparin in unstable angina patients who would have been excluded from randomized pivotal trials. *J Am Coll Cardiol.* 2003;41:8-14.

224. Collet JP, Montalescot G, Agnelli G, et al. Non-ST-segment elevation acute coronary syndrome in patients with renal dysfunction: benefit of low-molecular-weight heparin alone or with glycoprotein IIb/IIIa inhibitors on outcomes. The Global Registry of Acute Coronary Events. *Eur Heart J.* 2005;26:2285-2293.

Chapter 2
Vasopressors and Inotropes

Scott W. Mueller and Robert MacLaren

Introduction

Medication errors and adverse drug events occur more frequently in the intensive care unit compared to general care units.[1] Adverse drug events become more likely as patients receive more medications. Sentinel events and medication errors are more common as the number of failing organs increases.[2,3] Vasopressors are frequently associated with adverse drug events and they are considered high-alert drugs by the Institute of Safe Medication Practices due to their increased potential to cause harm.[4-6] Vasopressors and inotropes are used in patients with the highest acuity and under stressful situations which adds to the potential for errors. In addition, dosing guidelines, ranges and units are not always standardized across agents at specific institutions or for a certain agent across institutions. The literature is disparate with respect to dosing recommendations. With the exception of vasopressin, we report the dosing of these agents in a weight-based manner. This should enhance dosing consistency to help minimize errors. We encourage institutions to adopt this dosing scheme to reduce discrepancies associated with their administration. Moreover, using a weight based dosing strategy in an era of increasing obesity raises the question of whether actual, adjusted or ideal body weight should be used when administering vasopressors. No data are available to select an appropriate weight and trials evaluating the use of vasopressors rarely report the body weight used in cases of obesity. With the exception of milrinone, we encourage the use of ideal body weight for all weight-based dosing strategies because these agents possess short half-lives, rapid onsets, and low volumes of distribution but may be associated with severe adverse events when higher weights are used resulting in higher

R. MacLaren (✉)
Department of Clinical Pharmacy, University of Colorado
Denver School of Pharmacy, Aurora, CO, USA
e-mail: rob.maclaren@ucdenver.edu

S.L. Kane-Gill and J. Dasta (eds.),
High-Risk IV Medications in Special Patient Populations,
DOI: 10.1007/978-0-85729-606-1_2, © Springer-Verlag London Limited 2011

doses in heavier patients. Moreover, these agents are rapidly titrated to clinical response, so starting at lower doses based on ideal body weight is prudent.

This chapter discusses the safety concerns of select vasopressors and inotropes encountered in intensive care units. Published adverse reactions with these agents are summarized.

Dobutamine (DOB)

Dosing Considerations

Dobutamine's (DOB) clinical activity is primarily mediated by beta (β)-receptor agonism. Frequently observed effects of DOB include increased cardiac output (CO), decreased systemic vascular resistance (SVR), and tachycardia. Commonly cited dosing ranges of 2–20 mcg/kg/min may need to be exceeded to achieve adequate response which may enhance the likelihood of adverse events. DOB doses of 40 mcg/kg/min have been reported but higher doses may be needed depending on the clinical situation.[7] The increased risk of adverse events at elevated doses must be balanced with potential benefits of the higher dose. Lack of adequate fluid resuscitation prior to or concomitant use of other inotropes may increase the risk of adverse events.

Obesity: Data are not available for use in critically ill obese patients. However, since many institutions use weight based dosing for DOB, ideal body weight should be used to avoid excessive dosing of a drug with low volume of distribution and short half-life in over weight patients. The rate should be verified to ensure the correct dose is being administered.

Thinness/emaciation: There are no reports of dosing considerations in underweight or nutritionally depleted patients. Dobutamine doses should be titrated to the lowest dose required for goal hemodynamic response.

Kidney Injury: Dobutamine is mainly metabolized by the liver and catechol-O-methyl transferase (COMT). The pharmacokinetics of DOB in patients with renal insufficiency has not been studied. Dobutamine does not require specific dose changes for renal insufficiency.

Hemodialysis/Continuous Renal Replacement Therapy: The pharmacokinetics of DOB has not been studied. Dose adjustments should be titrated to hemodynamic response.

Liver Dysfunction: Dobutamine is metabolized by COMT and by conjugation to inactive metabolites. Dose adjustments are not necessary for hepatic insufficiency.

Hypothermia: Therapeutic hypothermia may decrease enzymatic metabolism of medications including DOB leading to higher serum concentrations. The clinical significance of this is unknown, therefore no initial dose adjustments are recommended and dose adjustments should be based on hemodynamic response.[8]

Safety Concerns

Safety concern	Rationale	Comments/recommendations
Extravasation	While DOB displays β-selective inotropic and vasodilatory properties, the L-enantiomer possesses α-agonistic properties.[9] Therefore, extravasation may cause vasoconstrictive related adverse events. Few case reports have been published regarding DOB extravasation, treatment, and outcomes[10]	DOB should be administered via a central catheter whenever possible. If not readily available, a central catheter should be placed as soon as possible. If extravasation and vasoconstriction are evident, phentolamine (10 mg/10 ml NS) may be given in and around the extravasation site via hypodermic syringe[11]
Tachyarrhythmia/ myocardial ischemia	β-adrenergic effects may contribute to tachycardia, tachyarrhythmia, and potentially myocardial ischemia. Effects may be greater in the elderly, those with preexisting cardiac ischemia or dysrhythmias, hypovolemia, or when used in combination with other inotropes and vasopressors[12,13]	Dose related increases in heart rate are predictable. Doses exceeding 20 mcg/kg/min are more likely to cause tachyarrhythmias and produce ischemic changes on electrocardiogram. When DOB was used in combination with norepinephrine (NE), lower heart rates were noted compared with other vasopressors alone.[14] Cardiac monitoring should include telemetry for heart rate and rhythm and serial troponin concentrations if ischemia is suspected. Echocardiography may be required
Glucose abnormalities	Administration of sympathomimetics may cause gluconeogenesis and insulin resistance[15]	DOB has been shown to cause hyperglycemia in animal studies. Serum glucose should be monitored and corrected with insulin as clinically indicated[15,16]
Hypotension	DOB may cause hypotension due to β-agonist induced vasodilation	Hypotension may occur in states of hypovolemia leading to rebound tachycardia.[12] Blood pressure should be frequently monitored and verified
Allergic reaction	DOB contains sodium bisulfite	Allergic reactions to bisulfite may occur. Eosinophilic myocarditis has been linked to DOB use.[17] White blood cell count with differential should be monitored

(continued)

Safety concern	Rationale	Comments/recommendations
Drug-drug interactions	DOB is metabolized by COMT. While pharmacokinetic drug interactions between COMT inhibitors (entacapone, tolcapone) may enhance DOB activity, close monitoring and frequent dose titration to the lowest effective dose is recommended DOB is alkaline labile. Caution should be used when coadministering medications through shared lines with DOB	Pharmacodynamic interactions such as the concomitant administration of other vasopressors and inotropes may increase DOB activity and enhance the likelihood of adverse effects. Interactions should not deter the use of additional agents in patients requiring supplemental therapy to reach hemodynamic goals. Medications that alter blood pressure (vasodilators, negative inotropes, etc.) may enhance or reduce the effectiveness of DOB. DOB should be administered through a dedicated lumen of a central venous catheter

Dopamine (DA)

Dosing Considerations

Dopamine's (DA) clinical activity is dose-dependent. Lower doses of 0.5–3 mcg/kg/min primarily stimulate dopamine receptors, intermediate doses of 3–10 mcg/kg/min stimulate beta (β)-receptors, and higher doses 10–20 mcg/kg/min stimulate alpha (α)-receptors.[7] Mixed actions may occur at doses above or below these commonly cited ranges. DA doses in excess of 50 mcg/kg/min have been reported but higher doses may be needed depending on the clinical situation. The increased risk of adverse events at elevated doses must be balanced with diminishing potential benefits of the higher dose. Additional or alternative vasopressor support may be needed if cardiovascular goals are not met within the standard dosing range. Lack of adequate fluid resuscitation prior to or concomitant vasopressor use may increase the risk of adverse events.

Obesity: Data are not available regarding dosing in critically ill obese patients. However, since DA is dosed in units based on weight, ideal body weight should be used to avoid excessive dosing of a drug with low volume of distribution and short half-life in over weight patients. The rate should be verified to ensure the correct dose is being administered.

Thinness/emaciation: There are no reports of dosing considerations in underweight or nutritionally depleted patients. Dopamine doses should be titrated to the lowest dose required for goal hemodynamic response.

Kidney Injury: Only a small amount of DA is excreted unchanged in the urine. Dopamine has been used at low doses in cases of acute or chronic renal insufficiency in attempts to increase urine production or prevent worsening renal function. The results of a large study of critically ill patients with acutely worsening renal function showed no benefit to "low-dose" or "renal-dose" DA.[18] Dopamine does not require specific dose adjustments for renal insufficiency. The dose should be titrated to hemodynamic response.

Hemodialysis/Continuous Renal Replacement Therapy: Dopamine does not require specific dosage adjustments and should be titrated to hemodynamic response during dialysis.

Liver Dysfunction: Dopamine is metabolized by COMT and monoamine oxidase (MAO) to inactive metabolites. Dose adjustments are not necessary for hepatic insufficiency.

Hypothermia: Therapeutic hypothermia may decrease enzymatic metabolism of medications including DA leading to higher serum concentrations. The clinical significance of this is unknown, therefore no initial dose adjustments are recommended and dose adjustments should be based on hemodynamic response.[8]

Safety Concerns

Safety concern	Rationale	Comments/recommendations
Extravasation	DA possesses dopamine, β, and α receptor activity which can cause vasoconstriction and skin sloughing, ischemia, gangrene and necrosis if extravasation occurs. Reports of adverse events have been published regarding DA extravasation[19]	DA should be administered via a central catheter whenever possible. If not readily available, a central catheter should be placed as soon as possible. Only dosages ≤5 mcg/kg/min should be administered peripherally. If extravasation is noted, phentolamine (10 mg/10 ml NS) may be given in and around the extravasation site via hypodermic syringe[11]
Peripheral ischemia	Higher dose DA (≥10 mcg/kg/min) acts as a potent vasoconstrictor that can cause peripheral ischemia (digits, skin, etc.) via α-adrenergic effects. Ischemia has been reported at lower doses as well. Inadequate volume resuscitation prior to and during vasopressor administration may increase the risk of ischemia	Fluid assessment and adequate resuscitation should be initiated prior to and during DA administration. Assessment of peripheral circulation and ischemia should be done frequently while receiving DA. Venous oxygen saturation should be maintained at ≥70%. The lowest effective dose of DA should be used to achieve hemodynamic goals and tapered off as soon as possible

Safety concern	Rationale	Comments/recommendations
Gastrointestinal ischemia and impaired motility	DA may increase hepato-splanchnic blood flow in septic patients by enhancing CO but DA impairs hepato-splanchnic metabolism leading to impaired hepatic energy balance when compared to norepinephrine. DA may contribute to mesenteric ischemia in septic shock and impedes gastrointestinal motility via DA-2 receptor stimulation[20-24]	DA impairs hepato-splanchnic and mesenteric mucosal perfusion in hypotensive patients. Serum lactate concentrations and liver function enzymes should be monitored frequently. Gastrointestinal function (e.g. aspirated gastric residual, bowel distension or pain, bowel movements) should be assessed routinely as DA decreases gastric motility
Glucose abnormalities	Administration of sympathomimetics may cause gluconeogenesis and insulin resistance	DA has been shown to increase serum glucose, glucagon and insulin even at low doses (i.e., 2 mcg/kg/min). Serum glucose concentrations should be monitored and corrected with insulin as clinically indicated[15,25]
Nephrotoxicity	"Low or renal-dose" DA is not renal protective and does not improve kidney function. Higher doses of DA may increase arterial constriction and decrease renal blood flow	Negative results found in a large prospective trial of "low-dose" DA suggest there is no renal protective benefit.[18] Fluid status, urine production and serum markers of renal function (BUN, creatinine) should be monitored frequently
Tachyarrhythmia/ myocardial ischemia	β-adrenergic receptor stimulation may contribute to tachycardia, tachyarrhythmia, and potentially myocardial ischemia. Effects may be greater in the elderly, those with preexisting cardiac ischemia or dysrhythmias, hypovolemia, or when used in combination with other inotropes and vasopressors[26]	Tachyarrhythmias may occur at doses as low as 3 mcg/kg/min. Sinus tachycardia, supraventricular tachycardia, and premature ventricular complexes may occur with DA. The largest trial of 1,679 patients in shock compared DA with NE and showed DA was associated with higher rates of atrial fibrillation (A-fib) and ventricular tachycardia leading to more patients being withdrawn from the DA group compared to NE (6.1% vs. 1.6%). Another trial of 252 patients with fluid resuscitated septic shock showed patients who received DA were more likely to develop sinus tachycardia, A-fib, and PVC compared to NE.[27,28] Cardiac monitoring should include telemetry for heart rate and rhythm and serial troponin concentrations if ischemia is suspected. Echocardiography may be required

Safety concern	Rationale	Comments/recommendations
Endocrine	DA suppresses prolactin secretion from the anterior pituitary gland.[29,30] DA has been reported to lower thyrotropin and thyroid hormone secretion in critically ill patients[30]	A 6 h DA infusion of 2.5 mcg/kg/min can decrease prolactin concentrations by 80%. Higher doses may suppress prolactin to a greater extent.[29,30] The clinical significance of prolactin suppression is unknown. A prospective study showed a three-fold decrease in TSH response to TRH in critically ill patients receiving DA.[30] TSH and T3/T4 should be intermittently monitored
Pulmonary	DA may increase pulmonary artery occlusive pressure, and cause pulmonary edema and intrapulmonary shunting	Studies confirm increased pulmonary pressures as well as increased pulmonary shunting in patients treated with DA.[31] Arterial blood gas analyses and the extent of respiratory support should be assessed routinely. In severe cases, echocardiography and/or pulmonary artery catheterization may aid monitoring
Drug-drug interactions	DA is metabolized by MAO and COMT. While pharmacokinetic drug interactions between MAO inhibitors (including linezolid, selegiline, phenelzine, isocarboxazid, tranylcypromine) and COMT inhibitors (entacapone, tolcapone) may enhance DA activity, close monitoring and frequent dose titration to the lowest effective dose is recommended DA is alkaline labile. Caution should be used when coadministering medications through shared lines with DA	Pharmacodynamic interactions such as the concomitant administration of other vasopressors and inotropes may increase DA activity and enhance the likelihood of adverse effects. Interactions should not deter the use of additional agents in patients requiring supplemental therapy to reach hemodynamic goals. Medications that lower blood pressure (vasodilators, negative inotropes, etc.) will decrease the effectiveness of DA. DA should be administered through a dedicated lumen of a central venous catheter

Epinephrine (EPI)

Dosing Considerations

Epinephrine's (EPI) clinical activity is mediated by alpha (α)-receptor and beta (β)-receptor agonism. Tachycardia, increased CO, and increased SVR are generally observed with EPI use. Commonly cited dose ranges of 0.01–3 mcg/kg/min may need to be exceeded to achieve adequate response which may enhance the likelihood of adverse events.[7] Lack of adequate fluid resuscitation prior to or concomitant vasopressor use may increase the risk of adverse events.

Obesity: Data are not available for use in critically ill obese patients. However, since many institutions use weight based dosing for EPI, ideal body weight should be used to avoid excessive dosing of a drug with low volume of distribution and short half-life in over weight patients. The mixed concentration and rate should be verified to ensure the correct dose is being administered.

Thinness/emaciation: There are no reports of dosing considerations in underweight or nutritionally depleted patients. Epinephrine doses should be titrated to the lowest dose required for goal hemodynamic response.

Kidney Injury: Only a small proportion of EPI is excreted unchanged in the urine. The pharmacokinetics of EPI in patients with renal insufficiency has not been studied. Epinephrine does not require specific dose changes for renal insufficiency.

Hemodialysis/Continuous Renal Replacement Therapy: The pharmacokinetics of EPI has not been studied. Doses should be titrated to hemodynamic response.

Liver Dysfunction: Epinephrine is metabolized by COMT and MAO to inactive metabolites. Dose adjustments are not necessary for hepatic insufficiency.

Hypothermia: Therapeutic hypothermia may decrease enzymatic metabolism of medications including EPI leading to higher serum concentrations. The clinical significance of this is unknown, therefore no initial dose adjustments are recommended and dose adjustments should be based on hemodynamic response.[8]

Safety Concerns

Safety concern	Rationale	Comments/recommendations
Extravasation	EPI is a potent vasoconstrictor that can cause skin sloughing, ischemia, gangrene and necrosis if extravasation occurs. Reports of adverse events have been published regarding EPI extravasation[19]	EPI should be administered via a central catheter. If not readily available, a central catheter should be placed as soon as possible. If extravasation is noted, phentolamine (10 mg/10 ml NS) may be given in and around the extravasation site via hypodermic syringe[11]

Safety concern	Rationale	Comments/recommendations
Peripheral ischemia	EPI is a potent vasoconstrictor that can cause peripheral ischemia (digits, skin, etc.) via α-adrenergic effects. Inadequate volume resuscitation prior to and during vasopressor administration may increase the risk of ischemia. Higher doses of EPI may increase the risk of peripheral ischemia	Fluid assessment and adequate resuscitation should be initiated prior to and during EPI administration. Assessment of peripheral circulation and ischemia should be done frequently while receiving EPI. Venous oxygen saturation should be maintained at ≥70%. The lowest effective dose of EPI should be used to achieve hemodynamic goals and tapered off as soon as possible
Tachyarrhythmia/ myocardial ischemia	β-adrenergic effects may cause tachycardia, tachyarrhythmia, and potentially myocardial ischemia. Dysrhythmias and/or ischemia occur irrespective of concomitant disease states or therapies; however, risk is greatest in those with preexisting cardiac disease or dysrhythmias, hypovolemia, or when used in combination with other inotropes and vasopressors[26]	In a large prospective trial of 277 patients, EPI significantly increased heart rate compared with NE.[32] Another study of 330 patients showed no difference in tachyarrhythmias between EPI and NE with DOB.[14] EPI may causes demand ischemia and ST segment deviations in patients after single doses as low as 0.1–0.3 mg.[33] Cardiac monitoring should include telemetry for heart rate and rhythm and serial troponin concentrations if ischemia is suspected. Echocardiography may be required
Gastrointestinal ischemia	EPI decreases hepato-splanchnic and mesenteric blood flow and oxygen delivery[20,21]	Serum lactate concentrations and liver function enzymes should be monitored frequently[20,21,34,35]
Lactic acidosis	EPI increases serum lactate concentration by decreasing hepato-splanchnic oxygenation, increasing calorigenesis, and enhancing the breakdown of glycogen leading to increased lactate concentrations[14,32]	Multiple clinical trials have shown statistically higher serum lactate concentrations in patients treated with EPI compared with other vasopressors. Increases in lactate are variable but significant acidosis is possible.[14,32,35] Arterial blood gas analyses and serum lactate concentrations should be monitored frequently
Glucose abnormalities	Administration of sympathomimetics may cause gluconeogenesis and insulin resistance[15]	EPI has the highest propensity to cause hyperglycemia compared to other vasopressors.[15,32,36] Serum glucose should be monitored and corrected with insulin as clinically indicated

(continued)

Safety concern	Rationale	Comments/recommendations
Nephrotoxicity	Vasopressors can cause renal artery constriction and decreased filtration via α-adrenergic receptors	Animal data suggest EPI may reduce renal blood flow but urine production may increase due to higher MAP in vasodilatory shock[37]
Drug-drug interactions	EPI is metabolized by MAO and COMT. While pharmacokinetic drug interactions between MAO inhibitors (including linezolid, selegiline, phenelzine, isocarboxazid, tranylcypromine) and COMT inhibitors (entacapone, tolcapone) may enhance EPI activity, close monitoring and frequent dose titration to the lowest effective dose is recommended EPI is alkaline labile. Caution should be used when coadministering medications through shared lines with EPI	Pharmacodynamic interactions such as the concomitant administration of other vasopressors and inotropes may increase EPI activity and enhance the likelihood of adverse effects. Interactions should not deter the use of additional agents in patients requiring supplemental therapy to reach hemodynamic goals. Medications that lower blood pressure (vasodilators, negative inotropes, etc.) will decrease the effectiveness of EPI. EPI should be administered through a dedicated lumen of a central venous catheter

Isoproterenol (ISO)

Dosing Considerations

Isoproterenol's (ISO) clinical activity is mediated by beta (β)-receptor agonism. ISO primarily acts as an inotrope causing increased CO, tachycardia, and vasodilation to decrease SVR. ISO possesses high arrhythmogenic potential and is not commonly used as an inotrope. Commonly cited dosing ranges of 0.01–0.3 mcg/kg/min may need to be exceeded to achieve adequate response which may enhance the likelihood of adverse events. Dose should be titrated to the lowest effective dose and only escalated as clinical or ventricular response allows. ISO infusions of 30 mcg/min have been reported. Lack of adequate fluid resuscitation prior to or concomitant inotrope use may increase the risk of adverse events.[38]

Obesity: Data are not available for use in critically ill obese patients. However, since many institutions use weight based dosing for ISO, ideal body weight should be used to avoid excessive dosing of a drug with low volume of distribution and short half-life in over weight patients. The rate should be verified to ensure the correct dose is being administered.

Thinness/emaciation: There are no reports of dosing considerations in underweight or nutritionally depleted patients. Isoproterenol doses should be titrated to the lowest dose required for goal hemodynamic response.

Kidney Injury: The pharmacokinetics of ISO in patients with renal insufficiency has not been studied. Isoproterenol does not require specific dose changes for renal insufficiency.

Hemodialysis/Continuous Renal Replacement Therapy: The pharmacokinetics of ISO has not been studied. Dose adjustments should be titrated to hemodynamic response.

Liver Dysfunction: Isoproterenol is metabolized by COMT to inactive metabolites. Dose adjustments are not necessary for hepatic insufficiency.[38]

Hypothermia: Therapeutic hypothermia may decrease enzymatic metabolism of medications including ISO leading to higher serum concentrations. The clinical significance of this is unknown, therefore no initial dose adjustments are recommended and dose adjustments should be based on hemodynamic response.

Safety Concerns

Safety concern	Rationale	Comments/recommendations
Cardiac dysrhythmias, tachyarrhythmias, ventricular arrhythmia, atrial arrhythmia/ myocardial ischemia	ISO causes increased heart rate and shortened atrioventricular nodal conduction. This may generate atrial and/or possibly serious ventricular arrhythmias. ISO decreases diastolic filling time and diastolic coronary perfusion. β-adrenergic effects may increase myocardial oxygen demand and induce ischemia	Dose related increases in heart rate are predictable. Increased risk of ventricular arrhythmia exists when ISO is dosed to a heart rate of 130 bpm. The ISO infusion rate should be decreased or temporarily discontinued if the heart rate reaches 110 bpm.[38] ISO is rarely used because it is associated with serious arrhythmias but it is used to treat slow prolonged QT-interval. The lowest effective dose of ISO should be used to reach goal clinical response and tapered off as soon as possible. Myocardial ischemia also occurs in adults and children after inhaled ISO. Intravenous use has been reported to cause myocardial ischemia and worsen myocardial injury. ISO is not recommended in patients with a history of cardiovascular disease or active myocardial ischemia.[38-40] Cardiac monitoring should include telemetry for heart rate and rhythm, blood pressure, and serial troponin concentrations if ischemia is suspected. Echocardiography may be required

(continued)

Safety concern	Rationale	Comments/recommendations
Gastrointestinal ischemia	ISO increases cardiac output but preferentially decreases hepato-splanchnic and mesenteric blood flow in favor of skeletal muscle blood flow[41]	Serum lactate concentrations and liver function enzymes should be monitored frequently[21]
Glucose abnormalities	Administration of sympath-omimetics may cause gluconeogenesis and insulin resistance[15,36]	ISO may cause hyperglycemia but not to the same extent as EPI. Serum glucose concentrations should be monitored and corrected with insulin as clinically indicated
Pulmonary	ISO decreases pulmonary vascular resistance and may overcome hypoxic pulmonary vasoconstriction[42,43]	ISO may increase intrapulmonary shunting especially in patients with parenchymal lung disease leading to decreased arterial oxygenation.[42,43] Arterial blood gas analyses and the extent of respiratory support should be assessed routinely. In severe cases, echocardiography and/or pulmonary artery catheterization may aid monitoring
Hypotension	ISO may cause hypotension due to β-agonist vasodilation	ISO increases pulse pressure and possibly systolic pressure but tends to cause an overall decrease in mean arterial and diastolic pressures due to vasodilation. Hypotension may be exacerbated by hypovolemia. Blood pressure should be frequently monitored and verified
Allergic reaction	ISO contains sodium bisulfite[38]	Allergic reactions to bisulfite may occur. White blood cell count with differential should be monitored
Drug-drug interactions	ISO is metabolized by COMT. While pharma-cokinetic drug interactions between COMT inhibitors (entacapone, tolcapone) may enhance ISO activity, close monitoring and frequent dose titration to the lowest effective dose is recommended	Pharmacodynamic interactions such as the concomitant administration of other vasopressors and inotropes may alter ISO activity and enhance the likelihood of adverse effects. Interactions should not deter the use of additional agents in patients requiring supplemental therapy to reach hemodynamic goals. Medications that alter blood pressure (vasodilators, negative inotropes, etc.) may enhance or reduce the effectiveness of ISO
	ISO is alkaline labile. Caution should be used when coadministering medications through shared lines with ISO	ISO should be administered through a dedicated lumen of a central venous catheter

Milrinone (MIL)

Dosing Considerations

Milrinone (MIL) is a phosphodiesterase III inhibitor which leads to increased cardiac contractility, CO, heart rate, and decreased SVR through vasodilation. A loading dose of 50 mcg/kg over 20 min may be administered, however many clinicians opt not to give a loading dose prior to the infusion due to concerns of hypotension. Commonly cited dosing ranges of 0.125–1 mcg/kg/min may need to be exceeded to achieve adequate response which may enhance the likelihood of adverse events. Lack of adequate fluid resuscitation prior to or concomitant inotrope use may increase the risk of adverse events.

Obesity: Data are not available for use in critically ill obese patients. Package labeling provides dosing recommendations for patients based on actual body weight to a maximum weight of 120 kg.[44] Given a published volume of distribution ranging 0.3–0.47 L/kg an adjusted body weight may be used for initiation in cases of morbid obesity with close titration to desired clinical response.

Thinness/emaciation: There are no reports of dosing considerations in underweight or nutritionally depleted patients. Milrinone doses should be titrated to the lowest dose required for goal hemodynamic response.

Kidney Injury: Milrinone is largely excreted unchanged in the urine (80–85%) therefore dose adjustments are needed for renal insufficiency. Package labeling recommends initial dose adjustments as follows: 0.2 mcg/kg/min for a calculated creatinine clearance <5 mL/min/1.73m^2, 0.23 mcg/kg/min for a calculated creatinine clearance of 5–10 mL/min/1.73m^2, 0.28 mcg/kg/min for a calculated creatinine clearance of 10–20 mL/min/1.73m^2, and further incremental rate increases of 0.05 mcg/kg/min for every increase in calculated creatinine clearance of 10 mL/min/1.73m^2 up to 0.5 mcg/kg/min for a calculated creatinine clearance >50 mL/min/1.73m^2.[35] Doses may be further adjusted based on hemodynamic response to a maximum of 0.75 mcg/kg/min in those without renal failure. No adjustment in loading dose is required (if given).[44]

Hemodialysis/Continuous Renal Replacement Therapy: While MIL is removed by continuous renal replacement therapy, pharmacokinetic analysis estimates the half-life of MIL to be 20 h (compared to 2.3 h in heart failure patients without renal failure).[45] No data are available to guide dosing in dialysis patients and extreme caution is advised due to the prolonged half-life.

Liver Dysfunction: Milrinone is minimally metabolized via conjugation and oxidation to inactive metabolites. Dose adjustments are not necessary for hepatic insufficiency.

Hypothermia: There are no reports of dosing considerations during therapeutic hypothermia, therefore dose adjustments should be based on hemodynamic response.

Safety Concerns

Safety concern	Rationale	Comments/recommendations
Hypotension	MIL is a phosphodiesterase III inhibitor which causes smooth muscle relaxation[12,13,46-48]	Hypotension requiring therapeutic intervention may occur with MIL.[12,13,46-50] Not administering a loading dose may lessen the occurrence of hypotension.[46,47] MIL should be decreased or stopped and vasopressors (NE, DA, EPI, phenylephrine, vasopressin) may need to be instituted if hypotension is severe.[50] Cardiac monitoring should include telemetry for heart rate and rhythm and blood pressure should be frequently verified. Echocardiography may be required
Tachyarrhythmia/ myocardial ischemia	MIL may cause increases in heart rate, atrial, and ventricular arrhythmias.[12,13,46,48,49] Inotropic and chronotropic properties of MIL may increase myocardial oxygen demand and induce ischemia[12,13,49]	Dose-related increases in heart rate are expected. MIL may lead to ischemic myocardial changes due to increasing oxygen demand. Caution should be used in patients with myocardial ischemia. Cardiac monitoring should include telemetry for heart rate and rhythm and serial troponin concentrations if ischemia is suspected. Echocardiography may be required
Glucose abnormalities	Animal models suggest MIL may cause insulin resistance[51]	Human data linking MIL to hyperglycemia are lacking. Serum glucose should be monitored and corrected with insulin as clinically indicated
Thrombocytopenia/ altered platelet activation	MIL is structurally related to amrinone, a medication that may cause thrombocytopenia via action of an acetylated metabolite. MIL does not share this metabolite. However, reports of thrombocytopenia have been published in clinical trials[44]	The reported incidence of thrombocytopenia with MIL use varies between studies from 0.4% in package labeling to 58% in a small pediatric trial used during open heart surgery. The majority of studies indicate a low risk of thrombocytopenia likely related to procedures or other medications and not directly linked to MIL[44,52,53]

Safety concern	Rationale	Comments/recommendations
	MIL increases cyclic adenosine monophosphate, which may inhibit platelet activation[48]	Conflicting data exist regarding altered platelet activity. Initial studies suggest platelet function and hemostatis was not inhibited by either amrinone or MIL.[52,54] However, a recent in vitro study suggests that higher MIL concentrations can inhibit adenosine diphosphate and arachidonic acid induced platelet activation[55]
		Patients should be monitored for signs and symptoms of bleeding. Hemoglobin, hematocrit, and platelets should be followed as clinically indicated
Drug-drug interactions	Pharmacokinetic drug interactions have not been reported with MIL. Pharmacodynamic interactions with other cardiovascular medications may occur	Concomitant use of other cardiovascular medications is common. Monitoring blood pressure and heart rate is standard of practice. Co-administration is often successful with close hemodynamic monitoring
	Intravenous compatibility should be checked prior to coadministering medications through shared lines with MIL	MIL should be administered through a dedicated lumen of a central venous catheter

Norepinephrine (NE)

Dosing Considerations

Norepinephrine's (NE) clinical activity is mediated by alpha (α)-receptor agonism and some beta (β)-1-receptor agonism although tachycardia is not generally seen with NE. NE primarily acts as a vasoconstrictor to increase SVR. Commonly cited dosing ranges of 0.05–3 mcg/kg/min may need to be exceeded to achieve adequate response, which may enhance the likelihood of adverse events.[7] Lack of adequate fluid resuscitation prior to or concomitant vasopressors use may increase the risk of adverse events.

Obesity: Data are not available for use in critically ill obese patients. However, since many institutions use weight based dosing for NE, ideal body weight should be used to avoid excessive dosing of a drug with low volume of distribution and short half-life in over weight patients. The mixed concentration and rate should be verified to ensure the correct dose is being administered.

Thinness/emaciation: There are no reports of dosing considerations in underweight or nutritionally depleted patients. Norepinephrine doses should be titrated to the lowest dose required for goal hemodynamic response.

Kidney Injury: 4–16% of NE is excreted unchanged in the urine. The pharmacokinetics of NE in patients with renal insufficiency has not been studied. Norepinephrine does not require specific dose changes for renal insufficiency. The dose should be titrated to hemodynamic response.

Hemodialysis/Continuous Renal Replacement Therapy: The pharmacokinetics of NE has not been studied; therefore no initial dose adjustments are required and titration should be based on clinical response. Norepinephrine has been used to increase MAP in patients who become hypotensive during dialysis.

Liver Dysfunction: Norepinephrine is metabolized by COMT and MAO to inactive metabolites. Dose adjustments are not necessary for hepatic insufficiency.

Hypothermia: Therapeutic hypothermia may decrease enzymatic metabolism of medications including NE leading to higher serum concentrations. The clinical significance of this is unknown, therefore no initial dose adjustments are recommended and dose adjustments should be based on hemodynamic response.[8]

Safety Concerns

Safety concern	Rationale	Comments/recommendations
Extravasation	NE is a potent vasoconstrictor that can cause skin sloughing, ischemia, gangrene and necrosis if extravasation occurs. Reports of adverse events have been published regarding NE extravasation[19]	NE should be administered via a central catheter. If not readily available, a central catheter should be placed as soon as possible. If extravasation is noted, phentolamine (10 mg/10 ml NS) may be given in and around the extravasation site via hypodermic syringe[11]
Peripheral ischemia	NE is a potent vasoconstrictor that can cause peripheral ischemia (digits, skin, etc.) via α-adrenergic effects. Inadequate volume resuscitation prior to and during vasopressor administration may increase the risk of ischemia. Higher doses of NE may increase the risk of peripheral ischemia	Fluid assessment and adequate resuscitation should be initiated prior to and during NE administration. Assessment of peripheral circulation and ischemia should be done frequently while receiving NE. Venous oxygen saturation should be maintained at ≥70%. The lowest effective dose of NE should be used to achieve hemodynamic goals and tapered off as soon as possible

Safety concern	Rationale	Comments/recommendations
Gastrointestinal ischemia	NE possesses variable effects on hepato-splanchnic and mesenteric blood flow in hypotensive patients. Most reports suggest minimal differences to improved blood flow and/or oxygen consumption when compared to EPI or DA[20-22]	NE alone or in combination with DOB improves hepato-splanchnic and mesenteric blood delivery compared to other agents in hypotensive patients. Serum lactate concentrations and liver function enzymes should be monitored frequently[21]
Glucose abnormalities	Administration of sympathomimetics may cause gluconeogenesis and insulin resistance[15,36]	NE dose correlates to hyperglycemic events. Serum glucose concentrations should be monitored and corrected with insulin as clinically indicated[15,36]
Nephrotoxicity	A decrease in creatinine clearance has been shown in healthy, non-hypotensive volunteers with NE administration. Vasopressors can cause renal artery constriction and decreased filtration. However, NE with fluid resuscitation may improve renal perfusion and filtration in hypotensive patients[37]	Decreased urine production in sepsis-related hypotension may be due to hypovolemia and efferent arteriole vasodilatation. This may be reversed by fluid resuscitation and NE. Compared to high dose DA, NE is more likely to achieve MAP goals and enhance urine production.[37] Fluid status, urine production and serum markers of renal function (BUN, creatinine) should be monitored frequently
Bradycardia or other arrhythmias	NE possesses β_1-agonist properties that may induce tachyarrhythmias. Increases in SVR may cause reflex bradycardia[26]	Studies of NE in shock report reflex bradycardia. CO remains constant or increases with NE. Tachycardia is most likely to occur at higher doses but tachyarrhythmias are less frequent than with DA or EPI.[27,28,32] Cardiac monitoring should include telemetry for heart rate and rhythm and serial troponin concentrations if ischemia is suspected. Echocardiography may be required

(continued)

Safety concern	Rationale	Comments/recommendations
Drug-drug interactions	NE is metabolized by MAO and COMT. While pharmacokinetic drug interactions between MAO inhibitors (including linezolid, selegiline, phenelzine, isocarboxazid, tranylcypromine) and COMT inhibitors (entacapone, tolcapone) may enhance NE activity, close monitoring and frequent dose titration to the lowest effective dose is recommended. NE is alkaline labile. Caution should be used when coadministering medications through shared lines with NE	Pharmacodynamic interactions such as the concomitant administration of other vasopressors and inotropes may increase NE activity and enhance the likelihood of adverse effects. Interactions should not deter the use of additional agents in patients requiring supplemental therapy to reach hemodynamic goals. Medications that lower blood pressure (vasodilators, negative inotropes, etc.) will decrease the effectiveness of NE. NE should be administered through a dedicated lumen of a central venous catheter

Phenylephrine

Dosing Considerations

Phenylephrine's clinical activity is mediated by alpha (α)-receptor agonism and acts mainly as a vasoconstrictor to increase SVR. Commonly cited dosing ranges of 0.2–5 mcg/kg/min may need to be exceeded to achieve adequate response, which may enhance the likelihood of adverse events.[7] Lack of adequate fluid resuscitation prior to or concomitant vasopressor use may increase the risk of adverse events.

Obesity: Data are not available for use in critically ill obese patients. However, since many institutions use weight based dosing for phenylephrine, ideal body weight should be used to avoid excessive dosing of a drug with low volume of distribution and short half-life in over weight patients. The mixed concentration and rate should be verified to ensure the correct dose is being administered.

Thinness/emaciation: There are no reports of dosing considerations in underweight or nutritionally depleted patients. Phenylephrine doses should be titrated to the lowest dose required for goal hemodynamic response.

Kidney Injury: Phenylephrine is mainly metabolized by MAO with up to 16% of an intravenous dose excreted in the urine unchanged. The pharmacokinetics of phenylephrine in patients with renal insufficiency has not been studied. Phenylephrine does not require specific dose changes for renal insufficiency.[56,57]

Hemodialysis/Continuous Renal Replacement Therapy: The pharmacokinetics of phenylephrine has not been studied; therefore no initial dose adjustments are required and titration should be based on clinical response. Phenylephrine may be used to increase MAP in patients who become hypotensive during dialysis.

Liver Dysfunction: Phenylephrine is primarily metabolized by MAO to inactive metabolites. Dose adjustments are not necessary for hepatic insufficiency.[56,57]

Hypothermia: Therapeutic hypothermia may decrease enzymatic metabolism of medications including phenylephrine leading to higher serum concentrations. The clinical significance of this is unknown, therefore no initial dose adjustments are recommended and dose adjustments should be based on hemodynamic response.

Safety Concerns

Safety concern	Rationale	Comments/recommendations
Extravasation	Phenylephrine is a potent vasoconstrictor that can cause skin sloughing, ischemia, gangrene and necrosis if extravasation occurs. Phenylephrine extravasation may lead to tissue ischemia and necrosis[19]	Phenylephrine should be administered via a central line. If not readily available, a central catheter should be placed as soon as possible. If extravasation is noted, phentolamine (10 mg/10 ml NS) may be given in and around the extravasation site via hypodermic syringe[11]
Peripheral ischemia	Phenylephrine is a potent vasoconstrictor that can cause peripheral ischemia (digits, skin, etc.) via α-adrenergic effects. Inadequate volume resuscitation prior to and during vasopressor administration may increase the risk of ischemia. Higher doses of phenylephrine may increase the risk of peripheral ischemia	Fluid assessment and adequate resuscitation should be initiated prior to and during phenylephrine administration. Assessment of peripheral circulation and ischemia should be done frequently while on phenylephrine. Venous oxygen saturation should be maintained at $\geq 70\%$. The lowest effective dose of phenylephrine should be used to achieve hemodynamic goals and tapered off as soon as possible

(continued)

Safety concern	Rationale	Comments/recommendations
Gastrointestinal ischemia	Phenylephrine may decrease hepato-splanchnic and mesenteric blood flow and oxygen delivery	When NE was changed to phenylephrine in late septic shock, decreases in splanchnic blood flow, oxygen delivery and intramucosal pH were noted which reversed when NE was reinstated. Increased serum lactate concentrations and decreased lactate uptake have been noted. Conversely, the same investigators found no differences in regional perfusion between NE and phenylephrine in early phase septic shock.[58,59] Despite mixed data, signs of hepato-splanchnic and mesenteric ischemia should be assessed. Serum lactate concentrations and liver function enzymes should be monitored frequently[21]
Glucose abnormalities	Phenylephrine is selective for α-receptors and therefore carries the lowest risk for hyperglycemia of the catecholamines[15]	Phenylephrine may precipitate hyperglycemic events. Serum glucose concentrations should be monitored and corrected with insulin as clinically indicated
Nephrotoxicity	Vasopressors can cause renal artery constriction and decreased filtration via α-adrenergic receptors. However, phenylephrine with fluid resuscitation may improve renal perfusion and filtration in hypotensive patients[37]	Decreased urine production in sepsis related hypotension may be due to hypovolemia and efferent arteriole vasodilatation. This may be reversed by fluid resuscitation and phenylephrine. In late septic shock, creatinine clearance was decreased when NE was changed to phenylephrine. The same authors found no difference in creatinine clearance when phenylephrine was compared to NE in early septic shock.[37,59] Fluid status, urine production and serum markers of renal function (BUN, creatinine) should be monitored frequently

Safety concern	Rationale	Comments/recommendations
Bradycardia and cardiac function	Phenylephrine does not stimulate β-adrenergic receptors. Increases in SVR may cause reflex bradycardia. Of all vasopressors, phenylephrine is the least likely to cause arrhythmias[26,56]	Reflex bradycardia may occur with phenylephrine. CO remains constant or increases with phenylephrine in septic shock. Because phenylephrine may decrease cardiac index in cardiac patients, caution is warranted when used in cases of severe cardiac dysfunction and impaired myocardial performance. Phenylephrine is less likely to cause arrhythmias when compared to DA or NE and is indicated to terminate paroxysmal supraventricular tachycardia.[26,56] Cardiac monitoring should include telemetry for heart rate and rhythm and serial troponin concentrations if ischemia is suspected. Echocardiography may be required
Drug-drug interactions	Phenylephrine is metabolized by MAO.[57] While pharmacokinetic drug interactions between MAO inhibitors (including linezolid, selegiline, phenelzine, isocarboxazid, tranylcypromine) may enhance phenylephrine activity, close monitoring and frequent dose titration to the lowest effective dose is recommended Phenylephrine is alkaline labile. Caution should be used when coadministering medications through shared lines with phenylephrine	Pharmacodynamic interactions such as the concomitant administration of other vasopressors and inotropes may increase phenylephrine activity and enhance the likelihood of adverse effects. Interactions should not deter the use of additional agents in patients requiring supplemental therapy to reach hemodynamic goals. Medications that lower blood pressure (vasodilators, negative inotropes, etc.) will decrease the effectiveness of phenylephrine. Phenylephrine should be administered through a dedicated lumen of a central venous catheter

Vasopressin (VASO)

Dosing Considerations

Vasopressin's (VASO) vasoconstrictive activity is mediated by agonism of vaso-pressin (V)-1 receptors to increase SVR. In septic shock, VASO is often used as adjunctive therapy to catecholamine vasopressors at doses of 0.01–0.04 units/min that reflect physiologic replacement of a relative vasopressin deficiency. In cases of hepatorenal syndrome, VASO is commonly titrated by 0.04 units/min to achieve an increase in MAP of 10 mmHg, urine production, or a maximum dose of 0.4 units/min. Close attention to infusion rates is needed, as dosing in the USA is in units per minute while dosing in many other countries is in units per hour.

Obesity: Data are not available for the use of VASO in critically ill obese patients. Vasopressin is not dosed based on weight and is not titrated when used as a vaso-pressor in septic shock. The mixed concentration and rate should be verified to ensure the correct dose is being administered

Thinness/emaciation: There are no reports of dosing considerations in underweight or nutritionally depleted patients.

Kidney Injury: Vasopressin is mainly metabolized by vasopressinase with only 5–10% excreted unchanged the urine. The pharmacokinetics of VASO in patients with renal insufficiency are not significantly altered and do not require dose adjustment.[56] Vasopressin may be used at moderate to high doses to improve renal function in hepatorenal syndrome.

Hemodialysis/Continuous Renal Replacement Therapy: Vasopressin is not removed by hemodialysis and requires no specific dose adjustments. Vasopressin has been used to increase tolerability of fluid removal during dialysis.[56]

Liver Dysfunction: No specific dose adjustments are required for patients with liver dysfunction. Vasopressin may be used in high doses in patients with hepatorenal syndrome.

Hypothermia: Therapeutic hypothermia may decrease enzymatic metabolism of medications including VASO leading to higher serum concentrations. The clinical significance of this is unknown, therefore no initial dose adjustments are recommended and dose adjustments should be based on hemodynamic response.[8]

Safety Concerns

Safety concern	Rationale	Comments/recommendations
Extravasation	VASO is a potent vasoconstrictor that can cause skin sloughing, ischemia, gangrene and necrosis if extravasation occurs. Reports of adverse events have been published regarding VASO extravasation	Although VASO may be administered subcutaneously for other indications, it should be given via a central catheter whenever possible when it is administered intravenously. If not readily available, a central catheter should be placed as soon as possible. If extravasation occurs, the infusion should be stopped, warm compresses applied, and the site of administration elevated. A trial of local vasodilator may be considered, however this presents a risk in the hypotensive patient
Peripheral ischemia	VASO is a potent vasoconstrictor that may cause peripheral ischemia (digits, skin, etc.) via V_1-receptor effects. Inadequate volume resuscitation prior to and during vasopressor administration may increase the risk of ischemia. Higher doses of VASO may increase the risk of peripheral ischemia[60]	Fluid assessment and adequate resuscitation should be initiated prior to and during VASO administration. Assessment of peripheral circulation and ischemia should be done frequently while on VASO. Ischemic skin lesions have been reported to occur at rates as high as 30% when VASO is added to NE in resistant shock.[61] In a randomized trial of 776 septic shock patients, ischemic digits occurred more frequently with VASO compared to NE but not statistically higher and infrequently overall[62]
Gastrointestinal ischemia	VASO decreases hepato-splanchnic and mesenteric perfusion. VASO has been used to treat variceal hemorrhage and hepatorenal syndrome because it constricts the hepato-splanchnic vasculature to decrease perfusion[21,60,63]	Hepato-splanchnic ischemia and decreased gastric blood flow is usually observed with doses exceeding 0.04 units/min; however, lower doses of VASO may cause mesenteric vasoconstriction. Increased transaminases and total bilirubin have been reported with VASO likely due to impaired hepato-splanchnic blood flow.[21,63] Serum lactate concentrations and liver function enzymes should be monitored frequently[21]

(continued)

Safety concern	Rationale	Comments/recommendations
Cardiac ischemia and function	VASO may decrease CO as a result of reduced stroke volume. Animal and human models show mixed data suggesting a potential to cause cardiac ischemia at doses ≥ 0.04 units/min[64,65]	While animal models suggest VASO causes cardiac ischemia, human trials have not shown this adverse effect when compared to other agents.[62,65] Use as an adjunct vasopressor in septic shock may lower heart rate compared to NE alone.[62] Decreased stroke volume and CO may occur in hyperdynamic vasodilatory shock. Caution is warranted in patients with severe cardiac dysfunction, ischemic cardiac disease, coronary artery disease, atherosclerosis, cardiomyopathies, or congestive heart failure. In patients requiring high doses of VASO for indications other than shock, adding nitroglycerin may be used to decrease myocardial ischemia and improve cardiovascular function. Cardiac monitoring should include telemetry for heart rate and rhythm and serial troponin concentrations if ischemia is suspected. Echocardiography may be required
Hematological	VASO receptors are found on platelets and may contribute to the release of von Willebrand factor and enhanced platelet aggregation[60]	Multiple studies have shown an association between VASO treatment and decreased platelet counts. No change is evident in global coagulation at an infusion of 0.067 units/min.[60,63,66] Platelet count and coagulation parameters should be monitored serially
Endocrine	Stimulation of VASO receptors may lead to increased prolactin concentrations[60]	Serum prolactin concentrations in vasodilatory shock are higher when patients are treated with VASO and NE compared to NE or VASO alone. The clinical significance of this finding is unknown[60]
Electrolyte imbalance	VASO is also an agonist of V_2 receptors which may lead to decreased free water excretion and hyponatremia[60]	Although doses used for vasoconstriction are higher than those needed to decrease free water excretion in the kidney, hyponatremia has been reported as a rare adverse event in clinical trials. Many case reports of serious hyponatremia using VASO analogs have been reported.[60,62] Fluid status and serum sodium concentration should be routinely monitored

Safety concern	Rationale	Comments/recommendations
Drug-drug interactions	Pharmacokinetic drug-drug interactions are minimal with VASO. Pharmacodynamic interactions leading to additive toxicities are a concern when VASO is added to other vasopressor agents. The risk of increased ischemic events due to enhanced vasoconstriction needs to be considered versus prolonged hypotension when adjunctive VASO is being contemplated Caution should be used when coadministering medications through shared catheters with VASO	Additive vasoconstriction and ischemia must be considered when adding VASO to other vasopressors. The risk of excessive vasoconstriction should be weighed against the benefit of increased MAP and decreased NE dose to maintain adequate hemodynamic response. VASO should be administered through a dedicated lumen of a central venous catheter

References

1. Bates DW, Cullen DJ, Laird N, et al. Incidence of adverse drug events and potential adverse drug events. Implications for prevention. ADE Prevention Study Group. *JAMA*. 1995;274: 29-34.
2. Giraud T, Dhainaut JF, Vaxelaire JF, et al. Iatrogenic complications in adult intensive care units: a prospective two-center study. *Crit Care Med*. 1993;21:40-51.
3. Valentin A, Capuzzo M, Guidet B, et al. Errors in administration of parenteral drugs in intensive care units: multinational prospective study. *BMJ*. 2009;338:b814.
4. Rothschild JM, Landrigan CP, Cronin JW, et al. The critical care safety study: the incidence and nature of adverse events and serious medical errors in intensive care. *Crit Care Med*. 2005;33:1694-1700.
5. Kopp BJ, Erstad BL, Allen ME, et al. Medication errors and adverse drug events in an intensive care unit: direct observation approach for detection. *Crit Care Med*. 2006;34:415-425.
6. Kane-Gill SL, Jacobi J, Rothschild JM. Adverse drug events in intensive care units: risk factors, impact and the role of team care. *Crit Care Med*. 2010;38(suppl):S38-S89.
7. Overgaard CB, Dzavik V. Inotropes and vasopressors. *Circulation*. 2008;118:1047-1056.
8. Polderman KH. Mechanism of action, physiological effects and complications of hypothermia. *Crit Care Med*. 2009;37(suppl):S186-S202. doi:10.1097/ccm.0b013e3181aa5241.
9. Ruffolo RR, Massick K. Systemic hemodynamic effects of dopamine, (+/−) dobutamine and the (+) and (−) enantiomers of dobutamine in anesthetized normotensive rats. *Eur J Pharmacol*. 1985;109:173-181.
10. Reed WP, Newman KA, Applefeld MM, Sutton FJ. Drug extravasation as a complication of venous access ports. *Ann Intern Med*. 1985;102:788-789.
11. Phentolamine [package insert]. Bedford: Bedford Laboratories; 1999.
12. Teerlin JR, Metra M, Zacà V, et al. Agents with inotropic properties for the management of acute heart failure syndromes. Traditional agents and beyond. *Heart Fail Rev*. 2009;14: 243-253.

13. Endoh M, Hori M. Acute heart failure: inotropic agents and their clinical uses. *Expert Opin Pharmacother.* 2006;7:2179-2202.

14. Annane D, Vignon P, Renault A, et al. Norepinephrine plus dobutamine versus epinephrine alone for the management of septic shock: a randomised trial. *Lancet.* 2007;370:678-684.

15. Barth E, Albuszies G, Baumgart K, et al. Glucose metabolism and catecholamines. *Crit Care Med.* 2007;35(suppl):S508-S518.

16. Rousseau-Migneron S, Nadeau S, Nadeau A. Hyperglycemic effect of high doses of dobutamine in the rate: studies of insulin and glucagon secretion. *Can J Physiol Pharmacol.* 1985;63:1308-1311.

17. Ginsberg F, Parrillo JE. Eosinophilic myocarditis. *Heart Fail Clin.* 2005;1:419-429.

18. Bellomo R, Chapman M, Finfer S, et al. Low-dose dopamine in patients with early renal dysfunction: a placebo-controlled randomized trial. Australian and New Zealand Intensive Care Society (ANZICS) Clinical Trials Group. *Lancet.* 2000;356:2139-2143.

19. Montgomery LA, Hanrahan K, Kottman K, Otto A, Barrett T, Hermiston B. Guideline for IV infiltrations in pediatric patients. *Pediatr Nurs.* 1999;25:167-180.

20. De Backer D, Creteur J, Silva E, Vincent JL. Effects of dopamine, norepinephrine, and epinephrine on the splanchnic circulation in septic shock: which is best? *Crit Care Med.* 2003;31:1659-1667.

21. Woolsey CA, Coopersmith CM. Vasoactive drugs and the gut: is there anything new? *Curr Opin Crit Care.* 2006;12:155-159.

22. Guérin JP, Levraut J, Samat-Long C, Leverve X, Grimaud D, Ichai C. Effects of dopamine and norepinephrine on systemic and hepatosplanchnic hemodynamics, oxygen exchange, and energy balance in vasoplegic septic patients. *Shock.* 2005;23:18-24.

23. Marzio L, Neri M, Pieramico O, Delle Donne M, Peeters TL, Cuccurullo F. Dopamine interrupts gastrointestinal fed motility pattern in humans. Effect on motilin and somatostatin blood levels. *Dig Dis Sci.* 1990;35:327-332.

24. Dive A, Foret F, Jamart J, Bulpa P, Installé E. Effect of dopamine on gastrointestinal motility during critical illness. *Intensive Care Med.* 2000;26:901-907.

25. Leblanc H, Lachelin GC, Abu-Fadil S, Yen SS. The effect of dopamine infusion on insulin and glucagon secretion in man. *J Clin Endocrinol Metab.* 1977;44:196-198.

26. Tisdale JE, Patel RV, Webb CR, Borzak S, Zarowitz BJ. Proarrhythmic effects of intravenous vasopressors. *Ann Pharmacother.* 1995;29:269-281.

27. Patel GP, Grahe JS, Sperry M, et al. Efficacy and safety of dopamine versus norepinephrine in the management of septic shock. *Shock.* 2010;33:375-380.

28. De Backer D, Biston P, Devriendt J, et al. Comparison of dopamine and norepinephrine in the treatment of shock. *N Engl J Med.* 2010;362:779-789.

29. Bailer AR, Burchett KR. Effect of low-dose dopamine on serum concentrations of prolactin in critically ill patients. *Br J Anaesth.* 1997;78:97-99.

30. Schilling T, Strang CM, Wilhelm L, et al. Endocrine effects of dopexamine vs. dopamine in high-risk surgical patients. *Intensive Care Med.* 2001;27:1908-1915.

31. Regnier B, Rapin M, Gory G, Lemaire F, Teisseire B, Harari A. Haemodynamic effects of dopamine in septic shock. *Intensive Care Med.* 1977;3:47-53.

32. Myburgh JA, Higgins A, Jovanovska A, et al. A comparison of epinephrine and norepinephrine in critically ill patients. *Intensive Care Med.* 2008;34:2226-2234.

33. Shaver KJ, Adams C, Weiss SJ. Acute myocardial infarction after administration of low-dose intravenous epinephrine for anaphylaxis. *CJEM.* 2006;8:289-294.

34. Sakka SG, Hofmann D, Thuemer O, Schelenz C, van Hout N. Increasing cardiac output by epinephrine after cardiac surgery: effects on indocyanine green plasma disappearance rate and splanchnic microcirculation. *J Cardiothorac Vasc Anesth.* 2007;21:351-356.

35. Martikainen TJ, Tenhunen JJ, Giovannini I, Uusaro A, Ruokonen E. Epinephrine induces tissue perfusion deficit in porcine endotoxin shock: evaluation by regional CO_2 content gradients and lactate-to-pyruvate ratios. *Am J Physiol Gastrointest Liver Physiol.* 2005;288: G586-G592.

36. Sacca L, Morrone G, Cicala M, Corso G, Ungaro B. Influence of epinephrine, norepinephrine and isoproterenol on glucose homeostasis in normal man. *J Clin Endocrinol Metab.* 1980;50:680-684.
37. Bellomo R, Wan L, May C. Vasoactive drugs and acute kidney injury. *Crit Care Med.* 2008;36(suppl):S179-S186.
38. Isoproterenol [package insert]. Lake Forest: Hospira Inc.; 2004.
39. Mueller H, Ayres SM, Gregory JJ, et al. Hemodynamics, coronary blood flow and myocardial metabolism in coronary shock: response to *l*-norepinephrine and isoproterenol. *J Clin Invest.* 1970;49:1885-1902.
40. Lekven J, Kjekshun JK, Mjös OD. Cardiac effects of isoproterenol during graded myocardial ischemia. *J Clin Lab Invest.* 1974;33:161-171.
41. Halloway EL, Stinson EB, Derby GC, Harison DC. Action of drugs in patients early after cardiac surgery. I. Comparison of isoproterenol and dopamine. *Am J Cardiol.* 1975;35:656-659.
42. Furman WR, Summer WR, Kennedy TP, Sylvester JT. Comparison of the effects of dobutamine, dopamine, and isoproterenol on hypoxic pulmonary vasoconstriction in the pig. *Crit Care Med.* 1982;10:371-374.
43. Russel WJ, James MF. The effects on increasing cardiac output with adrenaline or isoprenaline on arterial haemoglobin oxygen saturation and shunt during one-lung ventilation. *Anaesth Intensive Care.* 2000;28:636-641.
44. Milrinone [package insert]. Irvine: SICOR Pharmaceuticals, Inc.; 2003
45. Taniguchi T, Shibata K, Saito S, Matsumoto H, Okeie K. Pharmacokinetics of milrinone in patients with congestive heart failure during continuous venovenous hemofiltration. *Intensive Care Med.* 2000;26:1089-1093.
46. Cuffe MS, Calliff RM, Adams KF, et al. Short-term intravenous milrinone for acute exacerbation of chronic heart failure: a randomized controlled trial. *JAMA.* 2002;287:1541-1547.
47. Baruch L, Patacsil P, Hameed A, Pina I, Loh E. Pharmacodynamic effects of milrinone with and without a bolus loading infusion. *Am Heart J.* 2000;141:e6.
48. Levy JH, Bailey JM, Deeb GM. Intravenous milrinone in cardiac surgery. *Ann Thorac Surg.* 2002;73:325-330.
49. Parissis JT, Farmakis D, Nieminen M. Classical inotropes and new cardiac enhancers. *Heart Fail Rev.* 2007;12:149-156.
50. Jeon Y, Ryu JH, Lim YJ, et al. Comparative hemodynamic effects of vasopressin and norepinephrine after milrinone-induced hypotension in off-pump coronary artery bypass surgical patients. *Eur J Cardiothorac Surg.* 2006;29:952-956.
51. Yang G, Li L. In vivo effects of phosphodiesterase III inhibitors on glucose metabolism and insulin sensitivity. *J Chin Med Assoc.* 2003;66:210-216.
52. Kikura M, Lee MK, Safon R, Bailry JM, Levy JH. The effects of milrinone on platelets in patients undergoing cardiac surgery. *Anesth Analg.* 1995;81:44-48.
53. Ramamoorthy C, Anderson GD, Williams GD, Lynn AM. Pharmacokinetics and side effects of milrinone in infants and children after open heart surgery. *Anesth Analg.* 1998;86:283-289.
54. Kikura M, Sato S. Effects of preemptive therapy with milrinone or amrinone on perioperative platelet function and haemostasis in patients undergoing coronary bypass grafting. *Platelets.* 2003;14:277-282.
55. Wesley MC, McGowan FX, Castro RA, Dissanayake S, Zurakowski D, Dinardo JA. The effect of milrinone on platelet activation as determined by TEG platelet mapping. *Anesth Analg.* 2009;108:1425-1429.
56. Phenylephrine [package insert]. Deerfield: Baxter Healthcare Corporation; 2005.
57. Hengstmann JH, Goronzy J. Pharmacokinetics of ^{3}H-phenylephrine in man. *Eur J Clin Pharmacol.* 1982;21:335-341.
58. Morelli A, Ertmer C, Rehberg S, et al. Phenylephrine versus norepinephrine for initial hemodynamic support of patients with septic shock: a randomized, controlled trial. *Crit Care.* 2008;12:R143. doi:10.1186/cc7121.

59. Morelli A, Lange M, Ertmer C, et al. Short-term effects of phenylephrine on systemic and regional hemodynamics in patients with septic shock: a crossover pilot study. *Shock.* 2008;29:446-451.
60. van der Zee S, Thompson A, Zimmerman R, et al. Vasopressin administration facilitates fluid removal during hemodialysis. *Kidney Int.* 2007;71:318-324.
61. Russel JA. Vasopressin in vasodilatory and septic shock. *Curr Opin Crit Care.* 2007;13:383-391.
62. Dünser MW, Mayr AJ, Tür A, et al. Ischemic skin lesions as a complication of continuous vasopressin infusion in catecholamine-resistant vasodilatory shock: incidence and risk factors. *Crit Care Med.* 2003;31:1394-1398.
63. Russel JA, Walley KR, Singer J, et al. Vasopressin versus norepinephrine infusion in patients with septic shock. *N Engl J Med.* 2008;358:877-887.
64. Luckner G, Dünser MW, Jochberger S, et al. Arginine vasopressin in 316 patients with advanced vasodilatory shock. *Crit Care Med.* 2005;33:2659-2666.
65. Asfar P, Radermacher P. Vasopressin and ischaemic heart disease: more than coronary vaso-constriction? *Crit Care.* 2009;13:169. doi:10.1186/cc7954.
66. Indrambarya T, Boyd JH, Wang Y, McConechy M, Walley KR. Low-dose vasopressin infusion results in increased mortality and cardiac dysfunction following ischemia-reperfusion injury in mice. *Crit Care.* 2009;13:R98.
67. Dünser MW, Fries DR, Schobersberger W, et al. Does arginine vasopressin influence the coagulation system in advanced vasodilatory shock with severe multiorgan dysfunction syndrome? *Anesth Analg.* 2004;99:201-206.

Chapter 3
Sedatives

John W. Devlin

Introduction

Most critically ill patients undergoing mechanical ventilation require the administration of at least two different sedative agents for a median of 3 (interquartile range 2–6) days to optimize patient comfort and safety, facilitate patient-ventilator synchrony and optimize oxygenation.[1,2] With an increasing number of safety concerns associated with the administration of sedatives, the likelihood of patients experiencing an adverse drug event during their ICU admission is high.[3] While many adverse effects are common pharmacologic manifestations of an agent (e.g., dexmedetomidine-associated bradycardia) and therefore frequently reversible, others are idiosyncratic (e.g., propofol-related infusion syndrome), unexpected, and may be associated with substantial morbidity and mortality.[4,5]

Many factors, common among critically ill patients, increase the risk for adverse events related to sedative therapy. These include the much higher sedative doses that are administered to patients in the ICU compared to the non-ICU setting and the frequent presence of hepatic and renal dysfunction that may lead to reduced drug clearance and higher than desired drug concentrations.[3] Factors such as altered post-receptor binding, down-regulation of receptors, and brain dysfunction may dramatically alter the response of patients to these agents. Cardiac dysfunction may increase the risk for dysrhythmias and hypotension.

This chapter will review the most common and serious adverse drug events reported to occur with the use of sedatives in the ICU, highlight the pharmacokinetic, pharmacodynamic and pharmacogenetic factors that can influence sedative

J.W. Devlin
Pharmacy Practice, Northeastern University,
Boston, MA, USA
e-mail: j.devlin@neu.edu

S.L. Kane-Gill and J. Dasta (eds.),
High-Risk IV Medications in Special Patient Populations,
DOI: 10.1007/978-0-85729-606-1_3, © Springer-Verlag London Limited 2011

response and safety in the critically ill, and identify strategies that can be used to minimize toxicity with these agents.

Dexmedetomidine

Dosing Considerations

Obesity: Dexmedetomidine is highly lipophilic and widely distributed in the body thus suggesting that actual body weight be used when an initial dose is calculated. The dose should then be titrated to the desired level of sedation.[4] There are a paucity of data surrounding the use of dexmedetomidine in critically ill obese patients. Current data surrounding its use in the obese is limited to procedural sedation and bariatric surgery.

Thinness/emaciation: There are no reports of dosing considerations in underweight or nutritionally depleted patients.

Kidney Injury: Following metabolism in the liver, most of dexmedetomidine (80–95%) is recovered in the urine as inactive metabolites. The pharmacokinetics of dexmedetomidine have been studied in volunteers with severe renal impairment.[6-8] The elimination half-life is longer in patients with renal disease compared to healthy volunteers without renal disease. One study analyzed the relationship between the clearance of dexmedetomidine metabolites and renal function in a series of mechanically ventilated ICU patients who received a dexmedetomidine infusion for ≥24 h and found that the clearance of metabolites decreased as renal function worsened.[7] A second study found that the concentration of dexmedetomidine metabolites in the patients with renal impairment (CrCL ≤ 30 mL/min) were elevated but were not associated with a risk for toxicity.[6] Based on these two studies it appears dosing adjustments are not required for patients with renal dysfunction.

Hemodialysis/Continuous Renal Replacement Therapy: While there is no information available for dexmedetomidine administration in patients receiving hemodialysis or continuous renal replacement therapy it would be expected that accumulation will not occur and thus this population should receive dexmedetomidine that is dosed to the desired level of sedation.

Liver Dysfunction: Dexmedetomidine is metabolized in the liver to inactive metabolites; however, there are a lack of data regarding whether doses should be reduced in patients with end stage liver disease.[4] Therefore, dexmedetomidine should be dosed to the desired level of sedation in this population.

Elderly: While studies evaluating whether pharmacokinetic parameters and therapeutic response to dexmedetomidine are altered in the elderly have not yet been completed, the elderly would be expected to require lower doses of dexmedetomidine given the age-related changes in liver and renal function and the greater sensitivity of the elderly to sedative agents in general.[4] Furthermore, given that the elderly are at increased risk for experiencing delirium and that use of dexmedetomidine is associated with less delirium than either benzodiazepines or propofol, dexmedetomidine may be the preferred sedative agent in the elderly population.[9-12]

Pharmacogenomic: Pharmacogenomic factors have not been shown to influence either dexmedetomidine clearance or response.[4]

Hypothermia: While dexmedetomidine has been shown to reduce shivering during therapeutic hypothermia, its pharmacokinetics during therapeutic hypothermia has not yet been investigated.[13]

Safety Concerns

Safety concern	Rationale	Comments/recommendations
Bradycardia	Bradycardia is common with the alpha-2 agonist class of drugs (dexmedetomidine and clonidine) via reflex responses from vasoconstriction, direct sympatholytic effects, and augmentation of cardiac vagal activity.[14,15] Unlike the biphasic response seen with blood pressure, healthy volunteers receiving high doses of dexmedetomidine experience a consistent drop in heart rate.[14,15] While not incorporating a standard definition for bradycardia, clinical trials comparing dexmedetomidine to benzodiazepines or propofol, showed a greater incidence of bradycardia with dexmedetomidine compared to lorazepam or midazolam.[9,10] However, severe bradycardia or a requirement for intervention for bradycardia was rare in each group although tending to be slightly more common with dexmedetomidine than comparators	Dexmedetomidine should be avoided in patients with active myocardial ischemia, second or third degree heart block, severe ventricular dysfunction and baseline a heart rate ≤50 beats/min Bradycardia usually resolves when the dexmedetomidine dose is reduced. In some instances, the infusion will need to be discontinued The simultaneous administration of negative chronotropic medications (e.g., beta-blockers, calcium channel blockers) with dexmedetomidine may have an additive effect on both the occurrence and severity of bradycardia[4,16]
Hypotension	Dexmedetomidine may induce a dose-dependent decrease in blood pressure due to its inhibitory effects on the sympathetic nervous system. Rapid upward titration of infusions appears to increase the risk for hypotension.[4,7] However two large studies comparing dexmedetomidine (median duration of 3.5–4.2 days) with continuous benzodizapine therapy identified a similar incidence of hypotension (i.e., systolic blood pressure <80 mmHg) between the dexmedetomidine and benzodiazepine-treated groups[9,10]	Caution should be used when administering dexmedetomidine to patients that are hypovolemic, have a labile blood pressure or are receiving a vasopressor agent A recent study limited dose increases to 30-min intervals allowing more time for distribution of the drug resulting in a significant reduction in hypotensive episodes compared to historic controls[17]

(continued)

Safety concern	Rationale	Comments/recommendations
Hypertension	Hypertension appears to be correlated with the administration of a loading dose of dexmedetomidine.[18] The rate of administration may contribute to the hypertensive effect, in addition to the dose	Loading doses of dexmedetomidine have been used for procedural sedation studies. However, studies conducted in the intensive care unit either do not use a loading dose or refer to loading doses as optional.[9,10] In clinical practice, loading doses were not frequently used[18]
Deep sedation	Deep sedation, that includes total amnesia, is the desired goal in certain subsets of ICU patients (e.g., patients requiring continuous neuromuscular blockade)[1]	Dexemedetomidine will not achieve deep sedation in many patients nor are its amnestic effects predictable. Therefore, dexmedetomidine should not be used as the sole sedative agent when deep sedation is required. In these situations, sedation with a benzodiazepine agent should be considered[4]
Administration >24 h	Dexmedetomidine is currently labeled by the FDA for duration of administration of ≤24 h based on a potential concern for rebound hypertension after stopping dexmedetomidine. However, rebound hypertension has not been reported when infusions >24 h have been used in both case series and clinical trials[4,9,10,19]	Adverse effects (including rebound hypertension) have not been shown to occur in clinical studies at a greater frequency with dexmedetomidine, even when administered for up to 30 days Hypertension that develops in a patient who has recently received dexmedetomidine (assuming that the hypertension is not related to rebound agitation or pain) can be treated with clonidine
Drug-drug interactions	Pharmacokinetic-based drug-drug interactions such as cytochrome P450 inhibition is not a concern with dexmedetomidine[4] Pharmacodynamic interactions could be a concern in patients who receive a drug that has similar pharmacologic effects to dexmedetomidine	Drugs with chronotropic, vasodilatory or sedative effects should be used with caution in patients receiving dexmedetomidine[4,18]

Lorazepam

Dosing Considerations

Initiation of Therapy: Lorazepam therapy should be initiated using a series of IV loading doses. When agitation persists despite multiple IV loading doses (e.g., five or more) then a continuous IV infusion may be considered. However, given the association between use of lorazepam infusions and a prolonged duration of mechanical ventilation, daily interruption therapy should be considered.[1,20]

Obesity: Sedative effects may be increased in the obese patient administered a lorazepam infusion although these effects are far less than that observed with midazolam given midazolam's greater lipid solubility and higher volume of distribution.[21]

Thinness/emaciation: There are no reports of dosing considerations in underweight or nutritionally depleted patients.

Kidney Injury: Lorazepam is metabolized to inactive metabolites that are excreted unchanged in the urine and thus dosage adjustments are not required in this population.[21] Patients with severe kidney injury are at greater risk for experiencing propylene glycol toxicity (see Safety Concerns) and thus the serum osmolality should be checked more frequently in patients receiving lorazepam infusions >8 mg/h than patients without severe kidney injury.[22]

Hemodialysis/Continuous Renal Replacement Therapy: Dose adjustments are not required.

Liver Dysfunction: Lorazepam clearance is reduced in patients with liver disease although not to the same degree as midazolam given that the glucuronidation system (that metabolizes lorazepam) is better preserved in the face of hepatic dysfunction than the oxidative system (that metabolizes midazolam).[21] In all cases, however, patients with liver dysfunction should receive lower doses of lorazepam.

Hypothermia: The pharmacokinetics of lorazepam has not been investigated.

Elderly: Benzodiazepine dosing requirements are generally lower in the elderly, given the greater Vd and lower clearance seen in this population. In addition, older patients require lower benzodiazepine plasma concentrations to achieve levels of sedation comparable to those in younger patients.[23] Patient-related factors that affect the benzodiazepine pharmacodynamic response are numerous and include age, concurrent organ dysfunction, prior alcohol use and concurrent therapy with other sedative drugs.[1]

Pharmacogenomic: The lorazepam dose that is required in ICU patients is not dependent on pharmacogenomic factors.[24]

Tolerance and Withdrawal: Tolerance to benzodiazepines may occur after only a few hours of therapy and thus dosing requirements may increase.[25] Benzodiazepines must be withdrawn slowly, particularly after high-dose, long-term therapy.

Safety Concerns

Safety concern	Rationale	Comments/recommendations
Precipitation of IV drug	Lorazepam is far less water soluble than midazolam and thus may precipitate in either the bottle or at the IV site when it is administered in high concentrations. The risk for precipitation is greater when it is infused via a peripheral line or through a line where a drug known to precipitate with lorazepam is being infused[1]	Lorazepam infusions should be diluted to a concentration of <1 mg/mL and not administered through the same line that other drugs known to precipitate with lorazepam are infusing[26]
Hypotension	Hypotension is likely multifactorial, related to decreased environmental stimulation as sedation occurs, decreased sympathetic tone, and vasodilation and is more likely to occur in patients that are hypovolemic or already hemodynamically unstable[3]	Caution should be used with the administration of lorazepam to hypovolemic patients that are not adequately fluid resuscitated
Propylene glycol toxicity	Propylene glycol is a diluent used to facilitate drug solubility. Recent reports have alerted clinicians to the risks for toxicity related to propylene glycol accumulation in patients receiving intravenous lorazepam.[22,27] Toxicity from the direct effects of propylene glycol and its metabolites (i.e. lactate, pyruvate) may result in hyperosmolar states, cellular toxicity, metabolic acidosis and acute tubular necrosis. In addition to long-term and high-dose lorazepam therapy, other identified risk factors for propylene glycol toxicity include renal and hepatic dysfunction, pregnancy, age less than 4 years and treatment with metronidazole	Monitoring propylene glycol serum concentrations is impractical in most institutions because these assays are rarely available. Instead, clinicians should monitor a daily serum osmol gap in patients who have received a daily lorazepam dose that exceeds 50 mg or 1 mg/kg based on several studies demonstrating that an osmol gap greater than 10–15 reflects significant propylene glycol accumulation.[28] Hemodialysis effectively removes propylene glycol and corrects hyperosmolar states, but generally discontinuing the parenteral lorazepam is all that is required[29]
Paradoxical agitation	Parodoxical agitation has been described with lorazepam more than other benzodiazepines that may be the result of drug-induced amnesia or disorientation[1]	An alternate sedative non-benzodiazepine should be considered in a patient where this occurs

Safety concern	Rationale	Comments/recommendations
Deep sedation	Deep sedation is the goal of certain critically ill patients. For example, patients requiring chemical paralysis are provided deep sedation[1]	A benzodiazepine like lorazepam will achieve deep sedation in patients and its amnestic effects are predictable.[1] Therefore lorazepam is a sedative of choice in this situation
Delirium	There is emerging evidence that delirium in ICU patients is related to the administration of anxiolytic drugs, particularly lorazepam, thus strategies that can avoid this class of agents may help avoid delirium and its numerous negative sequelae.[30] It should be noted that delirium may be associated with alterations in level of consciousness and that the agitation that is sometimes present with delirium may lead to the administration of sedative agents, particularly if delirium is not recognized.[31] Although the mechanism by which benzodiazepines predispose patients to delirium remains unclear, the GABA receptor activation that this class of agents induces alters levels of potentially deliriogenic neurotransmitters such as dopamine, serotonin, acetylcholine, norepinephrine and glutamate	Benzodiazepines, such are lorazepam, should be avoided in patients at high risk for delirium or who develop delirium. Instead, sedation with dexmedetomidine should be considered since it has not been shown to cause delirium and in fact, may reduce the incidence and duration of delirium[9,10]
Drug-drug interactions	Pharmacokinetic-based drug-drug interactions such as cytochrome P450 inhibition is not a concern with lorazepam[21] Pharmacodynamic interactions could be a concern in patients who receive a drug that has similar pharmacologic effects to lorazepam	Drugs with sedative effects should be used with caution in a patient who is receiving lorazepam

Midazolam

Dosing Considerations

Initiation of Therapy: Midazolam therapy should only be initiated using a series of IV loading doses and an infusion should only being initiated when scheduled intermittent IV dosing does not reach the desired clinical endpoint given the association between a prolonged duration of mechanical ventilation and the use of continuous infusions.[32] Interruption of benzodiazepine sedation on a daily basis has been shown to shorten the duration of mechanical ventilation without compromising patient safety.[20]

Obesity: Patients who are obese are at particularly high risk for prolonged sedative effects when prolonged (>48 h) of infusions of midazolam are administered and should receive lower doses of midalam and be managed with a daily sedation interruption protocol.[21,33]

Thinness/emaciation: There are no reports of dosing considerations in underweight or nutritionally depleted patients.

Kidney Injury: Midazolam is a short-acting, water-soluble benzodiazepine that undergoes extensive oxidation in the liver via the CYP450 enzyme system to form water-soluble hydroxylated metabolites, which are excreted in the urine.[33] The primary metabolite of midazolam, 1-hydroxymidazolam glucuronide, has CNS depressant effects and may accumulate in the critically ill patient, especially in the presence of kidney failure. In one series of patients with prolonged sedation >36 h after cessation of a midazolam infusion, elevated concentrations of 1-hydroxymidazolam glucuronide were detected an average of 67 h after the midazolam infusion was discontinued.[34] Lorazepam should considered an alternative to midazolam in patients with kidney injury.

Hemodialysis/Continuous Renal Replacement Therapy: While accumulation of midazolam's 1-hydroxymidazolam glucuronide is likely less in the patient with end stage kidney when renal replacement therapy is used, it still may occur. Therefore, lorazepam should be considered an alternative to midazolam in this population.

Liver Dysfunction: Midazolam clearance is reduced in patients with liver disease given that the oxidative (i.e., CYP450 enzyme) system is usually compromised in this population.[21,33] Midazolam should be used with care in this population. If it is used, it should generally be administered as an intermittent dose rather than an as a continuous infusion.

Hypothermia: The pharmacokinetics of midazolam in this population has not been investigated.[33]

Elderly: Benzodiazepine dosing requirements are generally lower in the elderly, given the greater Vd and lower clearance seen in this population. In addition, older patients require lower benzodiazepine plasma concentrations to achieve levels of sedation comparable to those in younger patients.[1,33] Patient-related factors that affect the benzodiazepine pharmacodynamic response are numerous and include age, concurrent pathology, prior alcohol use and concurrent therapy with other sedative drugs.[1]

Pharmacogenomic: Increasing data suggested that the activity of CYP3A5, the primary isoenzyme that influences midazolam metabolism, is influenced by genetic polymorphism.[35] For example, individuals who are homozygotic for the *CYP3A5*1* allele will have increased hepatic CYP3A5 activity and will clear midazolam faster than patients who are homozygotic for the *CYP3A5*3* and *CYP3A5*6* allelic variants. It has been reported that individuals who are homozygotic for the *CYP3A5*1* allele have increased hepatic levels of the protein CYP3A5 compared to individuals who are homozygotic for the *CYP3A5*3* and *CYP3A5*6* allelic variants. It is also important to note that critical illness itself has been associated with a substantial decrease in CYP450 isoenzyme 3A4 activity, which could also further influence the risk for midazolam-related oversedation.[34]

Safety Concerns

Safety concern	Rationale	Comments/ recommendations
Hypotension	Hypotension is likely multifactorial, related to decreased environmental stimulation as sedation occurs, decreased sympathetic tone, and vasodilation and is more likely to occur in patients that are hypovolemic or already hemodynamically unstable[3]	Caution should be used with the administration of midazolam to hypovolemic patients that are not adequately fluid resuscitated
Infection	In vitro testing of clinically relevant concentrations of midazolam inhibits neutrophil chemotaxis, phagocytosis and the production of reactive oxygen species.[36] Randomized and blinded trials that have compared infection rates between mechanically ventilated ICU patients administered infusions ($\geq$24 h) of midazolam and dexmedetomidine have demonstrated a 100% increase in infections with midazolam[10]	Use of midazolam appears to be associated with a higher risk for infection than other sedative options (e.g., dexmedetomidine) in the ICU
Deep sedation	Deep sedation is the goal of certain critically ill patients such as patients requiring chemical paralysis[1]	A benzodiazepine like midazolam will achieve deep sedation in patients and its amnestic effects are predictable. Therefore midazolam is a sedative of choice in this situation[1]

(continued)

Safety concern	Rationale	Comments/ recommendations
Prolonged sedation	While the greater lipid solubility of midazolam compared to lorazepam will result in a faster onset of action after a single IV bolus dose, it is also associated with a greater likelihood to result in a prolonged sedative effect when it is administered for a prolonged period.[34,37] Prolonged sedative effects with midazolam have been observed in patients with renal dysfunction, who are obese or have lower serum albumin concentrations.[21] These differences lead to recommendations in the 2002 SCCM consensus guidelines that midazolam be used for only short-term (<48 h) therapy and that lorazepam be used for ICU patients requiring longer-term sedation.[1] While older randomized controlled trials that have compared lorazepam with midazolam for long-term sedation have found no difference in the time to awakening between the groups it should be noted that few of the patients in these comparative studies had renal, hepatic or neurologic impairment at baseline[23,38]	Patients receiving a continuous infusion of midazolam should be carefully monitored for signs of excessive sedation and the dosage should be decreased or held until the patient becomes arousable. Other sedation strategies (e.g., intermittent midazolam or use of a sedative shown to reduce the incidence of oversedation) should be considered. In addition, daily sedation interruption should be considered in all patients receiving midazolam infusions
Tolerance and withdrawal	Tolerance to benzodiazepines may occur after only a few hours of therapy and thus dosing requirements may increase[25]	Benzodiazepines must be withdrawn slowly (no more than 25%/day), particularly after high-dose, long-term therapy
Delirium	There is emerging evidence that ICU delirium is related to the administration of anxiolytic drugs, particularly the benzodiazepines, and thus strategies that can avoid this class of agents may help avoid delirium and its numerous negative sequelae.[30,39] It should be noted that delirium may be associated with alterations in level of consciousness and that the agitation that is sometimes present with delirium may lead to the administration of sedative agents, particularly if delirium is not recognized.[31] Although the mechanism by which benzodiazepines predispose patients to delirium remains unclear, the GABA receptor activation that this class of agents induces alters concentrations of potentially deliriogenic neurotransmitters such as dopamine, serotonin, acetylcholine, norepinephrine and glutamate	Benzodiazepines, such as midazolam, should be avoided in patients at high risk for delirium or who develop delirium. Instead, sedation with dexmedetomidine should be considered since it has not been shown to cause delirium and in fact, may reduce the incidence and duration of delirium[9,10]

Safety concern	Rationale	Comments/recommendations
Drug-drug interactions	Medications that interfere with CYP3A4 such as erythromycin, fluconazole, diltiazem and conivaptan may inhibit midazolam metabolism[33]	While co-administration of these medications is not necessarily a contraindication to their use, clinicians should carefully observe patients for signs of oversedation

Propofol

Dosing Considerations

Obesity: There are no reports of dosing considerations in obese patients.

Thinness/emaciation: There are no reports of dosing considerations in underweight or nutritionally depleted patients.

Kidney Injury: No dose adjustment is required.

Hemodialysis/Continuous Renal Replacement Therapy: Metabolism of propofol occurs primarily by conjugation in the liver to inactive metabolites which are eliminated in the kidneys. Clearance does not appear to be significantly altered by renal disease.[40]

Liver Dysfunction: Metabolism of propofol occurs primarily by conjugation in the liver to inactive metabolites, which are eliminated in the kidneys. Clearance does not appear to be significantly altered by hepatic disease although in critical care populations, clearance is generally slower than the general population due to decreases in hepatic blood flow.[40]

Severity of Illness: One recent study that evaluated the pharmacokinetics and pharmacodynamics of propofol in critically ill patients found that patients who were sicker (based on SOFA score) were more likely to have a deeper level of sedation that was felt to be related to decreased propofol clearance.[41]

Pharmacogenomic: Pharmacogenomic factors have not been shown to influence either propofol clearance or response.[3]

Use in non-intubated patients: Due to the potential for propofol to lead to rapid, profound changes in sedative/anesthetic depth and the resulting suppression of ventilation that can occur, propofol should be administered in a monitored setting only by anesthesia or non-anesthesia personnel who have the education and training to manage the potential complications of propofol.[42]

Safety Concerns

Safety concern	Rationale	Comments/recommendations
Bradycardia	Propofol may cause bradycardia that may be associated with the propofol-related infusion syndrome (see below)[3]	Should be avoided in patients with type II or III heart block. Consider changing to another sedative regimen in the patient who develops severe bradycardia (e.g., heart rate $\leq$50) that is not attributable to another cause
Hypotension	Hypotension is likely multifactorial, related to decreased environmental stimulation as sedation occurs, decreased sympathetic tone, and vasodilation and is more likely to occur in patients that are hypovolemic or already hemodynamically unstable.[3] Older studies comparing propofol and midazolam showed a similar incidence of hypotension between drugs.[43,44] Hypotension attributable to systemic vasodilation is a well-known adverse effect of propofol – particularly in hypovolemic patients. For this reason, and due to propofol's rapid onset of activity, it should not be administered as a bolus dose	Caution should be used with the administration of propofol to hypovolemic patients that are not adequately fluid resuscitated Given that propofol is one of the most "overridden" ICU drugs by nurses using smart pumps, these devices should be "locked" to prevent this practice with propofol[45]
Infection	Propofol, like any lipid-containing product, has been shown to have immunosuppressant effects, although the clinical importance of these effects remains unclear.[46] It has been shown to impair multiple aspects of the innate immune response, including reducing macrophage chemotaxis and phagocytosis, suppressing nitric oxide production, and limiting production of interferon, tumor necrosis factor, and various interleukins and reactive oxygen species (ROS).[47] In addition, at clinically relevant concentrations, propofol inhibited chemotaxis, phagocytosis, and ROS production from neutrophils. In rat models of sepsis, propofol blunts the increase in TNF and IL–6 concentrations after endotoxin administration whether given immediately or 1–2 h after endotoxin administration.[48,49] Following the detection of post-operative infections in patients receiving the old formulation of Diprivan (AstraZeneca) that did not contain a preservative, the FDA mandated that all propofol formulations be reformulated with a preservative and the vial not be infused for more than 12 h[1]	Despite the presence of a preservative in the currently marketed formulations of propofol (other than propoven), both the propofol bottle along with the IV infusion set should be changed every 12 h

Seizure-like activity	Propofol-associated hypertonicity and seizure-like movements have been reported and are felt to occur when cerebral concentrations of propofol rapidly change[50]	Despite these reports, propofol is recommended for the treatment of refractory status epilepticus[51]
Deep sedation	Deep sedation, that includes total amnesia, is the desired goal in certain subsets of ICU patients (e.g., patients requiring continuous neuromuscular blockade)[1]	Propofol will not reliably achieve the level of amnesia that is required during deep sedation and thus clinicians should consider adding a benzodiazepine to sedation regimens when this desired level of sedation is required[6]
Hypertri-glyceri-demia	Propofol's lipid vehicle introduces further risk for adverse drug events. The lipid formulation accounts for 1.1 kcal/mL, which has been reported to induce hypertriglyceridemia (triglyceride concentration ≥500 mg/dL) in up to 18% of ICU patients that may cause pancreatitis.[1,52] Hypertriglyceridemia in ICU patients receiving propofol is typically associated with high propofol infusion rates, concurrent administration of parenteral lipids for nutrition, or baseline hypertriglyceridemia[53]	A serum triglyceride concentration should be measured at least twice per week in patients receiving continuous propofol therapy. Patients with a serum triglyceride concentration ≥400 mg/dL should receive a reduced dose of propofol or an alternate sedation regimen[3]
Delirium	Delirium, characterized by fluctuations in mental status, inattention, disorganized thinking, hallucinations, disorientation, and altered level of consciousness, occurs frequently in the ICU.[39] Delirium is associated with higher mortality, a longer duration of mechanical ventilation, increased ICU and hospital lengths of stay and a number of adverse post-ICU sequelae.[39] Various sedative therapies (e.g., the benzodiazepines) have been shown to increase the risk for delirium[30]	While it is clear that propofol does not prevent or reduce delirium in the critically ill due to its activity within GABA receptors, it remains unclear whether its use is an independent factor for the development of delirium in the ICU[30]

(continued)

Safety concern	Rationale	Comments/recommendations
Propofol-related infusion syndrome (PRIS)	Propofol-related infusion syndrome (PRIS) has become a much more readily recognized consequence of propofol.[53] Reviews of this syndrome have identified metabolic acidosis, cardiac dysfunction, hyperkalemia, hyperlipidemia, elevated creatine kinase levels, rhabdomyolysis, myoglubinemia and/or myoglobinuria, and acute renal failure to be the most prominent characteristics identified in published cases.[53-55] Several pathological findings have been identified that may contribute to the development of PRIS leading to inhibition of the mitochondrial respiratory chain, impaired fatty-acid oxidation, and cardiac and peripheral muscle necrosis. Impaired liver metabolism and clearance of propofol's fat emulsion resulting in the accumulation of ketone bodies and lactate have been postulated to contribute to acidosis.[53-55] It is inconclusive whether the development of PRIS is a result of a disruption in the mitochondrial respiratory chain due to the propofol emulsion or a genetic predisposition, such as medium-chain acyl Co A dehydrogenase deficiency[55,56] Catecholamines are often required in critically ill patients due to propofol's reduction in inotropic activity; the resultant increase in cardiac output by catecholamines decreases propofol serum concentrations resulting in the need to increase propofol doses.[56] This cycle results in escalating doses of these agents in critically ill patients and may impact the development of PRIS. Additional identified risk factors for PRIS have been drawn mostly from retrospective evaluation of confidential safety data, and published cases to include poor oxygen delivery, sepsis, serious cerebral injury, and the administration of high-dose propofol to be risk factors of PRIS.[53] Dosage risk has been further described to be doses ≥ 83 µg/kg/min for greater than 48 h.[53,55,57]	To minimize the potential for PRIS, mechanisms to optimize hemodynamic and oxygen delivery parameters in critically ill patients should be employed. It is recommended for propofol infusions exceeding 48 h, duration should be limited to dosages less than 83 mcg/kg/min.[53,55,57] Carbohydrate administration at 6–8 mg/kg/min might prevent PRIS by suppressing fat metabolism.[55] Recognizing the risk factors and clinical manifestations mentioned above may be helpful in identifying patients developing PRIS. Monitoring parameters suggested by the FDA include blood pressure, electrocardiograms, and arterial blood gases to detect unexplained metabolic acidosis or arrhythmias. The American College of Critical Care Medicine provides further guidance to consider alternative sedative agents in patients with escalating vasopressor or inotropic requirements or in those with cardiac failure during high–dose propofol infusions.[1,52] Recommendations by the European Regulatory Authorities indicate monitoring for metabolic acidosis, hyperkalemia, rhabdomyolysis, or an elevated creatinine kinase concentration and/or the progression of heart failure.[53] If PRIS is suspected, propofol infusion should be discontinued immediately, and supportive care instituted to correct metabolic acidosis and other presenting symptoms. Hemodialysis or hemofiltration have reportedly been successfully used to increase the elimination of propofol[54,55]

	A recent large prospective observational study of 1,017 ICU patients at 11 academic centers who were prescribed propofol for >24 h identified an incidence of PRIS based on a conservative and evidence-based definition and using only new-onset PRIS symptoms of 1.1%.[5] Another large, retrospective analysis of the FDA's MEDWATCH database identified a mortality rate of 30%[57]	Propofol remains the sedative of choice in patients with a primary neurologic process (e.g., neurotrauma) because of its easy titratibility[1]
Rapid awakening	Its rapid onset and offset of action provides clinicians with a sedative option that is more titratable than that of the benzodiazepines and is considered the preferred sedative for patients where rapid awakening is important[1]	Propofol remains the sedative of choice in patients with a primary neurologic process (e.g., neurotrauma) because its beneficial effects on intracranial pressure and cerebral blood flow
Intracranial pressure	Propofol reduces intracranial pressure after traumatic brain injury more effectively than either morphine or fentanyl and also decreases cerebral blood flow and metabolism[58]	An example of a pharmacodynamic interaction is the concomitant administration of propofol and benzodiazepines midazolam[1]
Drug-drug interactions	Pharmacokinetic-based drug-drug interactions such as cytochrome P450 inhibition is not a concern with propofol.[52] Pharmacodynamic interactions could be a concern with the additive effect of other medications that cause sedation	

References

1. Jacobi J, Fraser GL, Coursin DB, et al. Clinical practice guidelines for the sustained use of sedatives and analgesics in the critically ill adult. *Crit Care Med*. 2002;30:119-141.
2. Arroliga A, Frutos-Vivar F, Hall J, et al. Use of sedatives and neuromuscular blockers in a cohort of patients receiving mechanical ventilation. *CHEST*. 2005;128:496-506.
3. Devlin JW, Mallow-Corbett S, Riker RR. Adverse drug events associated with the use of analgesics, sedatives and antipsychotics in the intensive care unit. *Crit Care Med*. 2010; 38(6 suppl):S231-S243.
4. Gerlach AT, Murphy CV, Dasta JF. An updated focused review of dexmedetomidine in adults. *Ann Pharmacother*. 2009;43:2064-2074.
5. Roberts RJ, Barletta JF, Fong JJ, et al. Incidence of propofol-related infusion syndrome in critically ill adults: a prospective, multicenter study. *Crit Care*. 2009;13(5):R169.
6. Dyck JB, Maze M, Haack C, et al. The pharmacokinetics and hemodynamic effects of intravenous and intramuscular dexmedetomidine hydrochloride in adult human volunteers. *Anesthesiology*. 1993;78(5):813-820.
7. Bokesch P, Riker R, Shehabi Y. Pharmacokinetics of dexmedetomidine for long-term infusion [abstract]. *Anesth Anal*. 2009;108:S298.
8. DeWolf AE, Fragen RJ, Avram MJ, et al. The pharmacokinetics of dexmedetomidine in volunteers with severe renal impairment. *Anesth Analg*. 2001;93:1205-1209.
9. Pandharipande PP, Pun BT, Herr DL, et al. Effect of sedation with dexmedetomidine vs lorazepam on acute brain dysfunction in mechanically ventilated patients: the MENDS randomized controlled trial. *JAMA*. 2007;298(22):2644-2653.
10. Riker RR, Shehabi Y, Bokesch PM, et al. Dexmedetomidine vs midazolam for sedation of critically ill patients: a randomized trial. *JAMA*. 2009;301:489-499.
11. Maldonado JR, Wysong A, van der Starre PJA, et al. Dexmedetomidine and the reduction of postoperative delirium after cardiac surgery. *Psychosomatics*. 2009;50:206-217.
12. Reade MC, O'Sullivan K, Bates S, et al. Dexmedetomidine vs. haloperidol in delirious, agitated, intubated patients: a randomized open-label trial. *Crit Care*. 2009;13:R75.
13. Talke P, Tayefeh F, Sessler DI, Jeffrey R, Noursalehi M, Richardson C. Dexmedetomidine does not alter the sweating threshold, but comparably and linearly decreases the vasoconstriction and shivering thresholds. *Anesthesiology*. 1997;87:835-841.
14. Gerlach At, Murphy CV. Dexmedetomidine-associated bradycardia progressing to pulseless electrical activity: case report and review of the literature. *Pharmacotherapy*. 2009;29:1492.
15. Ebert TJ, Hall JE, Barney JA, et al. The effects of increasing plasma concentrations of dexmedetomidine in humans. *Anesthesiology*. 2000;93:382-394.
16. Karol M, Maze M. Pharmacokinetics and interaction pharmacodynamics of dexmedetomidine in humans. *Best Pract Res Clin Anaesthesiol*. 2000;14(2):261-269.
17. Gerlach AT, Dasta JF, Steinberg S, et al. A new dosing protocol reduces dexmedetomidine-associated hypotension in critically ill surgical patients. *J Crit Care*. 2009;24:568-574.
18. Dasta JF, Kane-Gill SL, Durtschi AJ. Comapring dexmedetomidine prescribing patterns and safety in the naturalistic setting versus published data. *Ann Pharmacother*. 2004;38: 1130-1135.
19. Ruokonen E, Parviainen I, Jakob SM, et al. Dexmedetomidine versus propofol/midazolam for long-term sedation during mechanical ventilation. *Intensive Care Med*. 2009;35:282-290.
20. Kress JP, Pohlman AS, O'Connor MF, et al. Daily interruption of sedative infusions in critically ill patients undergoing mechanical ventilation. *N Engl J Med*. 2000;342(20):1471-1477.
21. Wagner BK, O'Hara DA. Pharmacokinetics and pharmacodynamics of sedatives and analgesics in the treatment of agitated critically ill patients. *Clin Pharmacokinet*. 1997;33(6): 426-453.
22. Yahwak JA, Riker RR, Fraser GL, et al. Determination of a lorazepam dose threshold for using the osmol gap to monitor for propylene glycol toxicity. *Pharmacotherapy*. 2008;28(8): 984-991.

23. Barr J, Zomorodi K, Bertaccini EJ, Shafer SL, Geller E. A double-blind, randomized comparison of IV lorazepam versus midazolam for sedation of ICU patients via a pharmacologic model. *Anesthesiology*. 2001;95(2):286-298.
24. Tiwari AK, Souza RP, Müller DJ. Pharmacogenetics of anxiolytic drugs. *J Neural Transm*. 2009;116(6):667-677.
25. Cammarano WB, Pittet JF, Weitz S, et al. Acute withdrawal syndrome related to the administration of analgesics and sedative medications in adult intensive care unit patients. *Crit Care Med*. 1998;26:676-684.
26. Trissel L. *Handbook on Injectable Drugs*. 16th ed. Bethesda, MD: American Society of Health-System Pharmacists; 2010.
27. Arroliga AC, Shehab N, McCarthy K, et al. Relationship of continuous infusion lorazepam to serum propylene glycol concentration in critically ill adults. *Crit Care Med*. 2004;32: 1709-1714.
28. Barnes BJ, Gerst C, Smith JR, et al. Osmol gap as a surrogate marker for serum propylene glycol concentrations in patients receiving lorazepam for sedation. *Pharmacotherapy*. 2006;26(1):23-33.
29. Parker MG, Fraser GL, Watson DM, Riker RR. Removal of propylene glycol and correction of increased osmolar gap by hemodialysis in a patient on high dose lorazepam infusion therapy. *Intensive Care Med*. 2002;28(1):81-84.
30. Pandharipande P, Shintani A, Peterson J, et al. Lorazepam is an independent risk factor for transitioning to delirium in intensive care unit patients. *Anesthesiology*. 2006;104(1):21-22.
31. Devlin JW, Fong JJ, Fraser GL, Riker RR. Delirium assessment in the critically ill. *Intensive Care Med*. 2007;33(6):929-940.
32. Kollef MH, Levy NT, Ahrens TS, Schaiff R, Prentice D, Sherman G. The use of continuous IV sedation is associated with prolongation of mechanical ventilation. *CHEST*. 1998;114(2): 541-548.
33. Spina SP, Ensom MH. Clinical pharmacokinetic monitoring of midazolam in critically ill patients. *Pharmacotherapy*. 2007;27(3):389-398.
34. Bauer TM, Ritz R, Haberthur C, et al. Prolonged sedation due to accumulation of conjugated metabolites of midazolam. *Lancet*. 1995;346(8968):145-147.
35. Fukasawa T, Suzuki A, Otani K. Effects of genetic polymorphism of cytochrome P450 enzymes on the pharmacokinetics of benzodiazepines. *J Clin Pharm Ther*. 2007;32(4): 333-341.
36. Nishina K, Akamatsu H, Mikawa K, et al. The effects of clonidine and dexmedetomidine on human neutrophil functions. *Anesth Analg*. 1999;88(2):452-458.
37. Venn RM, Karol MD, Grounds RM. Pharmacokinetics of dexmedetomidine infusions for sedation of postoperative patients requiring intensive care. *Br J Anaesth*. 2002;88:669-675.
38. Swart EL, van Schijndel RJ, van Loenen AC, et al. Continuous infusion of lorazepam versus midazolam in patients in the intensive care unit: sedation with lorazepam is easier to manage and is more cost-effective. *Crit Care Med*. 1999;27(8):1461-1465.
39. Skrobik Y. Delirium prevention and treatment. *Crit Care Clin*. 2009;25(3):585-591.
40. Bailie GR, Cockshott ID, Douglas EJ, Bowles BJ. Pharmacokinetics of propofol during and after long-term continuous infusion for maintenance of sedation in ICU patients. *Br J Anaesth*. 1992;68(5):486-491.
41. Peeters MY, Bras LJ, DeJongh J, et al. Disease severity is a major determinant for the pharmacodynamics of propofol in critically ill patients. *Clin Pharmacol Ther*. 2008;83(3):443-451.
42. https://www.asahq.org/For-Members/ClinicalInformation/~/media/For%2520Members/documents/Standards%2520Guidelines%2520Stmts/Safe%2520Use%2520of%2520Propofol. ashx. Accessed December 10, 2010.
43. Carrasco G, Molina R, Costa J, et al. Propofol versus midazolam in short-, medium-, and long-term sedation of critically ill patients. *CHEST*. 1993;103:557-564.
44. Chamorro C, DeLatorre FJ, Montero A, et al. Comparative study of propofol versus midazolam in the sedation of critically ill patients: results of a prospective, randomized, multicenter trial. *Crit Care Med*. 1996;24:932-939.

45. Williams C. Application of the IV medication harm index to assess the nature of harm averted by smart infusion safety systems. *J Patient Saf.* 2006;2:132-139.
46. Mikawa K, Akamatsu H, Nishina K, et al. Propofol inhibits human neutrophil functions. *Anesth Analg.* 1998;87(3):695-700.
47. Sanders RD, Hussell T, Maze M. Sedation & immunomodulation. *Crit Care Clin.* 2009;25: 551-570.
48. Taniguchi T, Yamamoto K, Ohmoto N, et al. Effects of propofol on hemodynamic and inflammatory responses to endotoxemia in rats. *Crit Care Med.* 2000;28(4):1101-1106.
49. Taniguchi T, Kanakura H, Yamamoto K. Effects of posttreatment with propofol on mortality and cytokine responses to endotoxin-induced shock in rats. *Crit Care Med.* 2002;30(4): 904-907.
50. Islander G, Vinge E. Severe neuroexcitatory symptoms after anaesthesia – with focus on propofol anaesthesia. *Acta Anaesthesiol Scand.* 2000;44(2):144-149.
51. Marik PE, Varon J. The management of status epilepticus. *CHEST.* 2004;126(2):582-591.
52. Devlin JW, Lau AK, Tanios MA. Propofol-associated hypertriglyceridemia and pancreatitis in the intensive care unit: an analysis of frequency and risk factors. *Pharmacotherapy.* 2005;25:1348-1352.
53. Corbett SM, Montoya ID, Moore FA. Propofol-related infusion syndrome in intensive care patients. *Pharmacotherapy.* 2008;28:250-258.
54. Kam PCA, Cardone D. Propofol infusion syndrome. *Anaesthesia.* 2007;62:690-701.
55. Fudickar A, Bein B. Propofol infusion syndrome: update on clinical manifestation and pathophysiology. *Minerva Anestesiol.* 2009;75:339-344.
56. Vasile B, Rasulo F, Candiani A, et al. The pathophysiology of propofol infusion syndrome: a simple name for a complex syndrome. *Intensive Care Med.* 2003;29(9):1417-1425.
57. Fong JJ, Sylvia L, Ruthazer R, et al. Predictors of mortality in patients with suspected propofol infusion syndrome. *Crit Care Med.* 2008;36:2281-2287.
58. Devlin JW, Roberts RJ. Pharmacology of commonly used analgesics and sedatives in the ICU: benzodiazepines, propofol, and opioids. *Crit Care Clin.* 2009;25(3):431-449. vii. Review.

Chapter 4
Analgesics and Neuromuscular Blocking Agents

Jaclyn M. LeBlanc and Marilee D. Obritsch

Introduction

Analgesic medications are used routinely in the ICU patient. In general, adverse drug events resulting from analgesic administration are common such as decreased gastrointestinal motility and hypotension. Clinicians are developing a better understanding of other adverse drug events such as delirium and infection. In addition, critically ill patients often have impairments in renal and hepatic function that increase the risk for adverse drug events due to pharmacokinetic alterations. As well, there are specific situations, such as hypothermia, that ICU patients experience which may affect drug dosing. While not used as routine care, neuromuscular blockers are high-risk medications that contribute to adverse events in a population already at high risk of adverse effects. This chapter will review the patient safety concerns associated with analgesics and neuromuscular blocking agents.

Acetaminophen

Dosing Considerations

Obesity: Lee et al. demonstrated that acetaminophen plasma concentrations and rate of elimination were similar in obese and non-obese persons; however, the rate of oral absorption was slower in obese subjects. These authors recommended basing the dose of this medication on ideal body weight.[1]

J.M. LeBlanc (✉)
Department of Pharmacy, Saint John Regional Hospital (Horizon Health Network),
Saint John, NB, Canada
e-mail: jaclynleblanc@hotmail.com

S.L. Kane-Gill and J. Dasta (eds.),
High-Risk IV Medications in Special Patient Populations,
DOI: 10.1007/978-0-85729-606-1_4, © Springer-Verlag London Limited 2011

Thinness/emaciation: No data regarding the use of acetaminophen in nutritionally depleted patients are available.

Kidney Injury: Acetaminophen is not cleared renally, therefore no dosage adjustments are needed if the patient has kidney impairment.[2] Since decreased renal function decreases liver blood flow, one author recommends limiting doses in this patient population to 40 mg/kg/day and monitoring for hepatic impairment.[3] The manufacturer of IV acetaminophen indicates that a longer dosing interval and decreased daily doses may be needed with severe renal impairment. The intravenous medication has been shown to have a prolonged half life in the setting of severe renal impairment (creatinine clearance 10–30 mL/min), and an increased dosage interval of 6 h is recommended for those patients.[4]

Hemodialysis/Continuous Renal Replacement Therapy: Acetaminophen and its conjugate metabolites were found not to accumulate in hemodialysis patients over a period of 10 days.[5] There is no information available regarding the use of acetaminophen in continuous renal replacement therapy.

Liver Dysfunction: In patients with cirrhosis, there is a prolongation of acetaminophen clearance, increasing the risk for toxicity and dose should be reduced.[3] Oral acetaminophen should be avoided in patients with moderate to severe liver failure.[3] A recent review of intravenous acetaminophen indicated no dosage adjustments were needed in patients with liver disease.[4] However, the manufacturer indicates that the intravenous form is contraindicated in patients with severe hepatic impairment or severe active liver disease, and it should be used with caution in hepatic impairment or active liver disease.[6]

Hypothermia: There are some reports of using acetaminophen in patients with hyperthermia in whom hypothermia is being attempted, but the decrease in temperature is modest (0.3–0.4°C) even with high doses (4–6 g/day).[7]

Safety Concerns

Safety concern	Rationale	Comments/recommendations
Administration of multiple acetaminophen products	Ingestions of acetaminophen exceeding the recommended 4,000 mg/day have the potential to cause toxicity. In the community setting, the FDA has recommended stronger warning labels for products containing multiple ingredients to highlight the maximum recommended dose of acetaminophen[2]	In the ICU, there is the potential for inadvertent administrations of multiple products containing acetaminophen. Patient's medication profiles should be screened such that the potential maximum dose of acetaminophen will not be exceeded
Drug-drug interactions	Medications inducing the CYP2E1 enzyme can lead to an overproduction of the N-acetyl-p-benzoquinone-imine, a toxic metabolite of acetaminophen[8]	Examples of medications that induce the CYP2E1 enzyme include phenytoin and phenobarbital

Safety concern	Rationale	Comments/recommendations
Hypotension	A study examining ICU and Medium Care Unit patients receiving IV paracetamol, found a clinically significant decrease in systolic blood pressure (at least 10 mmHg) in 22% and 33% of patients at 15 and 30 min post infusion, respectively.[9] Clinical interventions (noradrenaline infusion or fluid bolus) were needed in 16% of patients to increase pressure to an acceptable value. This finding has been documented with the oral formulation as well[10]	As the use of IV acetaminophen increases, there may be more data published with regards to this effect. In the interim, there should be careful monitoring when this agent is used in an already hypotensive patient

Ketamine

Dosing Considerations

Obesity: While there are data regarding the use of ketamine in morbidly obese patients, no studies were found specifically examining the pharmacokinetics and dose considerations of this agent in the obese population.

Thinness/emaciation: No data are available regarding the use of ketamine in nutritionally depleted patients.

Kidney Injury: One study examining the effects of low-dose ketamine in ICU patients with acute renal failure did not demonstrate a significant increase in ketamine concentrations during long-term infusions. There was an increase in the metabolite of ketamine; however, this has minimal potency as compared to the parent drug.[11]

Hemodialysis/Continuous Renal Replacement Therapy: Less than 10% of ketamine is removed by dialysis or hemofiltration; hence dosage adjustments should be unnecessary.[11] Small amounts of ketamine were removed by continuous renal replacement therapy in ICU patients with multiple organ dysfunction, with no effects on the degree of sedation measured by Ramsey Sedation Score or Glasgow Coma Scale.[12]

Liver Dysfunction: No studies with ketamine for sedation in the ICU have been published in patients with liver dysfunction.

Hypothermia: No data are available regarding dose considerations of ketamine during hypothermia.

Safety Concerns

Safety concern	Rationale	Comments/recommendations
Sympathomimetic effects	Ketamine is known to cause a cardiac stimulant effect, increasing myocardial oxygen demand[13]	This agent should be used with caution in patients with myocardial ischemia. If the agent is truly needed, administering a benzodiazepine will help to decrease the sympathomimetic effects[13]
Psychotropic effects	This agent is known to cause emergence delirium, unpleasant recall, hallucinations, and dysphoria. The dose needed for analgesia is much lower than the dose that causes these adverse effects. These effects are offset by concurrent use of a benzodiazepine or propofol[13]	The benefits of ketamine in providing analgesia for opioid sparing effects need to be balanced by the need to provide a sedative such as propofol or a benzodiazepine. The use of a lower "subdissociative" dose for analgesic purposes may decrease the need for and dose of additional medications to attenuate the psychotropic effects of ketamine

NSAIDS

Dosing Considerations

Obesity: No reports of NSAID dosing in obese patients are available.

Thinness/emaciation: No reports of NSAID dosing in nutritionally depleted patients are available.

Kidney Injury: NSAIDs should be used with caution in these patients since they can block prostaglandins and cause renal vasoconstriction. Indomethacin carries the highest risk, with aspirin yielding the lowest.[2] The half-life of ketorolac nearly doubles in patients with a creatinine clearance between 20 and 50 mL/min, with some authors suggesting a maximum dose of 60 mg/day in those patients and avoiding the drug in those with a clearance less than 20 mL/min.[3] Close monitoring of renal function is recommended with IV ibuprofen in patients with advanced renal disease.[14]

Hemodialysis/Continuous Renal Replacement Therapy: An older report of ibuprofen use for 2 weeks in seven chronic hemodialysis patients demonstrated a lack of accumulation of ibuprofen and metabolites.[15] There is no information available regarding the use of NSAIDs in continuous renal replacement therapy.

Liver Dysfunction: Studies with the newer NSAIDs, COX-2 specific inhibitors, have shown increased serum concentrations in patients with moderate hepatic impairment.[3] In patients with liver cirrhosis, ketorolac has shown a slightly prolonged clearance and higher risk of renal dysfunction.[3] If liver failure occurs during NSAID therapy, the drug should be stopped immediately.

Hypothermia: There is no information available regarding the use of NSAIDs in hypothermia.

Safety Concerns

Safety concern	Rationale	Comments/recommendations
Bleeding and thrombocytopenia	NSAIDs are known to increase bleeding risk secondary to inhibiting platelet cyclooxygenase[16]	Postoperative NSAIDs in children after tonsillectomy developed an increased risk of bleeding in a meta-analysis.[16] In ICU patients with thrombocytopenia, bleeding rates, number of required transfusions and mortality were higher; there were significantly more patients receiving NSAIDs who were thrombocytopenic[17]
Gastrointestinal bleeding	NSAIDs are known to predispose patients to gastrointestinal bleeding through reducing prostaglandin synthesis by cyclooxygenase inhibition	There are a lack of data consistently implicating the NSAIDs as a cause of gastrointestinal bleeding in ICU patients, but the potential risk should be acknowledged[8]
Acute renal failure	NSAIDs have multiple mechanisms to cause acute renal failure including inhibiting prostaglandin induced vasodilation in the kidney (prerenal), allergic interstitial nephritis, and glomerulonephritis[18]	Dose and duration of therapy are implicated in the propensity of these agents to cause renal failure.[19] The cyclooxygenase-2 inhibitors may also cause acute renal failure, specifically in high dosages, patients with preexisting renal disease, prerenal states, or concomitant nephrotoxins.[20] NSAIDs should be avoided in at risk patient groups if possible or used with caution[14,18]
Impaired bone healing	Unknown if mechanism of impairment of bone healing is secondary to inhibition of only cyclooxygenase-2 or seen with all cyclooxygenases[21]	There are a lack of data regarding the implications of this effect in ICU patients. A recent meta-analysis found a pooled odds ratio of 3.0 (95% confidence interval 1.6–5.6) with NSAID exposure and risk of non-union of fractures, osteotomies, or fusions.[22] However, there was a significant association of lower quality studies with high odds ratio for non-union. Analysis of only seven high-quality spine fusion studies yielded an odds ratio of 2.2 (95% confidence interval 0.8–6.3)

Opioids

Fentanyl

Dosing Considerations

Obesity: In peri-operative surgical patients, a non-linear relationship between total body weight and drug clearance was found, suggesting that fentanyl dose should be not be based upon this parameter.[23] Other reports suggest prolonged effects in repeated dosing or infusion, specifically in obese patients.[24]

Thinness/emaciation: No data are available for the intravenous or subcutaneous forms of this medication. Data have shown impaired absorption of the transdermal patch in cachectic cancer patients, which could be extrapolated to any emaciated patient.[25]

Kidney Injury: In some studies, fentanyl has been shown to have normal clearance values in the patients with renal dysfunction.[3] Clearance may be impaired in patients with high levels of uremia (blood urea nitrogen concentrations greater than 60 mg/dL) and a reduction of 30–50% of usual initial doses may be required.[3,26]

Hemodialysis/Continuous Renal Replacement Therapy: Fentanyl is poorly dialyzable, secondary to high protein binding, high molecular weight, and large volume of distribution.[26] One case report demonstrated that fentanyl was not removed by high-flux or high-efficiency hemodialysis membranes with the exception of one specific type of dialyzer membrane (CT 190), suggesting that no supplemental dose would be necessary.[27] There are no data available with regards to fentanyl dosing during continuous renal replacement therapy.

Liver Dysfunction: No specific studies are available regarding the use of fentanyl in liver failure; however, due to its high hepatic extraction ratio, a reduction in clearance would be expected, especially when liver blood flow is affected.[3]

Hypothermia: Studies of adult and pediatric patients requiring cardiac surgery undergoing hypothermia have demonstrated a reduction in fentanyl clearance related to inhibition of the CYP3A4 enzyme.[28]

Hydromorphone

Dosing Considerations

Obesity: No reports with regards to hydromorphone and use in obesity are available.

Thinness/emaciation: No reports with regards to hydromorphone and emaciation are available.

Kidney Injury: The metabolite of hydromorphone, hydromorphone-3-glucuronide, can accumulate in renal dysfunction, contributing to neuroexcitation and cognitive impairment.[3] A study of renally impaired and non-renally impaired palliative care patients found mean doses of hydromorphone similar between patient groups.[29] This opioid may be used with caution in renally impaired patients, monitoring for clinical effects secondary to accumulation of the metabolite.[26]

Hemodialysis/Continuous Renal Replacement Therapy: In patients with chronic renal failure requiring dialysis, hydromorphone does not accumulate; however, the hydromorphone metabolite, hydromorphone-3-glucuronide, does accumulate between dialysis sessions.[30] No data are available with regards to hydromorphone removal during continuous renal replacement, however, given the relatively quick conversion to the metabolite, the parent compound would not be expected to accumulate.

Liver Dysfunction: Because hydromorphone undergoes first-pass metabolism, patients with liver dysfunction may have increased bioavailability when this drug is administered orally.[3] Decreased metabolism of the drug may occur in patients with liver impairment and lower initial doses of oral hydromorphone are recommended in patients with liver dysfunction.[31] Recommendations for intravenous dosing are lacking; however, lower initial doses of the drug can be used and the patient monitored carefully for symptoms of accumulation.

Hypothermia: No data are available in human subjects who were hypothermic and receiving hydromorphone.

Meperidine

Dosing Considerations

Obesity: No data are available regarding the use of meperidine in obesity.

Thinness/emaciation: No data are available regarding the use of meperidine in emaciation.

Kidney Injury: The metabolite of meperidine (normeperidine) accumulates in renal failure due to a prolonged half life, and has been reported to cause myoclonus, seizures, and death.[3] Repeated doses are not recommended in this setting.

Hemodialysis/Continuous Renal Replacement Therapy: While meperidine is not recommended in renal failure, hemodialysis has been utilized in one case report for clearing the normeperidine metabolite in a patient who was experiencing toxicity secondary to the metabolite.[2,32] There is no information available regarding the use of meperidine in continuous renal replacement therapy.

Liver Dysfunction: No data are published with regards to the use of meperidine in the setting of liver dysfunction.

Hypothermia: Meperidine has been used as a bolus dose to control shivering in induced hypothermia.[7] No data regarding altered metabolism are available.

Morphine

Dosing Considerations

Obesity: A recent review regarding the use of morphine in obesity showed that although there are many expected pharmacokinetic and pharmacodynamic changes, there are a lack of data available in this population.[33] There are reports of use of morphine in obese post gastric bypass patients that demonstrates safety and efficacy in this population.[34]

Thinness/emaciation: There are no published reports of dosing considerations in underweight or nutritionally depleted patients. However, given that morphine is not highly protein bound, cachexia would not be expected to affect the free fraction of this drug.

Kidney Injury: Approximately 90% of morphine and its metabolites are cleared renally.[31] A study of the renal clearance of continuous infusion morphine in 15 intensive care patients with varying degrees of renal dysfunction demonstrated a significant linear relationship between creatinine clearance and renal clearance of morphine and its metabolites, morphine 3-glucuronide and morphine 6-glucuronide.[35] The metabolites of morphine are active and can lead to not only increased therapeutic effects, but also adverse effects. The 3-glucuronide metabolite has little analgesic effects, but may cause behavioral excitation and stimulate respiration; it may also decrease the seizure threshold.[3] The 6-glucuronide metabolite causes analgesia and respiratory depression; it crosses the blood brain barrier more slowly than the parent compound, potentially leading to prolonged somnolence and hallucinations.[3,26] It is recommended to give 75% or 50% of the recommended morphine dose for a creatinine clearance < 50 mL/min and > 10 mL/min, respectively.[31] In practice, it may be safer for the patient to use an alternative agent in the setting of impaired renal function.[26]

Hemodialysis/Continuous Renal Replacement Therapy: Both morphine and its metabolites may be removed by dialysis. This can lead to a rebound effect following discontinuance of dialysis.[26] Due to slow diffusion of the 6-glucuronide across the blood brain barrier, its effects may persist longer than morphine.[26] There is no information available regarding the use of morphine in continuous renal replacement therapy. The use of morphine may cause risk to the patient and an alternative agent would be suggested.[26]

Liver Dysfunction: Because approximately 90% of morphine is conjugated to the 3- and 6-glucuronide, patients with liver dysfunction would be expected to have higher serum concentrations of the drug.[31] Over a 50% reduction in morphine clearance and three-fold increase in half-life was noted by McNab et al. in shocked ICU patients with impaired hepatic perfusion.[36] Data are lacking for recommendations of dosing in patients with "shocked liver". Authors of a study examining accumulation of unchanged morphine in cirrhosis patients recommended an increase of 1.5–2 fold the dosing interval to account for a prolonged half-life and lower body clearance.[37]

Hypothermia: One study showed that morphine total clearance was decreased by 22% in pediatric patients with a targeted temperature of 33–34°C.[38] Animal studies found a decreased affinity of morphine for the mu receptors resulting in a need for higher concentrations for effect, however there are no human studies to substantiate this.[39,40] Affinity of morphine for the receptor increases during rewarming, increasing the risk for respiratory depression.[40]

Remifentanil

Dosing Considerations

Obesity: Although lipophilic, remifentanil is reported to have a constant volume of distribution regardless of the presence of obesity.[41] One report of the use of remifentanil in massively obese (body mass index 54.5 ± 12 kg/m^2) bariatric surgical patients suggested increasing tolerance to the opioid during surgery when the medication was titrated based on cardiovascular parameters via a target-site controlled infusion.[41] Egan et al. compared the pharmacokinetics of this agent in obese and lean subjects undergoing surgery and found insignificant differences between the two populations, with parameters more closely related to lean body mass.[42]

Thinness/emaciation: No data are available regarding dosing considerations of remifentanil in patients who were nutritionally depleted.

Kidney Injury: In ICU patients, the pharmacokinetics of remifentanil were not found to be significantly different in patients with moderate to severe renal impairment (mean creatinine clearance 14.7 ± 15.7 mL/min; half of these patients were receiving dialysis).[43] Although less supplemental propofol was needed in this group, this did not reach statistical significance. The major metabolite, remifentanil acid, was shown to have a decreased clearance of 25% in ICU patients with moderate to severe renal impairment, thought to be due to differences in volumes of distribution.[43] This metabolite does not have significant therapeutic effects at the concentrations accumulated, and no toxic effects were observed in this study.[43] Given these data, the dose of remifentantil does not need to be adjusted in renal impairment.

Hemodialysis/Continuous Renal Replacement Therapy: In patients with end stage renal disease receiving dialysis, remifentanil acid was shown to have a prolonged half-life and decreased clearance compared to patients with normal kidney function, most likely related to having hemodialysis with subsequent volume depletion the day prior to the study.[44] The clinical effects of this accumulation are not thought to be significant. There are data in patients receiving remifentanil while on continuous renal replacement, however these patients are grouped with other patients receiving dialysis, and subgroup data could not be extracted.[43]

Liver Dysfunction: Dosage adjustments are not required for remifentanil in patients with liver dysfunction, although these patients may be more susceptible to the respiratory depressant effects.[45] This latter effect was found in one study with ten subjects with stable hepatic disease and ten healthy volunteers, and the clinical significance was questionable.

Hypothermia: Data in patients undergoing cardiopulmonary bypass demonstrated a 20% reduction in remifentanil clearance that was attributed to a decrease in hydrolytic enzyme activity secondary to hypothermia.[46]

Safety Concerns

Safety concern	Rationale	Comments/recommendations
Bradycardia	Fentanyl and remifentanil may cause bradycardia secondary to decreased vagal tone[47]	The minimal dose needed should be used, as bradycardia is more common with higher doses
Decreased respiratory rate	All opioids cause respiratory depression	This effect can be compounded when opioids are used concomitantly with other agents that suppress the respiratory drive. Extreme caution should be used in this instance if patients are not ventilated
Delirium	The opioids cause many clinical symptoms that have been shown to be associated with the development of delirium, such as hallucinations and sleep disturbances.[48] A clear association between opioid usage and delirium cannot be made. Although not discussed in this chapter, methadone may have the least risk of the all the opioids to cause delirium[24]	If patients exhibit symptoms associated with delirium or delirium itself, all efforts should be made to discontinue the offending agents
Gastrointestinal complications	All of the opioids decrease gastric motility secondary to altered neurotransmitter release through activation of the μ receptors[49]	Morphine administration has been shown to lead not only to constipation but also postoperative ileus, which can significantly prolong ICU stay.[49] All opioids should be used at the lowest possible dose for the shortest period of time needed. As well, all patients should have a bowel regimen instituted if possible

Safety concern	Rationale	Comments/recommendations
Genetic polymorphisms	Certain genetic factors have been shown to affect opioid dosage and clearance. The A118G polymorphism of the mu opioid receptor is very common and is associated with a higher dose requirement for morphine.[50] Both fentanyl and morphine oral absorption and elimination may be affected by a P-glycoprotein encoded efflux pump that can remove opioids from the cell.[50,51] The CYP3A5 metabolic pathway is highly expressed in only 30% of Caucasians, which may result in a lower clearance in non-Caucasian patients[24]	All of these genetic factors may alter serum concentrations of opioids, and may account for some variability of effect in different patients[24]
Hypotension	Multiple mechanisms are implicated in morphine induced hypotension including increased vagal tone, decrease in cardiac sympathetic nerve activity, histamine release, and venous and arterial vasodilation.[52] Morphine exhibits more hypotension than fentanyl and remifentanil secondary to more histamine release[47]	Caution should be used when administering morphine to patients receiving vasodilatory agents, especially in patients with labile blood pressures
Infection susceptibility	In animal and human models, morphine has been shown to alter numerous macrophage functions, including a decrease in macrophage nitric oxide formation and phagocytosis, as well as decreasing natural killer cell activity.[53] Effects upon B and T cells are more controversial, but decreased T helper cell function, CD4/CD8 population, and antibody production have been documented.[53] Published data shows that fentanyl exhibits a dose-dependant effect upon human immune modulation[54]	Although in vivo and in vitro data support the chemical basis for effects on the innate and adaptive immune functions, there are limited clinical data to support the clinical relevance. More evidence is needed before recommendations can be given to either avoid or decrease the dose morphine in the setting of infection
Muscle rigidity	Bolus doses of remifentanil and fentanyl may cause thoracic muscle rigidity[24,55]	High bolus doses may lead to difficulty in ventilation of patients and should be avoided if possible

(continued)

Safety concern	Rationale	Comments/recommendations
Nausea and vomiting	All of the opioids can cause nausea and vomiting due to their effects at the chemoreceptor trigger zone in stimulating serotonin and dopamine receptors. Their action at the μ_2 receptors also causes delayed gastric transit, which may contribute to the nausea and vomiting	Gastric motility agents or serotonin receptor antagonists may be helpful if needed
Oversedation	Oversedation and slower recovery of neurologic function is most often seen in patients where opioids accumulate	Opioids may accumulate in patients receiving scheduled administration (infusion or intermittent). Other at risk patients include patients with end-stage renal disease receiving morphine (secondary to morphine-6-glucuronide accumulation) or obese patients receiving fentanyl (due to its high lipophilicity).[24] Because of its short duration of action, remifentanil should have the least propensity to accumulate. In comparison with morphine, patients receiving remifentanil spent more time in the desired sedation range and less time receiving mechanical ventilation[56]
Route of administration	The oral equivalent dose of an IV dose of morphine is higher and will therefore produce a higher metabolite load, with possible additional toxicity.[57] As well, the doses of hydromorphone and morphine are not equivalent, and medication errors have occurred due to incorrect conversions	In patients with renal failure, one author recommends decreasing the equivalence dosing up to a factor of three or to use another agent that doesn't have active metabolites.[3] Careful attention should be paid when switching from morphine to hydromorphone or vice versa, given the two agents are not equivalent and the propensity for errors
Seizures	Seizures are documented to occur secondary to the metabolite of meperidine, normeperidine	Although this metabolite accumulates in renal failure, patients receiving high doses with normal renal function or long term therapy may also be at risk for accumulation and subsequent seizures[3]

Safety concern	Rationale	Comments/recommendations
Tachycardia	Meperidine can cause tachycardia directly; this is not seen with other opioids[47]	With low doses of meperidine used in ICU patients, the clinical significance of induced tachycardia is questionable. In patients for whom an increased heart rate is intolerable, an alternative agent should be sought
Drug-Drug Interactions	Further respiratory depression may occur when opioids are administered in conjunction with other respiratory or central nervous system depressants, such as benzodiazepines and propofol	When administering agents with similar effects on the central nervous system or respirations, patients should be closely monitored for adverse effects

Neuromuscular Blocking Agents

Succinylcholine

Dosing Considerations

Obesity: In a group of morbidly obese (body mass index greater than 40 kg/m^2), intubating conditions were most favorable when succinylcholine was dosed using total body weight instead of ideal or lean body weight.[58]

Thinness/emaciation: No reports with regards to succinylcholine and emaciation were found.

Elderly: No evidence of altered effects in elderly patients.[59]

Kidney Injury: Metabolism of succinylcholine is not affected by renal failure.[60]

Hemodialysis/Continuous Renal Replacement Therapy: No reports in regards to succinylcholine and hemodialysis/CRRT were found.

Liver Dysfunction: Patients with liver dysfunction may have reduced levels of plasma cholinesterase which is responsible for succinylcholine metabolism potentially resulting in enhanced effects of the drug.[60]

Hypothermia: May prolong the duration of neuromuscular blockade.[61]

Safety Concerns

Safety concern	Rationale	Comments/recommendations
Qualified personnel	Pharmacologic response to these drugs results in respiratory muscle paralysis	Prescribers of these agents must be qualified to manage ventilation/intubation
Need for sedation and analgesia	None of these agents possess analgesic or anxiolytic properties	Administration of scheduled or continuous doses of opioids and benzodiazepines is necessary while neuromuscular blockade is administered
Hyperkalemia	Conditions which upregulate acetylcholine receptors (i.e., direct muscle trauma, tumor or inflammation; thermal injury; disuse atrophy; severe infection; upper/lower motor neuron defect; prolonged chemical denervation) can cause potassium efflux from muscle when depolarized by succinylcholine resulting in hyperkalemia	Increases in potassium ranging from 0.5 to 1 mEq/L. Monitor for electrocardiographic changes and cardiac instability; may occur within 2–5 min and may last for 10–15 min. Treatment includes calcium chloride or gluconate to stabilize cardiac membranes, and agents to increase cellular uptake of potassium (insulin with glucose, albuterol, sodium bicarbonate). Does appear to be dose-related. In susceptible states, nondepolarizing neuromuscular blocking agents would be preferred over succinylcholine[62]
Decreased pseudocholin-esterase activity	Condition seen in genetic mutation causing prolonged paralysis of 30 min. Other states with low pseudocholi-netsterase levels include cirrhosis, malnutrition, pregnancy, cancer, burns, uremia, or patients undergoing cardiopulmonary bypass.[60,63] Certain drugs may inhibit pseudocholinest-erase activity (cyclophosph-amide, monoamine oxidase inhibitors, organophos-phates, neostigmine)	Duration of blockade could be prolonged especially with high initial doses or repeated doses of succinylcholine[63]
Fasciculations	Caused by skeletal muscle depolarization	May be managed by small dose of non-depolarizing neuromuscular blocker prior to succinylcholine administra-tion. Dose of succinylcholine may need to be increased in this situation[63]

Safety concern	Rationale	Comments/recommendations
Malignant hyperthermia	Administration may trigger hypermetabolic response (hypercapnia, metabolic acidosis, muscle rigidity, rhabdomyolysis, arrhythmias, hyperpyrexia, and/or hyperkalemia) which may be lethal. Defect responsible may be sarcoplasmic reticulum calcium release channel causing excessive release of intracellular calcium with protracted contraction of the muscle[64]	Swift and aggressive treatment is required. Succinylcholine and other potential causative agents (inhaled anesthetics) should be immediately discontinued. Surgery may need to be stopped. Hyperventilation with 100% oxygen. Administration of dantrolene 2.5 mg/kg intravenous dose followed by an infusion to a total of 10 mg/kg should be initiated with repeat doses based on heart rate, muscle rigidity, and temperature for up to 48 h. Cold intravenous fluids at 15–45 mL/h may be administered as well as cooling by other methods (nasogastric lavage, bladder irrigation, cooling blankets). Sodium bicarbonate administration is dependent on arterial blood gas results. Close monitoring of patients for 48 h is warranted with the first 24 h in the intensive care unit
Myasthenia gravis	Functional reduction in number of postsynaptic acetylcholine receptors[60]	Results in decreased response to succinylcholine
Drug interactions	Magnesium	Inhibits effect of succinylcholine[60]
	Theophylline, aminophylline	Potentiates effect of succinylcholine

Cisatracurium

Dosing Considerations

Obesity: Dosing cisatracurium based on total body weight in morbidly obese women (body mass index greater than 40 kg/m^2) resulted in a prolonged duration of action compared to patients of normal weight and morbidly obese women with cisatracurium dosed based on ideal body weight.[65]

Thinness/emaciation: No reports with regards to cisatracurium and emaciation were found.

Gender: No difference in onset time or duration of clinical effect in females compared to males after single dose administration.[66]

Elderly: Reports of delay in onset of block but clinical duration of effect unaltered with advanced age.[59]

Kidney Injury: Renal failure has little effect on the pharmacokinetic profile of the drug.[67]

Hemodialysis/Continuous Renal Replacement Therapy: No reports in regards to cisatracurium and hemodialysis/CRRT were found.

Liver Dysfunction: Hepatic failure has little effect on the pharmacokinetic profile of the drug.[67]

Hypothermia: One study found the duration of action of cisatracurium to be predicted by lowest core body temperature.[68]

Rocuronium

Dosing Considerations

Obesity: Reduced infusion rates were required in one study comparing obese patients (body mass index greater than 26 kg/m^2) to non-obese patients.[69] Another study found reduced time to effect and prolonged duration of effect. Despite no statistical significance, some have recommended dosing based on ideal body weight for rocuronium.[70]

Thinness/emaciation: Use in these patients can cause profound neuromuscular blockade.[71]

Gender: It has been reported that onset time is shorter and duration of clinical effect is longer in female patients after administration of a single dose.[66]

Elderly: Reports of prolonged duration of effect due to decreased drug elimination in surgery patients 70 years of age and older.[72]

Kidney Injury: One study found a 32% reduction in clearance but no difference in volume of distribution at steady state or half life in patients with normal renal function and patients with end-stage renal disease.[67] One report of bolus dosing in renal patients demonstrated a significant increase in the duration of action of rocuronium compared to healthy controls.[73] A similar study with bolus dosing of rocuronium in severe to end-stage renal disease patients resulted in reduced clearance of the drug and decreased renal excretion of the drug.[74]

Hemodialysis/Continuous Renal Replacement Therapy: No reports in regards to rocuronium and hemodialysis/CRRT were found.

Liver Dysfunction: Reports demonstrate increased volume of distribution, increased half-life and slightly reduced clearance of the drug with hepatic failure which may result in slight prolongation of recovery parameters.[67] Patients with mild to moderate cirrhosis exhibited reduced clearance and prolonged half-life with prolongation of effect.[75]

Hypothermia: Use in neurosurgical and hypothermic cardiopulmonary bypass patients resulted in a reduced clearance and increased duration of action of the drug.[67]

Vecuronium

Dosing Considerations

Obesity: In a small study comparing obese surgical patients to non-obese patients, a prolonged duration of effect was observed due to the large dose administered based on total body weight. Ideal body weight may be used to calculate vecuronium dosing for obese patients.[76]

Thinness/emaciation: The effects of vecuronium may be prolonged in patients with cachexia.[77]

Gender: One report demonstrated reduced clearance of vecuronium in females.[78] An earlier study reported lower plasma concentrations and higher volume of distribution in male patients compared to female patients.[79]

Elderly: Reports of prolonged duration of effect.[59]

Kidney Injury: Patients with renal failure scheduled for transplant compared to patients with normal renal function have a decreased plasma clearance and prolonged elimination half-life resulting in longer duration of neuromuscular blockade with vecuronium.[80] An active metabolite, 3-desacetylvecuronium, can accumulate in patients with end-stage renal disease. Successive doses of vecuronium may result in prolonged duration of neuromuscular blockade in part due to accumulation of this active metabolite.[81]

Hemodialysis/Continuous Renal Replacement Therapy: No reports in regards to vecuronium and hemodialysis/CRRT were found.

Liver Dysfunction: Vecuronium bolus doses did not result in significantly different effects when administered to surgical patients with or without alcoholic liver disease.[82] Surgical patients with cirrhosis exhibited reduced drug clearance and prolonged neuromuscular blockade with vecuronium compared to patients without cirrhosis.[83]

Hypothermia: Decreased core temperature reduces plasma clearance of vecuronium resulting in a prolonged duration of action and prolonged time to recover.[40]

Safety Concerns

General safety concerns with the nondepolarizing neuromuscular blocking agents

Safety concern	Rationale	Comments/recommendations
Qualified personnel	Pharmacologic response to these drugs results in respiratory muscle paralysis	Prescribers of these agents must be qualified to manage ventilation/intubation

(continued)

Safety concern	Rationale	Comments/recommendations
Need for sedation and analgesia	None of these agents possess analgesic or anxiolytic properties	Administration of scheduled or continuous doses of opioids and benzodiazepines is necessary while neuromuscular blockade is utilized
Myasthenia gravis	Functional reduction in number of postsynaptic acetylcholine receptors[60]	Increased susceptibility to nondepolarizing neuromuscular blockers requiring a 50–75% reduction in dose[60]
Prolonged recovery and myopathy	Time necessary to recover 50–100% longer than expected; may be related to organ dysfunction for agents cleared renally or hepatically as well as drug-drug interactions[84]	Avoid indiscriminate use of neuromuscular blocking agents by maximizing use of sedatives and analgesics first. Try to avoid drug-drug interactions
		May need to choose alternative agents if organ dysfunction present
Acute quadriplegic myopathy syndrome	Involves acute paresis, myonecrosis and abnormal electromyography[84]	Consider screening patients with serial creatine phosphokinase measurements especially if patient receiving concurrent corticosteroid therapy. Consider drug holidays[84]
Drug interactions	Chronic phenytoin and carbamazepine therapy increases clearance of vecuronium and reduces patient sensitivity	Increased doses of vecuronium will be required in patients receiving phenytoin and carbamazepine[60]
	Inhalational anesthetics decrease time of openness of acetylcholine receptor[60]	Results in increased potency of agents and prolonged duration of blockade[60]
	Ketamine, meperidine, and propofol have potentiating effects[60]	Prolonged blockade at clinical concentrations possible[60]
	Aminoglycosides, tetracyclines, clindamycin all interfere with neuromuscular transmission	Neostigmine may be ineffective or only partially effective in reversing blockade[60]
	Aminophylline, theophylline	Antagonizes effect[84]
	Quinidine, procainamide, local anesthetics, calcium channel blockers	Prolongation of neuromuscular blockade[84]
	Magnesium	Dose dependent prolongation of neuromuscular blockade[60]
	Loop diuretics	Prolongs blockade at low doses and antagonizes blockade at high doses[84]

Safety concern	Rationale	Comments/recommendations
	Corticosteroids	Increases risk of steroid myopathy with both classes of neuromuscular blocking agents[84]
	Ranitidine	Antagonizes blockage[84]
	Lithium	Prolongation of blockade[84]
	Cyclosporine	Prolongation of blockade[60]
	Cyclophosphamide	Prolongation of blockade[68]
	Dantrolene	Prolongation of blockade[68]
Reversal	Mechanism of reversal agents is anticholinesterase activity	Initial doses of edrophonium 1,000 mcg/kg, pyridostigmine 300 mcg/kg, and neostigmine 60 mcg/kg may be administered and supplemental doses given as needed. Atropine and glycopyrrolate may be given adjunctively to prevent the cardiovascular effects of the reversal agents[85]

Safety concerns with specific nondepolarizing neuromuscular blocking agents

Safety concern	Rationale	Comments/recommendations
Vagolytic properties (specific to rocuronium)	Resultant tachycardia and hypertension possible at higher doses	Minimize doses of rocuronium to avoid this effect[60]
Laudanosine metabolite (specific to cisatracurium)	Since has three times the potency of atracurium, one-third of the laudanosine will be produced	Monitor for side effects of laudanosine (seizures) in patients on prolonged infusions of cisatracurium[60]

References

1. Lee WH, Kramer WG, Granville GE. The effect of obesity on acetaminophen pharmacokinetics in man. *J Clin Pharmacol*. 1981;21:284-287.
2. Kurella M, Bennett WM, Chertow GM. Analgesia in patients with ESRD: a review of available evidence. *Am J Kidney Dis*. 2003;42:217-228.
3. Murphy EJ. Acute pain management pharmacology for the patient with concurrent renal or hepatic disease. *Anaesth Intensive Care*. 2005;33:311-322.

4. Duggan ST, Scott LJ. Intravenous paracetamol (Acetaminophen). *Drugs.* 2009;69:101-113.
5. Martin U, Temple RM, Winney RJ, et al. The disposition of paracetamol and its conjugates during multiple dosing in patients with end-stage renal failure maintained on haemodialysis. *Eur J Clin Pharmacol.* 1993;45:141-145.
6. Ofirmev (acetaminophen) Injection Product Monograph. San Diego, CA: Cadence Pharmaceuticals, Inc. 2010 Nov. 8.
7. Polderman KH, Herold I. Therapeutic hypothermia and controlled normothermia in the intensive care unit: practical considerations, side effects, and cooling methods. *Crit Care Med.* 2009;37:1101-1120.
8. Lat I, Foster DR, Erstad B. Drug-induced acute liver failure and gastrointestinal complications. *Crit Care Med.* 2010;38:S175-S187.
9. de Maat MM, Tijssen TA, Brüggemann RJ, et al. Paracetamol for intravenous use in medium- and intensive care patients: pharmacokinetics and tolerance. *Eur J Clin Pharmacol.* 2010; 66:713-719.
10. Boyle M, Hundy S, Torda TA. Paracetamol administration is associated with hypotension in the critically ill. *Aust Crit Care.* 1997;10:120-122.
11. Köppel C, Arndt I, Ibe K. Effects of enzyme induction, renal and cardiac function on ketamine plasma kinetics in patients with ketamine long-term analgesosedation. *Eur J Drug Metab Pharmacokinet.* 1990;15:259-263.
12. Tsubo T, Sakai I, Okawa H, et al. Ketamine and midazolam kinetics during continuous hemodiafiltration in patients with multiple organ dysfunction syndrome. *Intensive Care Med.* 2001;27:1087-1090.
13. Panzer O, Moitra V, Sladen RN. Pharmacology of sedative-analgesic agents: dexmedetomidine, remifentanil, ketamine, volatile anesthetics, and the role of peripheral mu antagonists. *Crit Care Clin.* 2009;25:451-469.
14. Caldolor (Ibuprofen) Injection Product Monograph. Nashville, TN: Cumberland Pharmaceuticals Inc. 2009 June.
15. Antal EJ, Wright CE, Brown BL, et al. The influence of hemodialysis on the pharmacokinetics of ibuprofen and its major metabolites. *J Clin Pharmacol.* 1986;26:184-190.
16. Marret E, Flahault A, Samama C, et al. Effects of postoperative, nonsteroidal, antiinflammatory drugs on bleeding risk after tonsillectomy meta-analysis of randomized, controlled trials. *Anesthesiology.* 2003;98:1497-1502.
17. Strauss R, Wehler M, Mehler K, et al. Thrombocytopenia in patients in the medical intensive care unit: bleeding prevalence, transfusion requirements, and outcome. *Crit Care Med.* 2002;30:1765-1771.
18. Bentley ML, Corwin HL, Dasta JF. Drug-induced acute kidney injury in the critically ill adult: recognition and prevention strategies. *Crit Care Med.* 2010;38:S169-S174.
19. Whelton A. Nephrotoxicity of nonsteroidal anti-inflammatory drugs: physiologic foundations and clinical implications. *Am J Med.* 1999;106:13S-24S.
20. Swan SK, Rudy DW, Lasseter KC, et al. Effect of cyclooxygenase-2 inhibition on renal function in elderly persons receiving a low-salt diet. A randomized, controlled trial. *Ann Intern Med.* 2000;133:1-9.
21. Gerstenfeld LC, Einhorn TA. COX inhibitors and their effects on bone healing. *Expert Opin Drug Saf.* 2004;3:131-136.
22. Dodwell ER, Latorre JG, Parisini E, et al. NSAID exposure and risk of nonunion: a meta-analysis of case-control and cohort studies. *Calcif Tissue Int.* 2010;87(3):193-202.
23. Shibutani K, Inchiosa MA, Sawada K, et al. Pharmacokinetic mass of fentanyl for postoperative analgesia in lean and obese patients. *Br J Anaesth.* 2005;95:377-383.
24. Devlin JW, Roberts RJ. Pharmacology of commonly used analgesics and sedatives in the ICU: benzodiazepines, propofol, and opioids. *Crit Care Clin.* 2009;25:431-449.
25. Heiskanen T, Matzke S, Haakana S, et al. Transdermal fentanyl in cachectic cancer patients. *Pain.* 2009;144:218-222.
26. Dean M. Opioids in renal failure and dialysis patients. *J Pain Symptom Manage.* 2004;28: 497-504.

27. Joh J, Sila MK, Bastani B. Nondialyzability of fentanyl with high-efficiency and high-flux membranes. *Anesth Analg*. 1998;86:445-451.
28. Tortorici MA, Kochanek PM, Poloyac SM. Effects of hypothermia on drug disposition, metabolism, and response: a focus of hypothermia-mediated alterations on the cytochrome P450 enzyme system. *Crit Care Med*. 2007;35(9):2196-2204.
29. Lee MA, Leng MEF, Tiernan EJJ. Retrospective study of the use of hydromorphone in palliative care patients with normal and abnormal urea and creatinine. *Palliat Med*. 2001;15(1): 26-34. 27:4-419-4-421.
30. Davison SN, Mayo PR. Pain management in chronic kidney disease: the pharmacokinetics and pharmacodynamics of hydromorphone and hydromorphone-3-glucuronide in hemodialysis patients. *J Opioid Manag*. 2008;4(6):335-336. 339–44.
31. Micromedex® Healthcare Series [intranet database]. Version 5.1. Greenwood Village, Colo: Thomson Reuters (Healthcare) Inc.
32. Hassan H, Bastani B, Gellens M. Successful treatment of normeperidine neurotoxicity by hemodialysis. *Am J Kidney Dis*. 2000;35:146-149.
33. Linares CL, Decleves X, Oppert JM, et al. Pharmacology of morphine in obese patients clinical implications. *Clin Pharmacokinet*. 2009;48(10):635-651.
34. Choi YK, Brolin RE, Wagner BK, et al. Efficacy and safety of patient-controlled analgesia for morbidly obese patients following gastric bypass surgery. *Obes Surg*. 2000;10(2): 154-159.
35. Milne RW, Nation RL, Somogyi AA, et al. The influence of renal function on the renal clearance of morphine and its glucuronide metabolites in intensive-care patients. *Br J Clin Pharmacol*. 1992;34(1):53-59.
36. MacNab MS, Macrae DJ, Guy E, et al. Profound reduction in morphine clearance and liver blood flow in shock. *Intensive Care Med*. 1986;12:366-369.
37. Mazoit JX, Sandouk P, Zetlaoui P, et al. Pharmacokinetics of unchanged morphine in normal and cirrhotic subjects. *Anesth Analg*. 1987;66:293-298.
38. Roka A, Melinda KT, Vasarhelyi B, et al. Elevated morphine concentrations in neonates treated with morphine and prolonged hypothermia for hypoxic encephalopathy. *Pediatrics*. 2008; 121(4):e844-e849.
39. Puig MM, Warner W, Tang CK, et al. Effects of temperature on the interaction of morphine with opioid receptors. *Br J Anaesth*. 1987;59:1459-1464.
40. van den Broek MPH, Groenendaal F, Egberts ACG, et al. Effects of hypothermia on pharmacokinetics and pharmacodynamics a systematic review of preclinical and clinical studies. *Clin Pharmacokinet*. 2010;49:277-294.
41. Albertin A, La Colla G, La Colla L, et al. Effect site concentrations of remifentanil maintaining cardiovascular homeostasis in response to surgical stimuli during bispectral index guided propofol anesthesia in seriously obese patients. *Minerva Anestesiol*. 2006;72: 915-924.
42. Egan TD, Huizing B, Gupta SK, et al. Remifentanil pharmacokinetics in obese versus lean patients. *Anesthesiology*. 1998;89:562-573.
43. Pitsiu M, Wilmer A, Bodenham A, et al. Pharmacokinetics of remifentanil and its major metabolite, remifentanil acid, in ICU patients with renal impairment. *Br J Anaesth*. 2004; 92:493-503.
44. Dahaba AA, Oettl K, von Klobucar F, et al. End-stage renal failure reduces central clearance and prolongs the elimination half-life of remifentanil. *Can J Anaesth*. 2002;49: 369-374.
45. Dershwitz M, Hoke F, Rosow CE, et al. Pharmacokinetics and pharmacodynamics of remifentanil in volunteer subjects with severe liver disease. *Anesthesiology*. 1996;84: 812-820.
46. Russell D, Royston D, Rees PH, et al. Effect of temperature and cardiopulmonary bypass on the pharmacokinetics of remifentanil. *Br J Anaesth*. 1997;79:456-459.
47. Bowdle TA. Adverse effects of opioid agonists and agonist-antagonists in anaesthesia. *Drug Saf*. 1998;19:173-189.

48. Gaudreau JD, Gagnon P, Roy MA, et al. Opioid medications and longitudinal risk of delirium in hospitalized cancer patients. *Cancer.* 2007;109:2365-2373.
49. Viscusi ER, Gan TJ, Leslie JB, et al. Peripherally acting mu-opioid receptor antagonists and postoperative ileus: mechanisms of action and clinical applicability. *Anesth Analg.* 2009;108:1811-1822.
50. Somogyi AA, Barratt DT, Coller JK. Pharmacogenetics of opioids. *Clin Pharmacol Ther.* 2007;81:429-444.
51. Smith HS. Variations in opioid responsiveness. *Pain Physician.* 2008;11:237-248.
52. Darrouj J, Karma L, Arora R. Cardiovascular manifestations of sedatives and analgesics in the critical care unit. *Am J Ther.* 2009;16:339-353.
53. Roy S, Wang J, Kelshenbach J, et al. Modulation of immune function by morphine: implications for susceptibility to infection. *J Neuroimmune Pharmacol.* 2006;1:77-89.
54. Beilin B, Shavit Y, Hart J, et al. Effects of anesthesia based on large versus small doses of fentanyl on natural killer cell cytotoxicity in the perioperative period. *Anesth Analg.* 1996;82:492-497.
55. Wilhelm W, Kreuer S. The place for short-acting opioids: special emphasis on remifentanil. *Crit Care.* 2008;12(Suppl 3):S5.
56. Dahaba AA, Grabner T, Rehak PH, et al. Remifenatnil versus morphine analgesia and sedation for mechanically ventilated critically ill patients: a randomized double blind study. *Anesthesiology.* 2004;101:640-646.
57. D'Honeur GD, Gilton A, Sandouk P, et al. Plasma and cerebrospinal fluid concentrations of morphine and morphine glucuronides after oral morphine: the influence of renal failure. *Anesthesiology.* 1994;81:87-93.
58. Lemmens H, Brodsky J. The dose of succinylcholine in morbid obesity. *Anesth Analg.* 2006;102:438-442.
59. Cope T, Hunter J. Selecting neuromuscular-blocking drugs for elderly patients. *Drugs Aging.* 2003;20:125-140.
60. Booij L. Neuromuscular transmission and its pharmacological blockade Part 2: pharmacology of neuromuscular blocking agents. *Pharm World Sci.* 1997;19:13-34.
61. Merck Manual Professional. Succinylcholine monograph. http://www.merck.com/mmpe/print/lexicomp/succinylcholine.html. Accessed July 24, 2010.
62. Martyn J, Richtsfeld M. Succinylcholine-induced hyperkalemia in acquired pathologic states. *Anesthesiology.* 2006;104:158-169.
63. Orebaugh S. Succinylcholine: adverse effects and alternatives in emergency medicine. *Am J Emerg Med.* 1999;17:715-721.
64. Book W, Abel M, Eisenkraft J. Adverse effects of depolarizing neuromuscular blocking agents: incidence, prevention, and management. *Drug Saf.* 1994;10:331-349.
65. Leykin Y, Pellis T, Lucca M, et al. The effects of cisatracurium on morbidly obese women. *Anesth Analg.* 2004;99:1090-1094.
66. Adamus M, Gabrehelik T, Marek O. Influence of gender on the course of neuromuscular block following a single bolus dose of cisatracurium or rocuronium. *Eur J Anaesthesiol.* 2008;25:589-595.
67. Atherton D, Hunter J. Clinical pharmacokinetics of the newer neuromuscular blocking drugs. *Clin Pharmacokinet.* 1999;36:169-189.
68. Fassbender P, Geldner G, Blobner M, et al. Clinical predictors of duration of action of cisatracurium and rocuronium administered long-term. *Am J Crit Care.* 2009;18:439-445.
69. Mann R, Blibner M, Probst R, et al. Pharmacokinetics of rocuronium in obese and asthenic patients: reduced clearance in the obese. *Anesthesiology.* 1997;87:A85.
70. Puhringer F, Khuenl-Brady K, Mitterschiffhaler G. Rocuronium bromide: time-course of action in underweight, normal weight, overweight and obese patients. *Eur J Anaesthesiol Suppl.* 1995;11(Suppl 12):107-110.
71. Rocuronium package insert. Irvine, CA: Teva Parenteral Medicines, Inc; 2008 Nov.
72. Matteo R, Ornstein E, Schwartz A, et al. Pharmcokinetics and pharmacodynamics of rocuronium (Org 9426) in elderly surgical patients. *Anesth Analg.* 1993;77:1193-1197.

73. Robertson E, Driessen J, Booij H. Pharmacokinetics and pharmacodynamics of rocuronium in patients with and without renal failure. *Eur J Anaesthesiol*. 2005;22:4-10.
74. Staals L, Snoeck M, Driessen J, et al. Reduced clearance of rocuronium and sugammadex in patients with severe to end-stage renal failure: a pharmacokinetic study. *Br J Anaesth*. 2010;104: 31-39.
75. van Miert M, Eastwood N, Boyd A, et al. The pharmacokinetics and pharmacodynamics of rocuronium in patients with hepatic cirrhosis. *Br J Clin Pharmacol*. 1997;44:139-144.
76. Schwartz A, Matteo R, Ornstein E, et al. Pharmacokinetics and pharmacodynamics of vecuronium in the obese surgical patient. *Anesth Analg*. 1992;74:515-518.
77. Vecuronium package insert. Bedford, OH: Ben Venue Laboratories, Inc; 2007 June.
78. Caldwell J, Heier R, Wright P, et al. Temperature-dependent pharmacokinetics and pharmacodynamics of vecuronium. *Anesthesiology*. 2000;92:84-93.
79. Xue F, An G, Liao X, et al. The pharmacokinetics of vecuronium in male and female patients. *Anesth Analg*. 1998;86:1322-1327.
80. Lynam D, Cronnelly R, Castognoli K, et al. The pharmacodynamics and pharmacokinetics of vecuronium in patients anesthetized with isoflurane with normal renal function or renal failure. *Anesthesiology*. 1988;69:227-231.
81. Sakamota H, Takita K, Kemmotsu O, Morimoto Y, Mayumi T. Increased sensitivity to vecuronium and prolonged duration of its action in patients with end-stage renal failure. *J Clin Anesth*. 2001;13:193-197.
82. Arden J, Lynam D, Castagnoli K, et al. Vecuronium in alcoholic liver disease: a pharmacokinetic and pharmacodynamic analysis. *Anesthesiology*. 1988;68:771-776.
83. Lebrault C, Berger J, D'Hollander A, et al. Pharamacokinetics and pharmacodynamics of vecuronium (ORG NG 45) in patients with cirrhosis. *Anesthesiology*. 1985;62:601-605.
84. Murray M, Cowen J, DeBlock H, et al. Clinical practice guidelines for sustained neuromuscular blockade in the adult critically ill patient. *Crit Care Med*. 2002;30:142-156.
85. Booij L. Neuromuscular transmission and its pharmacological blockade Part 3: continuous infusion of relaxants and reversal and monitoring of relaxation. *Pharm World Sci*. 1997; 19:35-44.

Chapter 5
Hypertonic Saline, Electrolytes, and Insulin

Mitchell S. Buckley

Introduction

Hypertonic saline, insulin and electrolyte replacement are commonly used in the intensive care unit.[1-3] Hypertonic saline has several beneficial effects including volume-expanding properties, increased cardiac output, and intracranial pressure reduction.[4,5] The electrolytes play a pivotal role in maintaining several metabolic functions and processes.[1,6] Appropriate glucose management in the critically ill using insulin infusions has been associated with beneficial outcomes.[7-9]

Although these agents are cornerstone in the management of critically ill patients, each is associated with specific safety concerns.[3,10,11] The balance in maintaining targeted serum electrolyte as well as glucose concentrations involve complex homeostatic systems and are influenced by several factors including acid–base status, fluids, and organ function.[1,6] These factors can be further complicated in critically ill patients.[1] This chapter will discuss dosing considerations as well as safety issues for each of these therapies, including human factors affecting accurate drug delivery.

Hypertonic Saline (Sodium Chloride >0.9%)

Dosing Considerations

Obesity: There are no reports of dosing considerations in the obese patient population.

M.S. Buckley
Department of Pharmacy, Banner Good Samaritan Medical Center, Phoenix, AZ, USA
e-mail: mitchell.buckley@bannerhealth.com

S.L. Kane-Gill and J. Dasta (eds.),
High-Risk IV Medications in Special Patient Populations,
DOI: 10.1007/978-0-85729-606-1_5, © Springer-Verlag London Limited 2011

Thinness/emaciation: There are no reports of dosing considerations in underweight or nutritionally depleted patients.

Kidney Injury: Sodium is primarily excreted by the kidneys.[1] Although no published studies have evaluated appropriate dosing adjustments needed in patients with renal insufficiency, it is recommended to use hypertonic saline solutions with caution in this patient population.[12,13]

Hemodialysis/Continuous Renal Replacement Therapy: There are no published reports for patients receiving hemodialysis or continuous renal replacement therapy. Unfortunately, no dosing recommendations have been reported in renal replacement therapy. However, it may be appropriate to increase monitoring of sodium as well as chloride serum concentrations in these patients to avoid overcorrection or elevated concentrations. Overall, sodium removal in continuous renal replacement therapy is minimal. However, absolute impact on serum concentration is dependent upon several variables including the convection mode and dialysate sodium concentration.[14]

Liver Dysfunction: No published information is available regarding any considerations in liver dysfunction. However, it is recommended to use with caution in patients with liver cirrhosis.[12,13]

Hypothermia: No information is currently available.

Safety Concerns

Safety concern	Rationale	Comments/recommendations
Electrolyte & acid–base disturbances (Hypernatremia, Hypokalemia, Hyperchloremic acidemia)	Hypertonic saline administration is a potential source for the development of several electrolyte as well as acid–base disturbances as a result of an exogenous source of sodium chloride; volume expansion leading to hypokalemia[2,6,12,13]	Frequent monitoring serum sodium concentrations every 4–6 h for either bolus administration of hypertonic solutions or continuous infusions[5,6] Estimating water and sodium deficits when correcting severe hyponatremia may avoid overcorrection of serum sodium concentrations[6]
Pulmonary edema, congestive heart failure, respiratory failure	Rapid volume expansion can result from these solutions, which can either develop or exacerbate pre-existing conditions[4]	Caution should be used in patients with pre-existing cardiopulmonary conditions
Coagulopathy; Intracranial hematomas or effusions	Hypertonic saline may produce elevated activated prothrombin and partial thromboplastin times as well as platelet aggregation dysfunction[15]	Caution should be used when treating patients with active bleeding or coagulopathies
	Rapid volume expansion with hypertonic solutions may increase the rate of blood loss in patients with active bleeds or contribute to dilutional coagulopathy[4,5]	Recommended to monitor for signs and symptoms of bleeding. Consider monitoring coagulation studies and hemoglobin/hematocrit

Safety concern	Rationale	Comments/recommendations
Phlebitis	Peripheral administration of hypertonic saline may lead to irritation at the administration site[4]	Recommended to administer via central venous line to avoid complications
Renal dysfunction	Impaired renal function may develop as a result of hypernatremia or hyperosmolarity from hypertonic saline[11,14]	Caution should be used when administering in patients with pre-existing renal dysfunction
	Hypertonic saline-induced hypernatremia may lead to decreased renal function although this association is poorly understood[2]	Recommended to monitor renal function closely with those patients at risk for acute renal failure
Neurologic disturbances (central pontine myelinolysis, encephalopathy, seizures)	Rapid correction of hyponatremia with hypertonic saline may lead to neurologic injury. This condition could manifest within 1–6 days following rapid sodium serum increases[6]	The rate of correction within the first 24 h may be more predictive as a risk factor for demyelination than the maximum hourly rate of administration
	An increase in sodium serum concentrations by 35–40 mEq/L may induce myelinolysis[4]	Demyelination may be more common if the serum sodium concentration is increased >20 mEq/L within the first 24 h; less common if rate of increase is <10–12 mEq/L within 24 h.[15] Therefore, the maximum recommended increase in serum sodium concentrations is 8–12 mEq/L within the first 24 h with the goal of complete correction of sodium deficits over 2–4 days[6]
		Patients with severe or symptomatic hyponatremia should have serum sodium concentrations corrected at about 1–2 mEq/L every hour or 0.5 mEq/L every hour if the duration of hyponatremia is suspected of being a chronic condition[6]
		3% sodium chloride at a rate of 0.38 mL/kg/h would be expected to increase serum sodium concentrations by <0.5 mEq/L/h[11]
		Frequent serum sodium monitoring is recommended to avoid rapid sodium correction

(continued)

Safety concern	Rationale	Comments/recommendations
Rebound intracranial hypertension	May occur following rapid infusion withdrawal[4]	Caution should be used in patients with neurological or traumatic brain injury
		Gradual discontinuation or transition to isotonic solutions is recommended
Transient hypotension	May occur following rapid intravenous injections[4]	Caution should be used in hemodynamically unstable patients
		May require increased monitoring of intracranial pressure following bolus injections as transient lower blood pressures may affect intracranial pressures
Intravascular hemolysis	Hypertonic solutions may result in sudden fluctuations in the osmotic gradient leading to hemolysis[4]	Caution should be used in patients at risk for bleeding complications
		Recommended to administer hypertonic solutions as a slow infusion to avoid this potential complication[4]

Insulin (Short-, Intermediate-, and Long-Acting Agents)

Dosing Considerations

Obesity: There are no reports of dosing considerations in the obese patient population.

Thinness/emaciation: There are no reports of dosing considerations in underweight or nutritionally depleted patients.

Kidney Injury: Renal impairment may be associated with reduced insulin metabolism and/or elimination. Although no reports have evaluated specific insulin dosing regimens, dose reductions may be required in patients with renal dysfunction. However, suggested insulin dosing modifications may be based upon creatinine clearance (CrCl). About 75% of the estimated insulin dose requirements for patients with CrCl 10–50 mL/min and about 25–50% of the insulin dose for those with CrCl < 10 mL/min.[12,13,16]

Hemodialysis/Continuous Renal Replacement Therapy: Hemodialysis would not be expected to significantly remove insulin. Since hypoglycemia is frequent in hemodialysis, it may be reasonable to reduce the basal morning insulin by 50%.[17] However, dosing adjustments in dialysis patients may not be needed assuming appropriate dietary intake (glucose source) prior to dialysis.[12,13,17] In continuous renal replacement therapy, it is suggested to reduce the insulin dose by 25% in these patients.[12,13]

Liver Dysfunction: No published reports are available regarding any considerations in liver dysfunction. However, dose reductions may be required in patients with hepatic impairment.[12,13]

Hypothermia: No information is currently available.

Safety Concerns

Safety concern	Rationale	Comments/recommendations
Hypoglycemia	The most common adverse event often as a result of insufficient dietary modifications relative to timing of insulin administration as well as increase in activity level and acute illness[12,13,18]	Caution should be used in patients at risk for developing hypoglycemia (e.g., reduced oral dietary intake, emesis, NPO status, fluctuations in parenteral nutrition, and corticosteroid dose reductions)[18]
		The incidence of hypoglycemia associated with continuous insulin infusions have been reported as high as 19%.[19] Several major insulin infusion trials have shown an increased risk of hypoglycemia with strict glucose control compared to more liberal serum glucose ranges[7,8,19,20]
		Recommended to increase blood glucose monitoring
Drug interactions	Several medications may interfere with insulin's effects on blood glucose[13]	Increased insulin effects leading to hypoglycemia may be associated with the use of oral antihyperglycemics and quinolones, pramlintide, angiotensin converting enzyme inhibitors, disopyramide, fibrates, fluoxetine, monoamine oxidase inhibitors, propoxyphene, pentoxifylline, salicylates, somatostatin analogs, and sulfonamides[12,13]
		Recommended to increase blood glucose monitoring and adjust insulin requirements upon addition, removal as well as dose adjustment of these agents

(continued)

Safety concern	Rationale	Comments/recommendations
		Decreased insulin effects leading to hyperglycemia may be associated with the use of corticosteroids, thiazide diuretics, beta-adrenergic blocking agents, clonidine, corticosteroids, niacin, danazol, diuretics, sympathomimetic agents (e.g., epinephrine, albuterol, terbutaline), glucagon, isoniazid, phenothiazine derivatives, somatropin, thyroid hormones, estrogens, progestogens, protease inhibitors and atypical antipsychotic medications[12,13]
		Recommended to increase blood glucose monitoring and adjust insulin requirements upon addition, removal as well as dose adjustment of these agents
Cardiac dysfunction	Insulin administration may contribute to palpitations and tachycardia[13]	EKG monitoring and vital signs should be closely observed
		Caution should be exercised in patients with cardiac conditions
Hypokalemia	Insulin administration may lead to decreased serum potassium concentrations[12,13]	EKG monitoring and vital signs should be closely observed
		Potassium replacement should be administered prior to insulin use
		Caution should be used in patients at risk for hypokalemia

Magnesium Sulfate

Dosing Considerations

Obesity: There are no reports of dosing considerations in the obese patient population.

Thinness/emaciation: There are no reports of dosing considerations in underweight or nutritionally depleted patients.

Kidney Injury: About 75% of the magnesium is filtered through the kidneys, while most is reabsorbed.[21] Dose adjustments are recommended in patients with severe renal impairment (creatinine clearance <30 mL/min). The maximum dose should not exceed 10 g/24 h.[12,13]

Hemodialysis/Continuous Renal Replacement Therapy: There is no information available for patients receiving hemodialysis or continuous renal replacement therapy. It is recommended to increase monitoring serum magnesium serum concentrations and possibly reducing the dose.

Liver Dysfunction: No published information is available regarding any considerations in liver dysfunction. Furthermore, this patient population would not be expected to have any modifications in magnesium replacement therapy as the liver does not play a major role in homeostasis.

Hypothermia: No information is currently available.

Safety Concerns

Safety concern	Rationale	Comments/recommendations
Hypotension	Magnesium may cause an administration rate-related vasodilatory effect[12,13]	The recommended intravenous rate of administration should not exceed 2 g/h. However, 4 g/h may be considered in emergent clinical scenarios (e.g., seizures, eclampsia)[12,13]
		Caution should be used when administering to patients receiving vasodilatory agents
		Caution when administering to patients with labile blood pressure
		Caution when administering to hypovolemic patients
Neuromuscular dysfunction	Deep tendon reflexes decrease as magnesium serum levels exceed 4 mEq/L. Respiratory depression may occur as magnesium concentrations approach 10 mEq/L[12]	Recommended to increase monitoring for these signs and symptoms
Cardiac dysfunction	Hypermagnesemia may contribute to heart block, arrhythmias, including asystole[12]	EKG monitoring and vital signs should be closely observed
Central nervous system depression	Altered mental status may occur as a result of hypermagnesemia[12,13]	Recommended to increase monitoring for these signs and symptoms

(continued)

Safety concern	Rationale	Comments/recommendations
Drug-drug interactions	Significant drug-drug interactions are not well documented. However, several medications may exacerbate or contribute to the development of hypermagnesemia with magnesium replacement. These include lithium (toxicity), insulin, and the catecholamines[1] Lithium intoxication may interfere with magnesium renal excretion[22] Exogenous catecholamines (e.g., norepinephrine) and insulin therapy may contribute to hypermagnesemia as a result of causing transcellular shifts of magnesium into the extracellular space[23] Several medications may also contribute to hypomagnesemia including the aminoglycosides, cyclosporine, colony-stimulating factors, digoxin, and diuretics[1]	Caution should be used when replacing magnesium in patients with lithium intoxication Caution should be used when replacing magnesium in patients receiving vasopressors and aggressive insulin therapy (e.g., continuous insulin infusion)

Potassium Chloride

Dosing Considerations

Obesity: There are no reports of dosing considerations in the obese patient population.

Thinness/emaciation: There are no reports of dosing considerations in underweight or nutritionally depleted patients.

Kidney Injury: About 80% of potassium is filtered through the kidneys with over 90% reabsorbed within the renal tubules.[1] Dose adjustments are recommended for potassium supplementation in patients with renal impairment.[1-3] It is recommended to reduce the estimated replacement dose by 50% in this patient population to avoid hyperkalemia.[1-3]

Hemodialysis/Continuous Renal Replacement Therapy: There are no published reports for patients receiving hemodialysis or continuous renal replacement therapy since hypokalemia requiring potassium replacement is not common in this population. It is recommended to reduce the estimated replacement dose by 50% in this patient population to avoid electrolyte disturbances with potassium.[6,12,13] The potassium concentration used in the dialysate or replacement fluid should be considered when determining the potassium replacement dose.[6]

Liver Dysfunction: No published information is available regarding any considerations in liver dysfunction. Furthermore, this patient population would not be expected to have any modifications in potassium chloride as the liver does not play a major role in homeostasis.

Hypothermia: No information is currently available.

Safety Concerns

Safety concern	Rationale	Comments/recommendations
Cardiac arrhythmias	Arrhythmias, including asystole can develop due to hyperkalemia[6,12,13]	Caution should be used when replacing significant amounts of potassium chloride, especially in renal insufficiency
		EKG monitoring and vital signs should be closely observed
		Caution should be used in patients with acid–base disturbances
Neuromuscular dysfunction	Generalized weakness, paresthesias, and paralysis may result from hyperkalemia[6]	Caution should be used when replacing significant amounts of potassium chloride, especially in renal insufficiency
Administration infusion rates	Rapid infusions are associated with local pain and vein irritation[13]	Infusion pumps should be used in the administration of potassium chloride
		Recommended infusion rates should not exceed 10 mEq/h[13]
		Extreme caution should be used for higher than recommended infusion rates (20–40 mEq/h) for situations with significant potassium depletion. It is also recommended to have continuously EKG monitoring and central line administration[13]
Drug-drug interactions	Several medications may exacerbate or contribute to the development of hyperkalemia with potassium chloride replacement	Caution should be used in patients with potassium hyperalimentation
	Beta-adrenergic receptor blockers and digoxin can inhibit the Na+/K + ATPase pump possibly contributing to hyperkalemia[6]	

(continued)

Safety concern	Rationale	Comments/recommendations
	Angiotensin converting enzyme (ACE) and angiotensin receptor blockers (ARB) induce hyperkalemia by interfering with angiotensin I conversion to angiotensin II as well as inducing a state of hypoaldosteronism[1]	Caution should be used when administering concomitant medications identified as contributing to hyperkalemia such as beta-adrenergic receptor blockers, digoxin, ACE, ARBs, NSAIDs and potassium sparing diuretics
	Heparin and low molecular weight heparins can possibly decrease the affinity as well as the number of angiotension II receptors therefore reducing aldosterone synthesis contributing to hyperkalemia[1]	
	Nonsteroidal anti-inflammatory drugs and potassium-sparing diuretics can inhibit potassium excretion leading to hyperkalemia[6]	

Potassium Phosphate

Dosing Considerations

Obesity: There are no reports of dosing considerations in the obese patient population. However, it has been recommended adjusted body weight may be preferred in these patients when calculating the phosphorous replacement dose requirements to avoid.[6]

Thinness/emaciation: There are no reports of dosing considerations in underweight or nutritionally depleted patients.

Kidney Injury: About 80% of potassium is filtered through the kidneys with over 90% reabsorbed within the renal tubules.[6] Phosphorus is regulated primarily through the kidney.[24] Dose adjustments are recommended for potassium supplementation especially the phosphate salt preparation in patients with renal impairment.[12,13,24] It is recommended to reduce the estimated replacement dose by 50% in this patient population to avoid electrolyte disturbances with potassium and/or phosphorus.[6,12,13]

Hemodialysis/Continuous Renal Replacement Therapy: There are no published reports for patients receiving hemodialysis or continuous renal replacement therapy.

It is recommended to reduce the estimated replacement dose by 50% in this patient population to avoid electrolyte disturbances with potassium and/or phosphorus.[6,12,13] Patients receiving continuous renal replacement therapy may require standard replacement doses depending upon degree of hypophosphatemia. Also, the potassium and/or phosphorus concentrations used in the dialysate or replacement fluid should be considered when determining the potassium phosphate replacement dose.[6]

Liver Dysfunction: No published information is available regarding any considerations in liver dysfunction. Furthermore, this patient population would not be expected to have any modifications in potassium phosphate as the liver does not play a major role in homeostasis.

Hypothermia: No information is currently available.

Safety Concerns

Safety concern	Rationale	Comments/recommendations
Tetany	Hyperphosphatemia can contribute to hypocalcemia. These clinical manifestations are a result of calcium-phosphate precipitation[6,12,13]	Caution should be used when replacing significant amounts of potassium phosphate, especially in renal insufficiency
Cardiac arrhythmias	Arrhythmias, including asystole can develop due to hyperkalemia[6,12,13]	Caution should be used when replacing significant amounts of potassium phosphate, especially in renal insufficiency
		EKG monitoring and vital signs should be closely observed
		Caution should be used in patients with acid–base disturbances
Neuromuscular dysfunction	Generalized weakness, parathesias, and paralysis may result from hyperkalemia[6]	Caution should be used when replacing significant amounts of potassium phosphate, especially in renal insufficiency
Drug-drug interactions	Several medications may exacerbate or contribute to the development of hyperkalemia and hyperphosphatemia with potassium phosphate replacement	Caution should be used in patients with potassium or phosphorous hyperalimentation
	Beta-adrenergic receptor blockers and digoxin can inhibit the Na+/K + ATPase pump possibly contributing to hyperkalemia[6]	Caution should be used in patients receiving concomitant medications identified as contributing to hyperkalemia

(continued)

Safety concern	Rationale	Comments/recommendations
	ACE and ARBs induce hyperkalemia by interfering with angiotensin I conversion to angiotensin II as well as inducing a state of hypoaldosteronism[1]	Caution should be used in patients receiving concomitant medications containing phosphate including phosphate-containing enemas and laxatives; exogenous phosphate replacement therapies; parenteral nutrition; medications with phosphate salt formulations (oseltamivir phosphate, clindamycin phosphate, etc.) as well as medications with phosphate metabolites (fosphenytoin, fospropofol, etc.)
	Heparin and low molecular weight heparins can possibly decrease the affinity as well as the number of angiotension II receptors therefore reducing aldosterone synthesis contributing to hyperkalemia[1]	
	NSAIDs and potassium-sparing diuretics can inhibit potassium excretion leading to hyperkalemia[6]	

References

1. Buckley MS, LeBlanc JM, Cawley MJ. Electrolyte disturbances associated with commonly prescribed medications in the intensive care unit. *Crit Care Med.* 2010;38(6 Suppl): S253-S264.
2. Froelich M, Quanhong Ni, Wess C, Ougorets I, Härtl R. Continuous hypertonic saline therapy and the occurrence of complications in neurocritically ill patients. *Crit Care Med.* 2009;37(4):1433-1441.
3. Gunst J, Van den Berghe G. Blood glucose control in the intensive care unit: benefits and risks. *Semin Dial.* 2010;23:157-162.
4. Bhardwaj A, Ulatowski A. Hypertonic saline solutions in brain injury. *Curr Opin Crit Care.* 2004;10:126-131.
5. Strandvik GF. Hypertonic saline in critical care: a review of the literature and guidelines for use in hypotensive states and raised intracranial pressure. *Anaesthesia.* 2009;64:990-1003.
6. Kraft MD, Btaiche IF, Sacks GS, et al. Treatment of electrolyte disorders in adult patients in the intensive care unit. *Am J Health Syst Pharm.* 2005;62:1663-1682.
7. Van den Berghe G, Wouters P, Weekers F, et al. Intensive insulin therapy in critically ill patients. *N Engl J Med.* 2001;345:1359-1367.

8. NICE-SUGAR Study Investigators, Finfer S, Chittock DR, Su S, et al. Intensive versus conventional glucose control in critically ill patients. *N Engl J Med.* 2009;360:1283-1297.

9. Pittas AG, Siegel RD, Lau J. Insulin therapy and in-hospital mortality in critically ill patients: systematic review and meta-analysis of randomized controlled trials. *JPEN J Parenter Enteral Nutr.* 2006;30:164-172.

10. Lacherade JC, Jacqueminet S, Preiser JC. An overview of hypoglycemia in the critically ill. *J Diabetes Sci Technol.* 2009;3:1242-1249.

11. Hashim MK, Issa D, Ahmad Z, Cappuccio JD, Kouides RW, Sterns RH. Hypertonic saline for hyponatremia: risk of inadvertent overcorrection. *Clin J Am Soc Nephrol.* 2007;2:1110-1117.

12. Gahart BL, Nazareno AR. *Intravenous Medications: A Handbook for Nurses and Health Professionals.* 26th ed. St. Louis: Mosby; 2010.

13. Lacy CF, Armstrong LL, Goldman MP, Lance LL. *Drug Information Handbook: A Comprehensive Resource for All Clinicians and Healthcare Professionals.* 17th ed. Hudson: Lexi-comp; 2008.

14. Locatelli F, Pontoriero G, Di Filippo S. Electrolyte disorders and substitution fluid in continuous renal replacement therapy. *Kidney Int Suppl.* 1998;53:S151-S155.

15. Soupart A, Penninckx R, Stenuit A, Perier O, Decaux G. Treatment of chronic hyponatremia in rats by intravenous saline: comparison of rate versus magnitude of correction. *Kidney Int.* 1992;41:1662-1667.

16. Shrishrimal K, Hart P, Michota F. Managing diabetes in hemodialysis patients: observations and recommendations. *Cleve Clin J Med.* 2009;76:649-655.

17. Ahmed Z, Simon B, Choudhury D. Management of diabetes in patients with chronic kidney disease. *Postgrad Med.* 2009;121:52-60.

18. Clement S, Braithwaite SS, Magee MF, et al. Management of diabetes and hyperglycemia in hospitals. *Diabetes Care.* 2004;27:553-591.

19. Van den Berghe G, Wilmer A, Hermans G, et al. Intensive insulin therapy in the medical ICU. *N Engl J Med.* 2006;354:449-461.

20. Brunkhorst FM, Engel C, Bloos F, et al. Intensive insulin therapy and pentastarch resuscitation in severe sepsis. *N Engl J Med.* 2008;358:125-139.

21. Dube L, Granry JC. The therapeutic use of magnesium in anesthesiology, intensive care and emergency medicine: a review. *Can J Anaesth.* 2003;50:732-746.

22. Nanji AA. Drug-induced electrolyte disorders. *Drug Intell Clin Pharm.* 1983;17:175-185.

23. Dacey MJ. Hypomagnesemic disorders. *Crit Care Clin.* 2001;17:155-173.

24. Stoff JS. Phosphate homeostasis and hypophosphatemia. *Am J Med.* 1982;72:489-495.

Chapter 6
Anti-Infectives

Zachariah Thomas and Dorothy McCoy

Introduction

Anti-infectives have been credited with much of the improvement seen in the mortality rates due to infectious diseases over the last 100 years. Anti-infectives include antibiotics, antifungals, antivirals, and immunomodulating therapies such as drotrecogin alpha (activated). Although the benefits of most anti-infectives have been clearly established, certain agents have significant toxicities associated with their use. The risk of toxicity is likely higher in critically ill patients. An in-depth knowledge of the safety profile of these anti-infectives can help the clinician better balance the risks and benefits of treatment. In some cases, the risk may be alleviated by dose adjusting for renal or liver dysfunction or in anticipation of a drug–drug interaction. Measures such as providing adjunctive medications before, during, or after each dose may also be necessary to decrease the risk associated with a particular antimicrobial agent. The focus of this chapter is to review high-risk intravenous anti-infectives; however, we also discuss the oral anti-infectives flucytosine and voriconazole due to the difficulties in dosing these medications in the critically ill.

D. McCoy (✉)
Department of Pharmacy Practice and Administration,
Ernest Mario School of Pharmacy, Piscataway, NJ, USA
e-mail: dmccoy@humed.com

S.L. Kane-Gill and J. Dasta (eds.),
High-Risk IV Medications in Special Patient Populations,
DOI: 10.1007/978-0-85729-606-1_6, © Springer-Verlag London Limited 2011

Acyclovir-Intravenous (IV)

Dosing Considerations

Obesity: The reports of acyclovir use in obese patients are limited. There is one case report in a male patient weighing 108.9 kg (ideal body weight 66.1 kg). The patient was given acyclovir 1 g IV every 8 h (approximately 10 mg/kg/dose based on his actual body weight). On day 3 of his acyclovir therapy he developed reversible acute renal failure.[1] The case scored a 7 on the Naranjo adverse drug reaction scale, which is suggestive of acyclovir being the cause of the acute renal failure.[1,2] In another study, acyclovir pharmacokinetics were evaluated in seven obese and five normal weight females. The females were all given one dose of acyclovir 5 mg/kg IV based on total body weight. The obese females had similar half-lives, volumes of distribution, and clearances to the normal weight females; however, the maximum concentration (C_{max}) and concentration 12 h after the dose were doubled in the obese females. Based on these findings the authors concluded that acyclovir should be dosed based on ideal body weight in obese patients.[3] Further, the prescribing information recommends dosing IV acyclovir in obese patients based on ideal body weight.[4]

Thinness/emaciation: There are no reports of dosing considerations in underweight or nutritionally depleted patients.

Kidney Injury: The major route of elimination of acyclovir is renal excretion, via glomerular filtration and tubular secretion, of unchanged drug.[4,5] The dose used is based on the indication (Table 6.1) and dose adjustment is necessary in patients with renal dysfunction (Table 6.2)[4,5] The clinician must calculate the patient's creatinine clearance (CrCl) in <u>mL/min/1.73 m^2</u> before initiating therapy in order to choose the appropriate dose for renal dysfunction (Table 6.2).[4,5] Doses should be calculated using the patient's actual body weight, but ideal body weight is recommended for obese patients.[4]

Table 6.1 Dosing of IV acyclovir based on indication[4]

Indication	Dose[a]
• Mucosal and cutaneous herpes simplex virus in immunocompromised patients	5 mg/kg every 8 h
• Severe initial episodes of herpes genitalis	
• Herpes simplex virus encephalitis	10 mg/kg every 8 h
• Varicella zoster virus in immunocompromised patients	

[a]Maximum dose is 20 mg/kg/dose every 8 h[4]

Table 6.2 IV acyclovir dose adjustments for renal dysfunction[4,5]

CrCl (mL/min/1.73 m^2)	% of recommended dose	Dosing interval
>50	100	Every 8 h
25–50	100	Every 12 h
10–25	100	Every 24 h
0–10	50	Every 24 h

Hemodialysis/Continuous Renal Replacement Therapy (CRRT): About 60% of the acyclovir dose is removed by hemodialysis.[4,6] It is recommended to administer the patient's acyclovir dose after hemodialysis.[4,5,7]

Intravenous acyclovir has been used in patients on peritoneal dialysis. In one case report a patient on continuous ambulatory peritoneal dialysis (CAPD) received acyclovir 200 mg IV daily. The authors found that only 7.3% of the acyclovir was recovered in the dialysate, which lead them to conclude that peritoneal dialysis is not as efficient as hemodialysis in removing acyclovir.[8] A dose of acyclovir 2.5 mg/kg/day IV was recommended in another case series based on pharmacokinetic data from six patients on CAPD.[9] In another case report, a patient on CAPD received acyclovir 1000 mg orally (for an unspecified time) for cutaneous herpes zoster infection. The patient was then switched to acyclovir 10 mg/kg (750 mg) IV daily when herpes zoster encephalitis was suspected due to the patient's worsening neurologic status. The acyclovir serum concentration on day 8 of therapy (details regarding time drawn in relation to dose unavailable) was 11 mg/L. The authors suspected that the patient's neurologic symptoms may have been prolonged by acyclovir-induced neurotoxicity.[10] For patients on peritoneal dialysis, no supplemental dose is necessary after adjustment of the dose and dosing interval.[4]

There are limited data regarding the pharmacokinetics of acyclovir during CRRT. One study evaluated the pharmacokinetics in three patients undergoing continuous venovenous hemodialysis (CVVHD). One patient received acyclovir 5 mg/kg IV every 24 h and two patients received 10 mg/kg IV every 48 h. The steady-state peak and trough concentrations were similar to those reported for patients with normal renal function; however, the half-life was approximately 10 h (half of the reported half-life in anuric patients).[4,11] Another study found that the percent of acyclovir removed during 24 h of CVVHD or continuous veno-venous hemodiafiltration (CVVHDF) was 18–65% of the administered dose.[12]

Liver Dysfunction: The pharmacokinetics of acyclovir in patients with hepatic impairment has not been investigated.

Hypothermia: The pharmacokinetics of acyclovir in hypothermia has not been investigated.

Other: Not applicable.

Safety Concerns

Safety concern	Rationale	Comments/recommendations
Nephrotoxicity	Renal tubular damage from precipitation of acyclovir crystals[4]	Adequately hydrate patients before administration and monitor serum creatinine (SCr) and CrCl[4]
Neurotoxicity	Encephalopathic changes such as lethargy, obtundation, tremors, confusion, hallucinations, agitation, seizures, or coma have occurred in about 1% of patients[4,5]	Use caution in patients with underlying neurologic abnormalities, including hepatic encephalopathy, and with serious renal or electrolyte abnormalities or significant hypoxia[4,5]

(continued)

Safety concern	Rationale	Comments/recommendations
Hematologic abnormalities	Thrombotic thrombocytopenic purpura/hemolytic uremic syndrome, anemia, neutropenia, thrombocytopenia have been rarely reported[4,5]	Monitor complete blood cell count and renal function[4]
Drug–drug interactions	Probenecid	Increased acyclovir half-life and area under the concentration-time curve (AUC) by 18% and 40% respectively, and decreased acyclovir urinary excretion and renal clearance by 13% and 32%, respectively[4,5]
General issues		Must be given over 1 h to reduce the risk of renal tubular damage[4]
		Maximum infusion concentration is 7 mg/mL. Infusion concentrations >7 mg/mL may produce phlebitis or inflammation at the injection site[4]
		Cerebrospinal fluid concentrations are approximately 50% of the serum concentrations[4]

Aminoglycosides (Amikacin, Gentamicin, Tobramycin)

Dosing Considerations

Obesity: Although the volume of distribution (Vd) of aminoglycosides increases with body weight, dosing based on total body weight will result in elevated serum concentrations. Rather, a dosing weight (DW) should be determined that accounts for the patient's ideal body weight plus a fraction of their excess body weight (total body weight minus ideal body weight). Various correction factors ranging from 20% to 40% of excess body have been used.[13] The following formula represents the most commonly employed DW and should be used for empiric dosing in obese individuals, i.e., those whose actual body weight exceeds their ideal body weight by more than 20%: DW = ideal body weight + 0.4 (total body weight − ideal body weight).[14] When using extended interval dosing, use of a dosing weight may result in a very large (>1000 mg) dose of tobramycin/gentamicin for extremely obese individuals. Limited experience exists with doses of tobramycin/gentamicin greater than 1000 mg daily[15] and some experts recommended a maximum dose of 1000 mg for single doses of tobramycin/gentamicin.[14] Serum drug concentration monitoring should be considered when such large doses are used.

Thinness/emaciation: Actual body weight is often used in clinical practice when dosing aminoglycosides in underweight patients, however, Traynor et al. determined that dosing based on actual body weight slightly underestimates aminoglycoside requirements in these patients.[16] The authors recommended the following equation to determine DW in underweight patients: DW = Total body weight (1.13).

Kidney Injury: Aminoglycosides are eliminated primarily through glomerular filtration and thus dose reductions are needed in the setting of kidney injury/renal insufficiency. Dosing tools such as the Sarubbi-Hull method[17] or the Hartford nomogram[15] can be used to estimate aminoglycoside requirements in patients with renal insufficiency. The Hartford nomogram should not be used if the estimated CrCl is less than 20 mL/min.[15] The Sarubbi-Hull method suggests an initial loading dose of 1–2 mg/kg of gentamicin/tobramycin and a 5–7.5 mg/kg loading dose of amikacin.[17] Subsequent doses are given as percentage of the initial dose and are adjusted for CrCl and the desired dosing interval. The Sarubbi-Hull nomogram can be viewed at the following website: http://www.rxkinetics.com/glossary/sarrubi.html (accessed November 17, 2010). Dosing tools such as these are useful for the initiation of aminoglycoside therapy, but serum concentration monitoring and subsequent dosage adjustments are needed to ensure therapeutic concentrations and avoid toxicity, particularly in the critically ill.[18,19]

Hemodialysis/Continuous Renal Replacement Therapy: It is common practice to administer a low dose of aminoglycoside, approximately 50% of the standard dose, immediately after dialysis.[20-22] Recent data challenge this paradigm. Assuming similar mg/kg dosing, predialysis dosing or intradialytic dosing results in similar peak concentrations compared to traditional postdialysis dosing. However, a theoretical benefit of this approach is that subsequent predialysis concentrations will be significantly lower with predialysis/intradialytic dosing (Fig. 6.1).[23] The prolonged elevated concentrations that result from traditional postdialysis dosing may increase the potential of aminoglycoside toxicity.[21] Emerging data also suggest that the rapid and efficient removal of aminoglycosides via high flux dialysis membranes may allow for higher doses to be given predialysis, while still ensuring acceptable subsequent predialysis concentrations. Higher doses (~2.5–3 mg/kg) are more likely to achieve the necessary C_{max} to minimum inhibitory concentration (MIC) ratio necessary to ensure optimal efficacy.[21,24] Although additional data are needed for more definitive recommendations, predialysis dosing of aminoglycosides in hemodialysis seem likely to maximize efficacy and safety compared to postdialysis dosing.

Many different recommendations exist for gentamicin and tobramycin dosing in CRRT. A recent review recommends a loading dose of 2–3 mg/kg and maintenance doses of 1.0–2.5 mg/kg when serum concentrations fall below 3–5 mcg/mL.[7] The recommended amikacin dose in CRRT is 7.5 mg/kg every 24–48 h.[7]

Liver Dysfunction: The Vd of aminoglycosides is increased in patients with ascites. Higher doses are thus likely needed in order to achieve optimal drug concentrations.[25] However, the need for higher doses must be balanced against the risks of nephrotoxicity. Several studies have documented that cirrhotic patients tend to be at

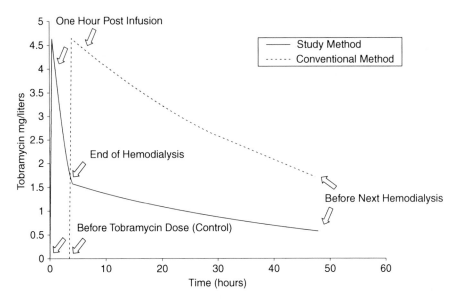

Fig. 6.1 The study method refers to administering tobramycin 1.5 mg/kg during the first 30 min of dialysis. The ensuing dialysis session results in a rapid decrease in tobramycin concentrations and a lower concentration before the next dialysis session, compared to the conventional method (postdialysis dosing) (Adapted with permission from Kamel Mohamed et al.[23])

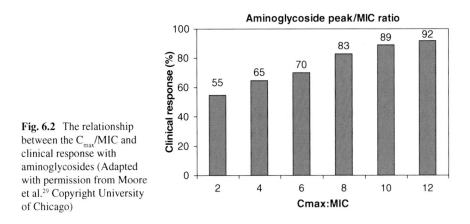

Fig. 6.2 The relationship between the C_{max}/MIC and clinical response with aminoglycosides (Adapted with permission from Moore et al.[29] Copyright University of Chicago)

high risk for aminoglycoside associated renal dysfunction.[26,27] If aminoglycoside therapy is warranted, serum drug concentrations should be monitored, and therapy limited to the shortest duration possible. Extended interval dosing has not been studied in these patients and thus should be avoided.

Hypothermia: Only one study has evaluated the impact of induced hypothermia on the pharmacokinetics of aminoglycosides.[28] The Vd and half-life of tobramycin were determined in three patients receiving induced hypothermia for the management of elevated intracranial pressures. In all three patients, the Vd and half-life were increased compared to predicted values based on population pharmacokinetic parameters. These data suggest that population pharmacokinetic parameters may be inaccurate during induced hypothermia and that serum monitoring should be considered.

Safety Concerns

Safety concern	Rationale	Comments/recommendation
De facto resistance	A C_{max}/MIC ratio of 8–10 has been correlated with aminoglycoside efficacy (Fig. 6.2).[29] Current Clinical and Laboratory Standards Institute guidelines state that organisms with gentamicin/ tobramycin MIC ≤4 mcg/mL are considered sensitive, however, it is unlikely that the necessary C_{max}/ MIC can be achieved when the MIC is >2 mcg/mL[30]	Conventional dosing of aminoglycosides (1–1.5 mg/kg q 8 h) is unlikely to achieve the necessary pharmacodynamic endpoints necessary to ensure efficacy.[15] Administering a relatively large dose (7 mg/kg) of gentamicin/tobramycin once daily results in peak concentrations of approximately 2 mcg/mL.[15] This would be sufficient to treat most organisms with an MIC of 2 mcg/mL. However, if the MIC were 4 mcg/mL, a 7 mg/kg dose would result in C_{max}/MIC ratio of only 5. Theoretically, a larger dose may be able to achieve the appropriate pharmacodynamic endpoints, but the safety of such large doses has not been established. Gentamicin/tobramycin should be avoided if the MIC is greater than 2 mcg/mL[30]
		Similarly, a 15 mg/kg dose of amikacin will result in peak concentrations of approximately 40 mcg/mL and a C_{max}/MIC ratio of 10 if the MIC is 4 mcg/mL.[15] A recent report suggests that an amikacin loading dose of 25 mg/kg can achieve peak concentrations of approximately 90 mcg/mL.[31] Limited experience exits with this higher dosing regimen and thus caution is advised before adapting this method into clinical practice. If using a standard dose of amikacin (15 mg/kg) the MIC should be 4 mcg/mL or less
Use in intraab-dominal infection	Aminoglycosides are associated with higher failures rates in intraabdominal infections.[32] This may be related to decreased activity of aminogly-cosides in settings of decreased pH[33]	Two meta-analyses have suggested that aminoglycosides are less likely to achieve clinical success compared to other standard agents in intra-abdominal infection.[32,34] Although the reasons for this finding are likely multifactorial, amino-glycosides should not be used preferen-tially in the treatment of intra-abdominal infections[32]

(continued)

Safety concern	Rationale	Comments/recommendation
Nephrotoxicity	Aminoglycoside nephrotoxicity is caused by uptake by proximal renal tubular epithelial cells. Tubular necrosis is the primary cause of nephrotoxicity[35]	Nephrotoxicity typically presents after several days of treatment and is usually non-oliguric.[35] The presence of increased urinary casts may be a harbinger of nephrotoxicity[36]
		Concurrent treatment with vancomycin may increase the likelihood of nephrotoxicity.[37] Other risk factors include age, pre-existing renal dysfunction, volume depletion, elevated trough concentrations, and use of concurrent nephrotoxic agents[36]
		Aminoglycoside-associated nephrotoxicity may even occur at low doses, i.e., 1 mg/kg every 8 h of gentamicin.[38] Since uptake of aminoglycoside is a saturable process, single large daily doses of aminoglycosides may be less nephrotoxic than multiple daily doses[39-41]
Ototoxicity	The ototoxicity of aminoglycosides is in part related to disruption of mitochondrial protein synthesis and the formation of free radicals. Aminoglycoside therapy can result in destruction of the cochlear hair cell[42]	The reported incidence of aminoglycoside related ototoxicity varies widely in the literature and is dependent upon the definition of ototoxicity used. An older study describing the use of aminoglycoside therapy for pseudomonal endocarditis reported a 43% incidence of ototoxicity[43]
		Animal experiments have demonstrated reduced nephrotoxicity with once daily dosing,[44,45] however, most clinical reports show similar rates of ototoxicity between single and multiple daily doses of aminoglycosides[46-48]
		Despite the risk of ototoxicity, in clinical practice most clinicians do not obtain audiograms during aminoglycoside therapy.[49] Audiometry testing has not been shown to benefit patients receiving aminoglycoside therapy and thus is not routinely recommended[49]
		Limited data suggests that antioxidants such as aspirin and N-acetylcysteine may have a role in mitigating aminoglycoside associated ototoxicity, but additional research is needed before these agents can be routinely recommended[50,51]

Safety concern	Rationale	Comments/recommendation
Once daily nomograms/ extended- interval dosing	Critically ill patients may require dose individu- alization to maximize efficacy and safety	In general, extended-interval nomograms, such as the Hartford nomogram, perform very well. However, limited data about the safety and efficacy of extended-interval dosing exists in the critically ill.[39] While the findings of Finnel et al.[52] suggest that nomogram-based daily dosing is effective, others have shown that nomograms perform poorly in the critically ill.[53-55] Dose individualization based on two serum drug concentrations may help improve the safety and efficacy of extended-interval aminoglycoside dosing in the critically ill[19]
General issues	Numerous factors may impact the pharma- cokinetics and pharmacodynamics of aminoglycosides. Individuals with specialized training may be better suited to manage these high-risk medications	Although aminoglycosides have been used for over 5 decades, there is still much uncertainty regarding dosing. A large database analysis found that institutions in which pharmacists were primarily responsible for aminoglycoside therapy had significantly lower rates of nephrotox- icity, ototoxicity, and even death.[56] Thus, consultation with a clinical pharmacist is encouraged when aminoglycosides are administered in critically ill

Amphotericin B

Dosing Considerations

Amphotericin B Products and Dosing

Product	Conventional (Fungizone®)	Cholesteryl sulfate complex (Amphotec®)	Lipid complex (Abelcet®)	Liposomal (AmBisome®)
Standard dosing	0.25–1 mg/kg IV every 24 h[57]	3–4 mg/kg IV every 24 h[58]	5 mg/kg IV every 24 h[59]	3–6 mg/kg IV every 24 h[60]
Dosing in obesity	No data	No data	No data	No data
Dosing in thin/ emaciated patients	No data	No data	No data	No data
Dosing in kidney injury	No dose adjustment required[61]	No data	No data	No data

(continued)

Product	Conventional (Fungizone®)	Cholesteryl sulfate complex (Amphotec®)	Lipid complex (Abelcet®)	Liposomal (AmBisome®)
Dosing in hemodialysis	Not dialyzable[62]	No data	No data	Not dialyzable[63]
Dosing in peritoneal dialysis	• 13 patients with CAPD and starting dose of 0.1 mg/kg/day and gradually increased to 0.75–1 mg/kg/day[64] • Not dialyzable[65]	No data	No data	No data
Dosing in CRRT	No dose adjustment required in continuous veno-venous hemofiltration (CVVHF)[66]	No dose adjustment required in CVVHF[66]	No data	No dose adjustment required in CVVHF[66,67]
Dosing in liver dysfunction	No data	No data	No data	No data
Dosing in hypothermia	No data	No data	No data	No data

Safety Concerns

Amphotericin B Products and Safety Concerns

Product	Conventional (Fungizone®)	Cholesteryl sulfate complex (Amphotec®)	Lipid complex (Abelcet®)	Liposomal (AmBisome®)
Infusion related toxicities (fever, chills, rigors, myalgias, nausea, headaches)	• Tolerance develops after 1–2 doses[57-59] • Liposomal formulation had decreased incidence of fevers, chills/rigors compared to conventional and lipid complex[60]			
Management/prevention of infusion related toxicities	• May slow down the rate of infusion for subsequent doses[68] • May pre-medicate with acetaminophen, aspirin, or a non-steroidal anti-inflammatory drug (NSAID) and diphenhydramine 30–60 min before subsequent doses[57,68,69] • Meperidine may be used to treat rigors and fever[57,68,69]			
Nephrotoxicity	• Cholesteryl sulfate had a lower incidence compared to conventional formulation[58] • Lipid complex had a lower incidence compared to conventional formulation[58,59] • Liposomal formulation had a lower incidence compared to conventional formulation and lipid complex[60]			

Product	Conventional (Fungizone®)	Cholesteryl sulfate complex (Amphotec®)	Lipid complex (Abelcet®)	Liposomal (AmBisome®)
Management/ prevention of nephrotoxicity	• May administer 0.5–1 L normal saline 30–60 min before and/or after each dose • Monitor SCr and blood urea nitrogen (BUN) closely[57,69,70]			
Electrolyte disturbances	• Hypernatremia, hypocalcemia, hypokalemia, hypomagnesemia • Monitor electrolytes closely[57-60]			
Cardiorespiratory (hypertension, hypotension, tachycardia, hypoxia)	• Liposomal formulation caused less hypertension, hypotension, tachycardia, and hypoxia compared to conventional formulation or lipid complex[60]			
Anaphylaxis (rare)	• If an anaphylactic reaction occurs, stop the infusion and treat accordingly • Do not rechallenge[57-60]			
Drug–drug interactions	• Antineoplastics may increase the risk for renal toxicity, bronchospasm, and hypotension • Corticosteroids and digoxin may increase the risk of hypokalemia • Concurrent use with flucyotosine may increase the risk of flucytosine toxicity • Potential for decreased efficacy or antagonism when combined with azoles • Use with other nephrotoxic agents may increase the risk for nephrotoxicity • Hypokalemia induced by amphotericin B may increase the risk of curariform effect of skeletal muscle relaxants[57-60]			
Additional drug–drug interactions	Concurrent use with leukocyte transfusions may increase the risk of acute pulmonary toxicity[57]	No additional drug–drug interactions reported[58]	Concurrent use with leukocyte transfusions may increase the risk of acute pulmonary toxicity Concurrent use with zidovudine may increase the risk of nephrotoxicity or myelotoxicity[59]	Concurrent use with leukocyte transfusions may increase the risk of acute pulmonary toxicity[60]

(continued)

Product	Conventional (Fungizone®)	Cholesteryl sulfate complex (Amphotec®)	Lipid complex (Abelcet®)	Liposomal (AmBisome®)
General issues: Administration	IV line must be flushed with 5% Dextrose Injection before and after each infusion	IV line must be flushed with 5% Dextrose Injection before and after each infusion	IV line must be flushed with 5% Dextrose Injection before and after each infusion	IV line must be flushed with 5% Dextrose Injection before and after each infusion
	An in-line membrane filter may be used for IV infusion with a mean pore diameter not less than 1 μm	Do not use an in-line filter	Do not use an in-line filter	An in-line membrane filter may be used for IV infusion with a mean pore diameter not less than 1 μm
	Administer as an IV infusion over 2–6 h, depending on the dose[57]	Administer as an IV infusion at a rate of 1 mg/kg/h	Administer as an IV infusion at a rate of 2.5 mg/kg/h	Administer as an IV infusion over 2 h
		Infusion time may be decreased to a minimum of 2 h in patients whom infusion is well-tolerated[58]	If the infusion time exceeds 2 h, mix the contents of the infusion bag every 2 h[59]	Infusion time may be decreased to 1 h in patients whom infusion is well-tolerated[60]
General issues: Reconstitution	Reconstitute with sterile water for injection and further dilute with 5% dextrose injection, with a pH above 4.2[57]	Do not filter	Does not have to be reconstituted	Reconstitute with sterile water for injection and further dilute with 5% dextrose injection[60]
		Reconstitute with sterile water for injection and further dilute with 5% dextrose injection[58]	Dilute with 5% dextrose injection[59]	
General issues: Compatibility	Do not mix with saline or other drugs due to risk of precipitation[57-60]			

Anidulafungin

Dosing Considerations

Obesity: There are no reports of anidulafungin use in obese patients.

Thinness/emaciation: There are no reports of dosing considerations in underweight or nutritionally depleted patients.

Kidney Injury: Dose adjustments for renal dysfunction are not required for anidulafungin.[71,72]

Hemodialysis/CRRT: Dose adjustments for hemodialysis or CRRT are not required for anidulafungin. It is not dialyzable.[71,72]

Liver Dysfunction: Dose adjustments for hepatic dysfunction are not required for anidulafungin.[71,72]

Hypothermia: The pharmacokinetics of anidulafungin in hypothermia has not been investigated.

Other: Anidulafungin undergoes slow chemical degradation at physiologic temperature and pH to a ring-opened peptide that does not have antifungal activity. It is eliminated in the feces. Dosing regimens are based on indication (Table 6.3).[71]

Table 6.3 Dose recommendations for anidulafungin per indication[71]

Indication	Dose of anidulafungin
Candidemia and other forms of *Candida* infections (intra-abdominal abscess, peritonitis)	200 mg loading dose on day 1, followed by 100 mg maintenance dose once daily thereafter
Esophageal candidiasis	100 mg loading dose on day 1, followed by 50 mg maintenance dose once daily thereafter

Safety Concerns

Safety concern	Rationale	Comments/recommendations
Preparation	Reconstitution with dehydrated alcohol[73,74]	When reconstituted with dehydrated alcohol, there is a concern in patients who are susceptible to disulfiram reactions (i.e. concurrent metronidazole use) or for recovering alcoholics.[73] However, the most recent prescribing information has instructions for reconstitution with sterile water for injection[71]

(continued)

Safety concern	Rationale	Comments/recommendations
Hepatic effects	Anidulafungin may cause abnormalities in liver function tests and clinically significant hepatic dysfunction, hepatitis, or hepatic failure[71]	Monitor liver function tests closely[71]
Histamine-mediated reactions	Rash, facial swelling, pruritus, sensation of warmth, and/ or bronchospasm[71,73,75]	Do not exceed infusion rates of 1.1 mg/min[71,73,75] Consider slowing the rate of the infusion or premedicating with an antihistamine[74]
Drug–drug interactions	There are no clinically significant drug interactions with anidulafungin[71,72]	
Practical issues	Rate of infusion should not exceed 1.1 mg/min (equivalent to 1.4 mL/min or 84 mL/h when reconstituted and diluted)[71,74]	Do not mix or co-infuse anidulafungin with other medications[71]

Caspofungin

Dosing Considerations

Obesity: There are no reports of caspofungin use in obese patients. However, there are discrepancies regarding dosing based on weight between the prescribing information in the United States compared to other countries.[76] For example, the prescribing information for the United Kingdom states that for patients >80 kg, the recommended dosing regimen is a 70 mg loading dose on day 1, followed by a 70 mg maintenance dose once daily. This was based on data that showed that in patients >80 kg the average exposure of caspofungin was 23% lower compared to patients weighing 60 kg.[77] Another study, which included patients weighing between 47 and 108 kg and a median of 75 kg, found similar results. Trough concentrations of caspofungin were below 1 mcg/mL (suggested target concentration for candidal infections) in 17 patients, ten of which were >75 kg. When the weight was >75 kg, the caspofungin trough concentration was decreased by 0.58 mcg/mL compared to patients who weighed less than <75 kg.[78]

Thinness/emaciation: There are no reports of dosing considerations in underweight or nutritionally depleted patients.

Kidney Injury: Dose adjustments for renal dysfunction are not required for caspofungin.[76]

Hemodialysis/CRRT: Dose adjustments for hemodialysis and CRRT are not required for caspofungin. It is not dialyzable.[76]

Liver Dysfunction: Caspofungin is metabolized by arylsulfatase and catechol-O-methyltransferase and excreted through bile. No dose adjustment is needed for mild hepatic impairment. For Child-Pugh scores of 7–9 (moderate hepatic insufficiency), the maintenance dose of caspofungin should be decreased to 35 mg once daily (Table 6.4). There are no data in patients with severe liver dysfunction (Child-Pugh score > 9).[76]

Hypothermia: The pharmacokinetics of caspofungin in hypothermia has not been investigated.

Other: Caspofungin concentrations may be influenced by albumin concentrations. In one study, hypoalbuminemia was associated with higher caspofungin concentrations (increased by 0.24 mcg/mL).[78]

Table 6.4 Dose recommendations for caspofungin[76]

Indication/hepatic dysfunction/drug interactions	Dose of caspofungin
• Empiric therapy for presumed fungal infections in febrile, neutropenic patients • Candidemia and intra-abdominal abscesses, peritonitis, and pleural space infections caused by *Candida* spp. • Invasive aspergillosis in patients refractory to or intolerant of other therapies	70 mg loading dose on day 1, followed by 50 mg maintenance dose once daily thereafter
Esophageal candidiasis	50 mg once daily
Dosing with rifampin and other enzyme inducers of drug clearance	• 70 mg once daily if given concurrently with rifampin • Consider a dose increase to 70 mg once daily if given concurrently with nevirapine, efavirenz, carbamazepine, dexamethasone, or phenytoin
Moderate hepatic impairment (Child-Pugh score 7–9)	Where recommended, a 70 mg loading dose on day 1 should be administered, followed by 35 mg maintenance dose once daily thereafter

Safety Concerns

Safety concern	Rationale	Comments/recommendations
Anaphylaxis	Anaphylaxis has been reported in patients receiving caspofungin[76,79]	If anaphylaxis is suspected, discontinue the caspofungin infusion and administer appropriate treatment

(continued)

Safety concern	Rationale	Comments/recommendations
Hepatic effects	Caspofungin may cause abnormalities in liver function tests and clinically significant hepatic dysfunction, hepatitis, or hepatic failure[76]	Monitor liver function tests closely[76]
Histamine-mediated reactions	Rash, facial swelling, pruritus, sensation of warmth, and/or bronchospasm[76,79]	Consider slowing the rate of the infusion or premedicating with an antihistamine[80]
Skin disorders	Erythema multiforme, Stevens-Johnson, skin exfoliation, and toxic epidermal necrolysis have been rarely reported[76,81]	If a serious skin disorder is suspected, discontinue the caspofungin and administer appropriate treatment
Drug–drug interactions	There may be an increased risk of developing abnormal liver function tests during concomitant therapy with cyclosporine[76]	Cyclosporine increased the AUC of caspofungin by about 35%. Limit concomitant use to patients for whom the benefit outweighs the potential risk. Monitor liver function tests closely[76]
	Rifampin induces caspofungin metabolism[76]	Caspofungin trough concentrations may be reduced by 30% when given concurrently with rifampin. A dose increase is recommended during concomitant administration with rifampin and should be considered with other enzyme inducers (Table 6.4)[76]
	Caspofungin reduces tacrolimus concentrations[76]	Co-administration with tacrolimus resulted in a 20% decrease in AUC_{0-12}, a 16% decrease in C_{max}, and a 26% decrease in 12-h concentrations of tacrolimus. Monitor tacrolimus concentrations closely during concomitant administration and appropriately adjust tacrolimus dose as needed[76]
Practical issues	Not for bolus administration	Infuse slowly over 1 h.
	There are no data on compatibility of caspofungin with other medications	Do not mix or co-infuse caspofungin with other medications
	Caspofungin is not stable in diluents containing dextrose[76]	Do not use diluents containing dextrose[76]

Table 6.5   Dosing of cidofovir based on the prescribing information[84]

Type of dosing	Recommended dose
Induction dosing	5 mg/kg once weekly for 2 consecutive weeks
Maintenance dosing	5 mg/kg once weekly every 2 weeks
Dose adjustments	• If SCr increases by 0.3–0.4 mg/dL above baseline during maintenance therapy, decrease the cidofovir dose to 3 mg/kg/dose • Discontinue cidofovir if SCr increases ≥0.5 mg/dL above baseline or development of ≥3+ proteinuria

Cidofovir-Intravenous

Dosing Considerations

Obesity: There are no reports of dosing considerations in obese patients.

Thinness/emaciation: There are no reports of dosing considerations in underweight or nutritionally-depleted patients.

Kidney Injury: Approximately 70–85% of cidofovir is excreted unchanged in the urine within 24 h when administered concurrently with probenecid. Cidofovir is cleared renally by active tubular secretion.[82,83] It is contraindicated if the SCr is >1.5 mg/dL, CrCl <55 mL/min, or urine protein ≥100 mg/dL (≥2+ proteinuria). Dose adjustments are recommended for patients who have SCr elevations during cidofovir therapy (Table 6.5).[84]

Alternative dosing recommendations have been proposed for cidofovir (Table 6.6). These suggested recommendations were extrapolated from a pharmacokinetic analysis of patients with varying degrees of renal dysfunction (n=24). Each patient received a single dose of cidofovir 0.5 mg/kg IV over 1 h. The patients were administered 1 L of normal saline and oral probenecid before the cidofovir dose. A dosing nomogram for renal dysfunction (Table 6.6) was developed using the correlation between cidofovir clearance and CrCl with a target AUC of 47–67 mg h/L.[85] It is important to note that the clinician must calculate the patient's CrCl in mL/min/kg. This nomogram has not been validated in any studies; however, it may be considered as a dosing guideline in the difficult clinical scenario when the benefit of using cidofovir outweighs the risk in a patient in whom the agent is contraindicated based on the prescribing information.

Hemodialysis/CRRT: Approximately 50–75% of the cidofovir dose is removed by high-flux hemodialysis.[84,85] As there are limited data in hemodialysis, it is not recommended to be used in patients on hemodialysis. Cidofovir is minimally removed by CAPD and it is suggested to administer a 0.5 mg/kg dose (similar to CrCl in mL/min/kg of 0.1 in Table 6.6).[85] This nomogram has not been validated in any studies; however, it may be considered as a dosing guideline in the difficult clinical scenario when the benefit of using cidofovir outweighs the risk in a patient in whom the agent is contraindicated based on the prescribing information.

Table 6.6 Cidofovir dosing nomogram
to maintain AUC of 47–67 mg h/L[85]

CrCl in mL/min/kg	Dose (mg/kg/dose)
1.3–1.8	5
1.0–1.2	4
0.8–0.9	3
0.7	2.5
0.5–0.6	2
0.4	1.5
0.2–0.3	1
0.1	0.5

Note: Induction doses once weekly for 2 consecutive weeks and maintenance doses once weekly every 2 weeks

There are no recommendations for dosing cidofovir in patients on CRRT.

Liver Dysfunction: The pharmacokinetics of cidofovir in patients with hepatic impairment has not been investigated.

Hypothermia: The pharmacokinetics of cidofovir in hypothermia has not been investigated.

Other: Cidofovir is converted to cidofovir diphosphate by cellular enzymes. Cidofovir diphosphate is the active intracellular metabolite and has a half-life of 17–65 h.[82] Due to the long half-life of this active metabolite, cidofovir should not be administered more frequently than once weekly.

Safety Concerns

Safety concern	Rationale	Comments/recommendations
Preparation	In animal studies, cidofovir was carcinogenic, teratogenic, and caused hypospermia (black box warning)[84]	Prepare in a Class II laminar flow biological safety cabinet
		Wear surgical gloves and a closed front surgical-type gown with knit cuffs
		If cidofovir contacts the skin or mucous membranes, flush thoroughly with water[84]
Nephrotoxicity (black box warning)	**Contraindicated if** SCr >1.5 mg/dL, CrCl<55 mL/min, urine protein≥100 mg/dL (≥2+ proteinuria), or use with or within 7 days of nephrotoxic drugs	**Must administer probenecid 2 g orally 3 h before each cidofovir dose and 1 g orally at 2 and 8 h after completion of the infusion (total 4 g)[82-84]**
	Hydration and oral probenecid must be given with each dose of cidofovir[84]	**Must administer 1 L of normal saline 1–2 h immediately before each cidofovir infusion; a second liter may be administered over 1–3 h at the start of each cidofovir infusion or immediately following each infusion, if tolerated[82-84]**

Safety concern	Rationale	Comments/recommendations
		Must be infused intravenously over 60 min[84]
		Ingestion of food or administration of an antiemetic **before** each dose of probenecid may reduce nausea and vomiting associated with probenecid[84]
		In patients who develop symptoms of hypersensitivity to probenecid, the use of an appropriate antihistamine and/or acetaminophen should be considered[84]
		Monitor urine protein and SCr within 48 h before each dose to monitor for renal dysfunction[84]
Neutropenia (black box warning)	In studies with the 5 mg/kg maintenance dose, neutropenia occurred in 24% of patients[84]	Monitor neutrophil count during therapy and within 48 h before each dose.[84]
Decreased intraocular pressure/ocular hypotony/ uveitis/iritis	Direct intraocular injection is contraindicated[84]	Monitor intraocular pressure and for signs and symptoms of uveitis/iritis and ocular disturbances periodically during therapy[84]
Drug–drug interactions		Concurrent administration with other nephrotoxic drugs is contraindicated and other nephrotoxic agents must be discontinued at least 7 days **before** starting cidofovir therapy due to the additive risk of nephrotoxicity
		Probenecid is known to inhibit the metabolism or renal tubular excretion of many drugs such as zidovudine, beta-lactams, dapsone, NSAIDS, and methotrexate
		Zidovudine should be temporarily discontinued or the dose decreased by 50% on the day cidofovir is administered
		Avoid use with methotrexate and ketorolac[84]
General issues	In animal studies, cidofovir was carcinogenic, teratogenic, and caused hypospermia (black box warning)[84]	Females with childbearing potential should use contraception during and for at least 1 month following therapy; males should use a barrier contraceptive during therapy and for 3 months following therapy[84]

Drotrecogin Alpha (Activated)

Dosing Considerations

Obesity: The FDA approval of Drotecogin alpha activated (DrotAA) was based on the results of the Protein C Worldwide Evaluation in Severe Sepsis (PROWESS) trial.[86] In this registration trial, DrotAA was administered as a fixed dose of 24 mcg/kg/h for 96 h based on actual body weight. Patients greater than 135 kg were excluded from this trial.[86] The lack of further data in patients with other body weights led clinicians to limit the dosing weight of DrotAA to 135 kg or to use an adjusted body weight for dosing in patients weighing more than 135 kg.[14,87] Subsequently in 2005, a phase IV trial of the pharmacokinetics of DrotAA found no major differences in steady-state drug concentration (Css) and half-life in patients weighing between 137 and 227 kg (mean = 158 kg), compared to those weighing less than 135 kg (mean = 93 kg).[88] These data suggest that the plasma clearance of DrotAA increases proportionally with body weight and that total body weight should be used when prescribing DrotAA in obese individuals.

Thinness/emaciation: Although there are no reports of dosing considerations specifically in thinness and emaciation, total body weight dosing is likely appropriate in these individuals as well.

Kidney Injury: Plasma clearance of DrotAA is reduced by 23.7% in patients with $CrCl < 20$ mL/min, compared to those with clearances >50 mL/min ($P \leq 0.001$).[89] However, this decrease is within the limits of interpatient variability and a dosage reduction is not recommended.[89,90]

Hemodialysis/Continuous renal replacement therapy: Plasma clearance of DrotAA did not differ significantly in patients receiving either hemodialysis or peritoneal dialysis compared to healthy volunteers.[90] Typical high flux dialysis membranes have a pore size between 20,000 and 30,000 Da.[91] DrotAA has a molecular weight of ~55,000 Da.[92] Dialysis filters do not usually remove molecules of this size and thus no dose adjustment is warranted in patients receiving dialysis. It should be noted that patients with chronic renal failure requiring renal replacement therapy were excluded in the PROWESS trial.[86]

Hepatic dysfunction: Hepatic dysfunction, defined as aspartate aminotransferase (AST) or alanine aminotransferase (ALT) greater than three times the upper limit of normal, results in a modest (~25%) increase in plasma concentrations of DrotAA.[89] Dose adjustment is likely unnecessary in these patients. Patients with chronic severe liver disease characterized by portosystemic hypertension, chronic jaundice, cirrhosis, or chronic ascites should not receive DrotAA since safety and efficacy have not been established in this population. Although severe liver disease is listed as a precaution to use in the product labeling,[90] patients such as these were excluded from trials with DrotAA.[86]

Hypothermia: DrotAA is unlikely to be used in the setting of induced hypothermia. No data are available.

Safety Concerns

Safety concern	Rationale	Comments/recommendation
Bleeding	DrotAA inactivates coagulation factors Va and VIIIa leading to decreased thrombin generation and also enhances fibrinolysis by inhibiting plasminogen activator inhibitor-1.[93] These properties likely contribute to the efficacy of DrotAA in the treatment of severe sepsis, but are also likely the cause of bleeding in patients receiving DrotAA	DrotAA increases the risk of serious bleeding compared to placebo (RR: 1.48; 95% CI: 1.07–2.06).[94] Thrombocytopenia (platelets $\leq 50,000/mm^3$) seems to increase the risk of serious bleeding.[95] Intracranial hemorrhage occurs in 1.1% of patients receiving DrotAA and has been linked to severe thrombocytopenia (platelets $\leq 30,000/mm^3$) and/or meningitis.[95] Although it has been theorized that maintaining platelet counts $> 30,000/mm^3$ via platelet transfusions can mitigate the risk of bleeding,[95,96] this approach has not been validated. DrotAA should be avoided in patients with severe thrombocytopenia and/or meningitis
Use in patients with bleeding precautions	Many of the exclusion criteria from the PROWESS trial are not listed as contraindications to therapy in the U.S. product labeling. Rather, they are listed as precautions.[97] Use of DrotAA in patients with these precautions likely increases the risk of bleeding[97,98]	Examples of clinical trial exclusion criteria that are listed as precautions in the product labeling include: platelet count $<30,000/mm^3$, platelet inhibitor use (aspirin > 650 mg/day or clopidogrel within 7 days), chronic severe hepatic disease, use of systemic thrombolytic therapy within 3 days, and concurrent use of heparin to treat an active thrombotic or embolic event.[86,90,97,98] Recent administration (within 7 days) of oral anticoagulants is listed as an additional precaution in the product labeling, however, warfarin (if used within 7 days before study entry and if the prothrombin time exceeded the upper limit of the normal) was an exclusion criteria in PROWESS.[86,90] In one trial, serious bleeding rates were higher in patients with precautions to therapy than in those without bleeding precautions (35% vs. 3.8% respectively, $p < 0.0001$).[97] The use of DrotAA should be highly scrutinized in patients with precautions to use

Safety concern	Rationale	Comments/recommendation
Use in surgical patients	The mortality benefit of DrotAA in critically ill surgical patients is questionable. Critically ill surgical patients may be more prone to bleeding with DrotAA therapy[99,100]	Subgroup analysis of surgical patients in the PROWESS trial failed to demonstrate a mortality benefit with DrotAA, even among those with APACHE II ≥ 25.[100] In addition, another clinical trial suggested that surgical patients with single organ dysfunction who receive DrotAA have an increased risk of death.[101] However, a large database analysis indicated a benefit of DrotAA in surgical patients with APACHE II ≥ 25 (RR 0.66: 95% CI 0.45–0.97).[102] The use of DrotAA in post-operative patients is given a weak (2C) recommendation by the Surviving Sepsis Campaign[103] Nearly 5% of surgical patients who receive DrotAA experience a serious bleeding event during infusion and 1.8% of patients experienced a fatal or life-threatening bleed during infusion.[102] Many of the bleeding complications with DrotAA are related to invasive procedures performed before or during the infusion.[95,99] DrotAA should be discontinued 2 h **before** undergoing an invasive surgical procedure.[90] DrotAA may be restarted 12 h after surgery and major invasive procedures or immediately after uncomplicated less invasive procedures[90]
Concomitant heparin use	The anticoagulant effects of therapeutic heparin may increase the bleeding risks of DrotAA.[97] Discontinuation of prophylactic heparin in patients receiving DrotAA may be harmful[104]	Patients receiving more than 15,000 units of heparin per day were excluded from clinical trials.[86] Although concurrent therapeutic heparin use is listed as a precaution to therapy,[90] preliminary data suggests that concomitant use of therapeutic heparin and DrotAA results in increased bleeding risks[97] The safety of subcutaneous heparin (5000 units every 12 h) and low molecular weight heparin (enoxaparin 40 mg daily) in patients being treated with DrotAA has been established.[104] The safety of doses greater than these is unknown

Safety concern	Rationale	Comments/recommendation
		In a randomized, placebo-controlled trial of the safety of concomitant prophylactic use of heparin with DrotAA, patients exposed to heparin before the initiation of DrotAA, who were subsequently randomized to placebo had higher mortality than those randomized to heparin (35.5% vs. 26.8%, respectively).[104] The reason for this increase in mortality is unclear but may be related to rebound thrombin production from abrupt heparin discontinuation.[105] Clinicians should continue prophylactic heparin in patients receiving DrotAA unless a clear contraindication exists
Use more than 48 h after organ failure onset	The benefits of DrotAA seem most apparent when started within the first 24 h after organ dysfunction failure onset.[106] In one study, patients receiving DrotAA ≥ 48 h after the onset of organ dysfunction were 2.5 times more likely to die than those patients who received DrotAA within 24 h of organ dysfunction[107]	Although patients in the PROWESS trial could be enrolled up to 48 h after the onset of sepsis induced organ dysfunction,[86] the median duration of organ dysfunction **before** initiation of DrotAA was only 18 h.[107] The European product labeling states that treatment should be started within 48 h, and preferably within 24 h from the onset of sepsis associated organ dysfunction.[108] The U.S. label makes no mention of time to initiation.[90] A retrospective observational study of patients treated with DrotAA at U.S. teaching hospitals demonstrated a trend between later initiation of DrotAA and higher mortality.[107] A large database analysis revealed that patients treated with DrotAA early (within 24 h of organ dysfunction) had improved survival compared to those treated later (>24 h after organ dysfunction).[106] Given the known risks of therapy, these data suggest that the most favorable risk to benefit ratio is achieved with early initiation of DrotAA. The use of DrotAA more than 24 h after the onset of severe sepsis should be discouraged since safety and efficacy has not been clearly established

Table 6.7 Flucytosine dosing in renal dysfunction[112]

CrCl (mL/min)	Flucytosine dose
20–40	12.5–37.5 mg/kg every 12 h
10–20	12.5–37.5 mg/kg every 24 h
<10	12.5–37.5 mg/kg every 24–48 h or longer based on concentrations

Flucytosine-Oral

Dosing Considerations

Obesity: The reports of flucytosine use in obese patients are limited to one case report. A 125 kg (ideal body weight 60 kg) female with normal renal function received 2500 mg orally every 6 h (167 mg/kg/day based on her ideal body weight). The 2-h post-dose serum concentration of flucytosine was approximately 0.08 mg/mL. The patient's half life was 6.5 h and total clearance was 1.5 mL/min/kg of ideal body weight. As these parameters were similar to those observed in non-obese patients, the authors concluded that ideal body weight should be used to dose flucytosine in obese patients.[109,110]

Thinness/emaciation: There are no reports of dosing considerations in underweight or nutritionally depleted patients.

Kidney Injury: The major route of elimination of flucytosine is renal excretion (> 90% unchanged in the urine by glomerular filtration).[110,111] The dose is 12.5–37.5 mg/kg given every 6 h. Monitoring of serum concentrations is recommended to avoid adverse effects. Maintain flucytosine peak serum concentrations (drawn 2 h after the dose is administered) between 40 and 100 mcg/mL.[111,112] Do not exceed 100 mcg/mL as this puts the patient at increased risk for adverse effects.[111,112] For patients with kidney impairment, the ideal method to adjust the dose of flucytosine is to base the dose on serum concentrations.[110] However, suggested empiric doses for patients with renal dysfunction are listed in Table 6.7.

Hemodialysis/CRRT: Flucytosine is removed by hemodialysis and concentrations of flucytosine decrease by approximately twofold.[62] Based on this information and the concentrations measured in the study in patients receiving hemodialysis, the authors concluded that single doses of 25–50 mg/kg/dose given every 48–72 h in patients undergoing hemodialysis are safe and effective.[62] A further study evaluating the pharmacokinetics of flucytosine in patients receiving hemodialysis using a computer model distinguished that a dose of 20 mg/kg after dialysis every 48–72 h would be appropriate.[113]

There are some reports of flucytosine use in patients on peritoneal dialysis. Muther et al. reported a case of a 48 year old male who received flucytosine 750 mg every 6 h while on peritoneal dialysis. The authors observed that flucytosine is removed by peritoneal dialysis at a rate of 14 mL/min and intraperitoneal concentrations ranged from 60–100% of the serum concentrations.[65] In one case series of 13 patients on CAPD, the patients received flucytosine 1 g daily as a single dose.[64]

There are two case reports on flucytosine dosing in CRRT. In the first, flucytosine was administered to a 17-year old male patient on continuous arterio-venous hemo-filtration (CAVHF). The patient was given 2.5 g of flucytosine every 24 h. The authors found that approximately 45–95% of the flucytosine dose was removed by CAVHF depending on the type of hemofilter membrane used and the ultrafiltration rate. As such, the authors concluded that serum concentration monitoring is necessary to optimize dosing in patients receiving CAVHF[114] In another report, a 21-year old female weighing 76 kg was started on CVVHF at a rate of 1 L/h. She received flucy-tosine 2500 mg (33 mg/kg) on day 1, then 3750 (50 mg/kg) on days 2 and 3. The concentration 13 h after the first dose on day 1 was 0.034 mg/mL and the concentra-tion on day 4 was 0.11 mg/mL. The authors concluded based on the pharmacokinetic estimates that 2500 mg every 48 h would have achieved target concentrations. However, the authors did not specify what they defined as target concentrations.[115]

Liver Dysfunction: The pharmacokinetics of flucytosine was investigated in one patient with mild to moderate liver dysfunction (postnecrotic cirrhosis). The patient was given flucytosine 25 mg/kg every 6 h. The flucytosine concentrations 1, 2, and 6 h after a dose were similar to those of patients with normal liver function given the same dose.[116]

Hypothermia: The pharmacokinetics of flucytosine in hypothermia has not been investigated.

Safety Concerns

Safety concern	Rationale	Comments/recommendations
Gastrointestinal issues	Nausea, vomiting, diarrhea, and abdominal pain in about 6% of patients[110,111]	May be reduced/avoided if flucytosine capsules are administered a few at a time over 15 min[110]
Hematologic toxicity (black box warning)	Potentially irreversible granulocytopenia, anemia, and thrombocytope-nia[110,111]	Monitor complete blood cell count for hematologic toxicity frequently during therapy Use extreme caution in patients with bone marrow suppression or receiving other agents that may cause bone marrow suppression[110]
Hepatic dysfunction (black box warning)[110,111]		Use extreme caution in patients with pre-existing hepatic impairment Monitor the patient's hepatic function (AST, ALT, alkaline phosphatase, bilirubin) fre-quently during therapy[110]

(continued)

Safety concern	Rationale	Comments/recommendations
Renal dysfunction (black box warning)	Use extreme caution in patients with renal impairment as they may accumulate flucytosine, putting them at higher risk for adverse effects[110]	Monitor renal function (SCr, CrCl) and flucytosine concentrations frequently during therapy[110]
Monotherapy	Flucytosine is generally not used as mono-therapy because resistance develops rapidly[110,111]	Flucytosine is usually combined with other antifungal agents, i.e. with amphotericin B for the treatment of cryptococcal meningitis[110]
Drug–drug interactions	Cytarabine[110]	Cytarabine may decrease flucytosine activity by competitive inhibition[110]
	Amphotericin B[112]	Flucytosine and amphotericin B have synergistic antifungal activity. Amphotericin B may increase the toxicity of flucytosine[111,112]
	Fluconazole[112]	Flucytosine and fluconazole may have synergistic antifungal activity[112]

Foscarnet

Dosing Considerations

Obesity: There are no reports of foscarnet use in obese patients.

Thinness/emaciation: There are no reports of dosing considerations in underweight or nutritionally depleted patients.

Kidney Injury: The major route of elimination of foscarnet is renal excretion by glomerular filtration and tubular secretion. Safety and efficacy data for patients with baseline SCr greater than 2.8 mg/dL or measured 24 h CrCl < 50 mL/min are limited.[117] The pharmacokinetics of foscarnet in 26 patients with varying degrees of renal insufficiency or on hemodialysis was studied. All patients received a single dose of 60 mg/kg IV. The mean half-life was about 2 h in patients with normal renal function (CrCl > 80 mL/min) and 25 h in patients with severe renal impairment (CrCl 10–25 mL/min).[118] Based on these results, the dosing nomogram for induction and maintenance dosing of foscarnet was developed.,[117,118] (Tables 6.8 and 6.9). It is important to note that the clinician must calculate the patient's CrCl in mL/min/kg using the equation shown below **before** initiating therapy in order to choose appropriate dose.[117] Even patients with a normal SCr may require dose adjustment

Table 6.8 Induction dosing of foscarnet in varying degrees of renal function[117]

CrCl in mL/min/kg	Dosing for Cytomegalovirus		Dosing for Herpes Simplex virus (acyclovir-resistant)	
	Dosing strategy: 90 mg/kg every 12 h	Dosing strategy: 60 mg/kg every 8 h	Dosing strategy: 40 mg/kg every 12 h	Dosing strategy: 40 mg/kg every 8 h
>1.4	90 mg/kg every 12 h	60 mg/kg every 8 h	40 mg/kg every 12 h	40 mg/kg every 8 h
>1–1.4	70 mg/kg every 12 h	45 mg/kg every 8 h	30 mg/kg every 12 h	30 mg/kg every 8 h
>0.8–1	50 mg/kg every 12 h	50 mg/kg every 12 h	20 mg/kg every 12 h	35 mg/kg every 12 h
>0.6–0.8	80 mg/kg every 24 h	40 mg/kg every 12 h	35 mg/kg every 24 h	25 mg/kg every 12 h
>0.5–0.6	60 mg/kg every 24 h	60 mg/kg every 24 h	25 mg/kg every 24 h	40 mg/kg every 24 h
≥0.4–0.5	50 mg/kg every 24 h	50 mg/kg every 24 h	20 mg/kg every 24 h	35 mg/kg every 24 h
<0.4	Not recommended	Not recommended	Not recommended	Not recommended

Table 6.9 Maintenance dosing of foscarnet in varying degrees of renal function[117]

CrCl in mL/min/kg	Dosing for Cytomegalovirus	
	Dosing strategy: 90 mg/kg every 24 h	Dosing strategy: 120 mg/kg every 24 h
>1.4	90 mg/kg every 24 h	120 mg/kg every 24 h
>1–1.4	70 mg/kg every 24 h	90 mg/kg every 24 h
>0.8–1	50 mg/kg every 24 h	65 mg/kg every 24 h
>0.6–0.8	80 mg/kg every 48 h	105 mg/kg every 48 h
>0.5–0.6	60 mg/kg every 48 h	80 mg/kg every 48 h
≥0.4–0.5	50 mg/kg every 48 h	65 mg/kg every 48 h
<0.4	Not recommended	Not recommended

using this equation. Doses should be calculated using the patient's actual body weight.

$$\text{CrCl in } \mathbf{mL/min/kg} \text{ for males} \geq 18 \text{ years old} = \frac{(140 - \text{patient's age in years})}{(72 \times \text{SCr in mg/dL})}$$

$$\text{CrCl in } \mathbf{mL/min/kg} \text{ for females} \geq 18 \text{ years old} = 0.85 \times \text{male value}$$

Hemodialysis/CRRT: Safety and efficacy data for patients with baseline SCr greater than 2.8 mg/dL or measured 24 h CrCl < 50 mL/min are limited.[117] The pharmacokinetics of foscarnet in 26 patients with varying degrees of renal insufficiency or on hemodialysis was studied. All patients received a single dose of 60 mg/kg IV. Conventional hemodialysis and high-flux hemodialysis removed 37% and 38% of the foscarnet dose, respectively.[118] Based on one study and two case reports, the recommended dose of foscarnet for patients on hemodialysis is 45–60 mg/kg following each hemodialysis session.[118-120]

There is one case report of a patient undergoing continuous cyclic peritoneal dialysis (CCPD) and CAPD while receiving foscarnet. The half-life on CCPD was 41.4 h and on CAPD 45.8 h (half-life in patients with normal renal function ranges from 3–4 h). CCPD and CAPD increased the total body clearance of foscarnet by 145% and 105%, respectively. The authors concluded that for CCPD or CAPD, foscarnet should be dosed as 45 mg/kg IV every 24 h.[121]

There is no information reported for dosing foscarnet in patients receiving CRRT.

Liver Dysfunction: Foscarnet does not undergo hepatic biotransformation

Hypothermia: The pharmacokinetics of foscarnet in hypothermia has not been investigated.

Other: Not applicable.

Safety Concerns

Safety concern	Rationale	Comments/recommendations
Preparation	Undiluted solution (24 mg/mL) can be administered without further dilution when administered through a central venous catheter.	Foscarnet solution must be used within 24 h after the seal of the glass bottle is broken and/or when transferred to plastic infusion bags[117]
	The solution must be diluted with normal saline or 5% dextrose solution to a final concentration ≤12 mg/mL when administering through a peripheral vein[117]	
Nephrotoxicity (black box warning)	There is a 33% incidence of acute tubular necrosis or tubular interstitial nephritis in patients not receiving hydration (defined as SCr ≥2 mg/dL)[117,122-126]	Hydrate patient with 750–1000 mL of normal saline or 5% dextrose solution before initial infusion
	Incidence decreased to 12% when 1000 mL normal saline or 5% dextrose solution given with each infusion of foscarnet[117]	For subsequent infusions, hydrate with 750–1000 mL normal saline or 5% dextrose solution for 90–120 mg/kg/dose or 500 mL normal saline or 5% dextrose solution for 40–60 mg/kg; give concurrently with each infusion

Safety concern	Rationale	Comments/recommendations
		Hydration may be decreased if clinically warranted. In patients at high risk of adverse effects from hydration (i.e. congestive heart failure), the lower recommended range of hydration should be considered[117]
Electrolyte disturbances and seizures (black box warning)	Foscarnet chelates divalent metal ions and alters electrolyte concentrations leading to hypocalcemia, hypo- or hyperphosphatemia, hypomagnesemia, and hypokalemia[117]	Use caution in patients with decreased total serum calcium or other electrolyte concentrations
		Use caution in patients with neurologic or cardiac abnormalities and if receiving other medications that alter calcium concentrations
		Correct any significant metabolic abnormality **before** initiating therapy
		Monitor serum calcium, magnesium, potassium, and phosphorus concentrations
		Monitor for perioral numbness, paresthesias, or seizures
		Slowing the infusion rate may decrease or prevent symptoms[117]
Drug–drug interactions		Avoid combining with other nephrotoxic agents unless potential benefits outweigh the risks
		Use caution with other agents known to influence serum calcium concentrations[117]
General issues	Toxicity can be increased as a result of excessive plasma concentrations	Do NOT administer by bolus intravenous injection
	Infuse only into veins with adequate blood flow[117]	Maximum infusion rate is 1 mg/kg/min, with doses usually administered over at least 120 min by an infusion pump
		Infusion through a peripheral vein: maximum solution concentration of 12 mg/mL
		Infusion through a central venous catheter: maximum solution concentration of 24 mg/mL[117]

Table 6.10 Induction dosing of ganciclovir[128]

CrCl (mL/min)	Induction dose for ganciclovir
≥ 70	5 mg/kg every 12 h
50–69	2.5 mg/kg every 12 h
25–49	2.5 mg/kg every 24 h
10–24	1.25 mg/kg every 24 h

Table 6.11 Maintenance dosing of ganciclovir[128]

CrCl (mL/min)	Maintenance dose for ganciclovir
≥70[a]	5 mg/kg every 24 h
50–69	2.5 mg/kg every 24 h
25–49	1.25 mg/kg every 24 h
10–24	0.625 mg/kg every 24 h

[a]Alternative maintenance therapy in patients with CrCl ≥ 70 mL/min is 6 mg/kg every 24 h 5 days/week[128]

Ganciclovir-Intravenous

Dosing Considerations

Obesity: There are no reports of ganciclovir use in obese patients.

Thinness/emaciation: There are no reports of dosing considerations in underweight or nutritionally depleted patients.

Kidney Injury: The major route of elimination of ganciclovir is renal excretion of unchanged drug by glomerular filtration and active tubular secretion.[127] Dose adjustment is necessary in patients with renal dysfunction (Tables 6.10 and 6.11) It is important to note that the clinician must calculate the patient's CrCl in mL/min using the **equation below** before initiating therapy in order to choose the appropriate dose. Doses should be calculated using the patient's actual body weight.[128]

$$\text{CrCl in } \underline{\text{mL} / \text{min}} \text{ for males} \geq 18 \text{ years old} = \frac{(140 - \text{patien's age in years})(\text{body weight in kg})}{(72 \times \text{SCr in mg/dL})}$$

$$\text{CrCl in } \underline{\text{mL} / \text{min}} \text{ for females} \geq 18 \text{ years old} = 0.85 \times \text{male value}$$

Hemodialysis/CRRT: The half-life of ganciclovir is prolonged from 3.5 h in healthy patients to 68.1 h in patients with end-stage renal disease on hemodialysis.[129] About 50% of the ganciclovir dose is removed by hemodialysis.[128-132] The dose in hemodialysis patients for induction therapy should not exceed 1.25 mg/kg administered three times per week shortly after the hemodialysis session. For maintenance therapy the dose in hemodialysis patients is 0.625 mg/kg administered three times per week shortly after the hemodialysis session.[128]

In a case report, one patient receiving ganciclovir 5 mg/kg IV every 12 h underwent continuous hemodiafiltration. The half-life was 12.6 h and the total body clearance was decreased (0.55 mL/min/kg compared to approximately 4 mL/min/kg in patients with normal renal function). The authors changed the ganciclovir dose to 5 mg/kg IV every 48 h based on their findings.[133]

Five heart transplant and one lung transplant patient received ganciclovir 5 mg/kg IV every 48 h while on CVVHD. The half-life was about 19 h, and a clearance of approximately 0.4 mL/min/kg. These authors concluded that 5 mg/kg IV every 48 h is an appropriate dose of ganciclovir in patients on CVVHD.[134,135]

Liver Dysfunction: The pharmacokinetics of ganciclovir in patients with hepatic impairment has not been investigated.

Hypothermia: The pharmacokinetics of ganciclovir in hypothermia has not been investigated.

Other: Not applicable.

Safety Concerns

Safety concern	Rationale	Comments/recommendations
Preparation	Carcinogenic, teratogenic, and caused aspermatogenesis in animal studies[128]	Caution should be exercised in the handling and preparation of ganciclovir products in a similar manner as antineoplastic drugs
		If ganciclovir contacts the skin or mucous membranes, wash thoroughly with soap and water for at least 15 min; for eye exposure rinse thoroughly with water[128]
Granulocytopenia, anemia, and thrombocytopenia (black box warning)	May occur at any time during therapy, but usually occurs in the first or second week of therapy	Monitor complete blood cell count for granulocytopenia, anemia, and thrombocytopenia frequently
	Should not be given if absolute neutrophil count is <500/mm³ or platelets <25,000/mm³,[128]	Use caution in patients with pre-existing cytopenias or with a history of cytopenic reactions to other drugs, chemicals, or irradiation[128]
Other adverse effects	Phlebitis and/or pain at the infusion site	Monitor patient for phlebitis/pain at the site of infusion and renal function frequently
	Increased SCr. In studies of transplant recipients, SCr elevations ≥2.5 mg/dL occurred in 18–20% of patients	Ophthalmologic follow-up evaluations every 4–6 weeks during treatment in patients being treated for cytomegalovirus retinitis

(continued)

Safety concern	Rationale	Comments/recommendations
	Retinal detachment (relationship to ganciclovir not established) Teratogenic[128]	Males and females with childbearing potential should use contraception during and for at least 90 days following therapy[128]
Drug–drug interactions		Ganciclovir increases didanosine concentrations. The didanosine AUC_{0-12} increased by 50–70% and the C_{max} increased by 36–49%
		Imipenem/cilastatin may increase seizure potential
		Probenecid decreases the renal clearance of ganciclovir
		Additive toxicity with other drugs known to cause granulocytopenia or renal impairment.[128]
General issues	Intramuscular or subcutaneous injection may result in severe tissue irritation due to high pH (pH 11)[128]	Must be infused intravenously over 60 min into a vein with adequate blood flow to permit rapid dilution and distribution
		Do not administer by rapid or bolus intravenous injection; intramuscular or subcutaneous injection may result in severe tissue irritation
		Monitor patient for phlebitis/pain at the site of infusion[128]

Micafungin

Dosing Considerations

Obesity: There are no reports of micafungin use in obese patients. However, one study identified weight as a factor that influences the clearance of micafungin. Patients weighing ≥ 66.3 kg had an increased mean clearance (1.23 L/h) compared to patients weighing <66.3 kg (0.83 L/h), suggesting that higher doses may potentially be needed in heavier patients.[136]

Thinness/emaciation: There are no reports of dosing considerations in underweight or nutritionally depleted patients.

Kidney Injury: Dose adjustments for renal dysfunction are not needed for micafungin.[137]

Hemodialysis/CRRT: Dose adjustments for hemodialysis or CRRT are not needed for micafungin. It is not dialyzable.[137]

Liver Dysfunction: Micafungin is metabolized by arylsulfatase to the M-1 catechol form. It is then further metabolized by catechol-O-methyltransferase to the M-2

Table 6.12 Dose recommendations per indication[137]

Indication	Dose of micafungin
Candidemia, acute disseminated candidiasis, *Candida* peritonitis and abscesses	100 mg once daily
Prophylaxis of *Candida* infections in patients undergoing hematopoietic stem cell transplantation	50 mg once daily
Esophageal candidiasis	150 mg once daily

methoxy form. The M-5 form occurs from hydroxylation at the side chain by cytochrome P450 (CYP) isozymes. Fecal excretion is the major route of elimination. No dose adjustment is needed for mild-moderate hepatic impairment. There are no data in patients with severe liver dysfunction.[137]

Hypothermia: The pharmacokinetics of micafungin in hypothermia has not been investigated.

Other: The dose of micafungin is based on the indication as listed in Table 6.12. A loading dose is not necessary.

Safety Concerns

Safety concern	Rationale	Comments/recommendations
Anaphylactic reactions	Serious hypersensitivity reactions (including shock) have been reported in patients receiving micafungin[137,138]	If anaphylaxis is suspected, discontinue the micafungin infusion and administer appropriate treatment[137,138]
Hepatic effects	Micafungin may cause abnormalities in liver function tests and clinically significant hepatic dysfunction, hepatitis, or hepatic failure[137,138]	Monitor liver function tests closely[137,138]
Histamine-mediated reactions	Rash, facial swelling, pruritus, sensation of warmth, and/or bronchospasm[79,137]	Consider slowing the rate of the infusion or premedicating with an antihistamine[137]
Hemolysis and hemolytic anemia	Hemolysis and hemolytic anemia have been reported in patients receiving micafungin[137-140]	Monitor for clinical or laboratory evidence of hemolysis or hemolytic anemia during micafungin therapy. If there is evidence of worsening of these conditions, evaluate the risk/benefit of continuing micafungin therapy[137,138]

(continued)

Safety concern	Rationale	Comments/recommendations
Renal effects	Elevations in SCr and BUN have been reported in patients receiving micafungin[137,138]	Monitor renal function closely[137]
Injection site reactions	Phlebitis and thrombophle-bitis have been reported in patients receiving micafungin[137]	Injection site reactions are more likely to occur in patients receiving mica-fungin through a peripheral IV line[137]
Drug–drug interactions	Micafungin is a substrate for and a weak inhibitor of CYP3A	Patients receiving micafungin concur-rently with sirolimus, nifedipine, and itraconazole should be monitored for adverse effects of these agents and their dose should be reduced if needed
	Concurrent administration with sirolimus increased the sirolimus AUC by 21%, with no effect on the maximum concen-tration C_{max} of sirolimus	
	Concurrent administration with nifedipine increased the nifedipine AUC and C_{max} by 18% and 42%, respectively	
	Concurrent administration with itraconazole increased the itracon-azole AUC and C_{max} by 22% and 11%, respectively	
	Concurrent administration with cyclosporine decreases the clearance of cyclosporine by 16%[137,138,141]	Monitor cyclosporine concentrations when using it concurrently with micafungin[137,138]
General Issues	Infuse over 1 h	Do not mix or co-infuse micafungin with other medications[137]
	Flush the IV line with 0.9% Sodium Chloride before infusion of micafungin[137]	

Vancomycin

Dosing Considerations

Obesity: According to published consensus guidelines, a loading dose of 25–30 mg/ kg of vancomycin is recommended for severely ill patients and initial maintenance doses should be between 15 and 20 mg/kg every 8–12 h.[142] These doses are based on total body weight. The use of total body weight for obese patients receiving vancomycin is supported by several small pharmacokinetic studies.[143-145] In general, these studies have shown that similar mg/kg dosing is required in obese and non-obese individuals to achieve therapeutic concentrations. However, limited safety data exists regarding the use of very large single doses of vancomycin and many institutions arbitrarily limit single doses of vancomycin to 2–3 g. Although controversial, single large doses of vancomycin may increase the likelihood of toxicity.[144] Some investigators have also shown that vancomycin half-life is decreased in obesity.[143,144] These observations, coupled with the time-dependent killing effects of vancomycin, suggest that frequent (every 6–8 h) dosing of relatively large (2 g) of vancomycin may be needed to maximize efficacy and safety.[14] Trough serum concentration monitoring of vancomycin is recommended in this setting.[142]

Thinness/emaciation: Although there are no studies of vancomycin specifically in underweight individuals, total body weight is likely appropriate.

Kidney Injury: Vancomycin is cleared predominantly via glomerular filtration and declining renal function is associated with a significant decrease in vancomycin elimination.[146] Thus, a dose reduction is necessary in the setting of renal impairment. Several nomograms exist for vancomycin dosing in renal insufficiency,[147-149] however, these nomograms were not intended to achieve the current recommended trough concentrations of 15–20 mg/L.[142] A recently validated nomogram, that includes recommendations for renal insufficiency, has been shown to achieve trough concentrations between 10 and 20 mg/L approximately 70% of the time (median trough concentration of 12 mg/L).[150] Importantly, this nomogram recognizes the need for a loading dose even in the presence of renal insufficiency. Similarly, Pea et al. have developed a nomogram that uses continuous infusion vancomycin after a 15 mg/kg loading dose.[151] The loading dose is administered over 2-h and the continuous infusion is started immediately thereafter. The daily dose of vancomycin is determined by renal function with the target Css (15 or 20 mg/L, Table 6.13). Although these nomogram-based recommendations represent a reasonable starting point for vancomycin dosing in renal insufficiency, serum drug concentration monitoring of vancomycin is highly recommended in the setting of renal insufficiency.[142]

Hemodialysis/Continuous renal replacement therapy: Vancomycin dose reductions are necessary in hemodialysis and during continuous renal replacement therapy. In patients with end-stage renal disease requiring dialysis, the half-life of vancomycin has been reported to be nearly 20 days.[152] Vancomycin is not significantly dialyzable when low flux membranes are used, but high flux membranes result in significant removal of vancomycin.[153] High flux membranes are likely used in the majority of patients receiving hemodialysis.[154] Vancomycin serum concentrations sampled immediately after hemodialysis are artificially low and do not account for the significant redistribution of vancomycin that occurs after dialysis.[155] Redistribution is usually complete 3 h following dialysis.[155] A variety of approaches have been studied for vancomycin dosing in hemodialysis including intradialytic dosing and post dialysis dosing.[156] Although there are likely many effective strategies for vancomycin dosing in hemodialysis, intradialytic dosing is usually preferred for convenience reasons.[154] Intradialytic dosing obviates the need for patients

Table 6.13 Vancomycin daily dose to be given as a continuous infusion to maintain a Css = 15 mg/L. The continuous infusion should be started immediately after a loading dose of 15 mg/kg is given[151]

Estimated CrCl (mL/min)	Recommended daily dose of vancomycin to be administered as continuous infusion (g)
10	0.44
20	0.54
30	0.65
40	0.76
50	0.86
60	0.96
70	1.07
80	1.17
90	1.28
100	1.38
120	1.59

Based on the following equation: Infusion rate (g/24 h) = [0.029 × CrCl (mL/min) + 0.94] × target Css × (24/1,000), where target Css is equal to 15 mg/L

to remain in the hemodialysis clinic for an additional 30–60 min in order to receive vancomycin. One commonly employed approach consists of administering a 1-g dose during the last hour of hemodialysis, followed by 500 mg in the last hour of every subsequent dialysis session. This method results in predialysis concentrations of 11 ± 3 mg/L.[157]

In situations where convenience is less important and more aggressive dosing of vancomycin is warranted, e.g., critically ill patients, postdialysis dosing may be preferred. Heintz et al. recommend administering an initial 15–25 mg/kg dose after dialysis, followed by a second dose of 5–10 mg/kg given after the second hemodialysis session.[7] A predialysis concentration should be obtained before the third dialysis session and subsequent doses should be administered as follows: <10 mg/L, give 1000 mg after hemodialysis; 10–25 mg/L, give 500–750 mg after hemodialysis; >25 mg/L, hold vancomycin.[7] Regardless of which approach is employed, frequent serum monitoring of vancomycin is needed in hemodialysis patients, especially those that are critically ill.[142]

Since clearance is constant in CRRT, following an initial loading dose of vancomycin, a vancomycin serum concentration can be obtained at any time.[153] Additional doses between 500 and 1000 mg should be administered when concentrations fall below 10–15 mg/L. Depending on the type of CRRT used, repeat doses may be required every 12–48 h.[7] Serum drug monitoring is recommended.

Hepatic dysfunction: Studies of vancomycin dosing in hepatic dysfunction have produced discordant results. One study demonstrated increased half-life and decreased clearance with hepatic failure[158]; conversely another study demonstrated no change.[159] In patients with hepatic failure and ascites, larger doses of vancomycin may be needed to compensate for an increased Vd. Serum drug concentrations should be monitored in order to ensure therapeutic concentrations.

Hypothermia: No data are available

Safety Concerns

Safety concern	Rationale	Comments/recommendations
Ototoxicity	Earlier reports of vancomycin-associated ototoxicity were attributed to impurities in the formulation, however, a recent pilot study reported a 12% rate of high-frequency hearing loss detected by audiometry in vancomycin treated patients.[160] The reported rate of vancomycin associated ototoxicity ranges from 1% to 12%[142,160]	A causal link between vancomycin administration and ototoxicity has not been established.[142,161] Vancomycin is not considered ototoxic by many experts, but has been shown to enhance the ototoxicity of other drugs such as aminoglycosides.[162] Although a clear link between vancomycin serum concentrations and ototoxicity has not been established, serum drug monitoring is recommended in the setting of concomitant ototoxic agents[142]
Nephrotoxicity	The exact mechanism of vancomycin-associated nephrotoxicity is unknown, but may be related to increased oxidative stress, altered mitochondrial function and/or cell proliferation in the renal tubule[142,163,164]	Vancomycin-associated kidney injury is more common when concomitant nephrotoxins such as aminoglycosides are given[37]
	Vancomycin associated-nephrotoxicity was commonly reported when the drug first became available and was attributed to impurities in the product. As purer formulations were developed, reports of nephrotoxicity became less frequent[165]	A series of recent reports have linked vancomycin trough concentrations greater than 15 mg/L and vancomycin daily doses greater than 4 g with nephrotoxicity.[166-168] Monitoring of trough concentrations is recommended in patients receiving aggressive dosing targeting concentrations of 15–20 mg/L, those receiving concurrent nephrotoxins, patients who are hemodynamically unstable, and in those with fluctuating renal function.[142] Continuous infusion of vancomycin may allow for lower daily doses while maintaining therapeutic concentrations. This approach may be able to reduce the likelihood of vancomycin-associated nephrotoxicity[151]
Use in patients with elevated MICs	An AUC/MIC ratio ≥400 is predictive of vancomycin efficacy.[169] This endpoint is not readily achievable in organisms with MIC's greater than 1 mcg/mL and thus may predispose patients to treatment failures[142]	Increased rates of vancomycin failure have been noted in the treatment of bacteremia and pneumonia when the organism MIC exceeds 1 mcg/mL. Alternative agents should be used if the MIC to vancomycin exceeds 1 mcg/mL[170-174]

(continued)

Safety concern	Rationale	Comments/recommendations
Red Man syndrome	Rapid infusion of vancomycin can result in profound histamine release causing skin rash (Fig. 6.3) and other adverse effects[175-177]	Common features of this syndrome are pruritus and rash. Less commonly patients can also present with hypotension, angioedema, and even cardiac arrest.[177] Vancomycin-related histamine release is minimized by limiting the rate of vancomycin administration to no more than 1 g/h. An even slower rate of infusion (such as 1 g over 2 h) results in even less histamine release and should be considered in patients with signs of Red Man syndrome.[178] A preemptive IV dose of 50 mg diphenhydramine can abort most of the reactions[177]
Thrombocytopenia	Vancomycin administration can induce the production of drug-dependent, platelet-reactive antibodies resulting in thrombocytopenia[179]	Vancomycin-dependent, platelet-reactive antibodies were detected in 20% of patients who were suspected of having vancomycin-associated thrombocytopenia.[179] Platelet recovery was usually complete within 8 days after drug discontinuation, but was delayed further in those with renal insufficiency. Serious bleeding occurred in some patients. It is important to note that only patients who were suspected of having vancomycin-associated thrombocytopenia were evaluated for immune thrombocytopenia. Thus the true incidence of this phenomenon is unknown, but is likely low. However, in the absence of other causes, clinicians should consider vancomycin as a possible cause of thrombocytopenia
Drug interaction with hemody-namically active agents	Concurrent use of vancomycin and drugs that enhance cardiac output and/or increase renal blood flow may enhance vancomycin clearance[180]	In one trial, cardiac surgery patients treated with hemodynamically active drugs (dopamine, dobutamine, and furosemide) demonstrated increased vancomycin clearance.[180] Of note, an increase in serum concentration of vancomycin was noted when the hemodynamically active agents were discontinued. Patients treated with drugs that enhance cardiac output/renal blood flow may require aggressive vancomycin dosing

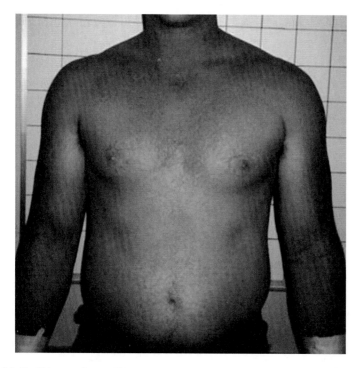

Fig. 6.3 Red Man syndrome: This pruritic reaction progressed to an erythematous rash appearing on the neck and upper torso at 30 min after administration of vancomycin (Reproduced with permission from Polk[175])

Voriconazole-Intravenous and Oral

Dosing Considerations

Obesity: There are no reports of voriconazole use in obese patients. Due to the non-linear pharmacokinetics, increasing the dose may lead to greater than proportional increases in voriconazole concentrations.[181]

Thinness/emaciation: There are no reports of dosing considerations in underweight or nutritionally depleted patients.

Kidney Injury: Less than 2% of the voriconazole dose is excreted unchanged in the urine; however, there is concern regarding the use of IV voriconazole in patients with kidney dysfunction.[181] The solvent for IV voriconazole, sulfobutyle-ther-beta-cyclodextrin (SBECD), may accumulate in patients with renal dysfunction since it is excreted by the kidney. In patients with renal dysfunction, there is a concern that SBECD may cause nephrotoxicity based on data from animal studies.[182] However, a review concluded that this is unlikely based on the amount of SBECD contained in IV voriconazole.[182] Contrary, a study found that the SBECD exposure is increased in patients on hemodialysis by a factor of 6.2.[183] IV voriconazole should not be used in patients with a CrCl < 50 mL/min. In clinical situations whereby IV voriconazole needs to be administered in these patients, it should only be used after determination of the risk versus benefit. If the decision is made to use IV voriconazole in this setting, the patient's SCr and CrCl should be closely monitored for nephrotoxicity.[181]

Hemodialysis/CRRT: IV voriconazole should not be used in patients with a CrCl < 50 mL/min.[181] No dose adjustments are needed in patients on hemodialysis.[181] In one case report a patient receiving CVVHDF was treated with IV voriconazole (6 mg/kg twice at a 14 h interval, followed by 4 mg/kg every 12 h). Based on the pharmacokinetic analysis, no dose adjustments of voriconazole are needed for CVVHDF.[184]

Liver Dysfunction: Voriconazole is eliminated extensively via hepatic metabolism. It is metabolized to the N-oxide (72%), which does not have any antifungal activity. For patients with mild to moderate cirrhosis (Child-Pugh Class A and B) it is recommended to give the standard loading dose regimen, but the maintenance dose should be halved (Table 6.14). Voriconazole has not been studied in patients with severe cirrhosis (Child-Pugh Class C) or in patients with chronic hepatitis B or C and should only be used in these patients if the benefit outweighs the risk.[181]

Hypothermia: The pharmacokinetics of voriconazole in hypothermia has not been investigated.

Other: Voriconazole has non-linear pharmacokinetics due to saturation of its metabolism, which results in high inter-individual variability in concentrations. As such, increasing the dose may lead to greater than proportional increases in voriconazole concentrations. Voriconazole is metabolized by CYP2C19, 2C9, and 3A4, with the major pathway being through CYP2C19. The CYP2C19 isoenzyme has genetic polymorphisms leading to increased variability in the metabolism of the drug.[181]

- Poor metabolizers have fourfold higher voriconazole exposure compared to homozygous extensive metabolizers[181]
  - Poor metabolizers: 15–20% of Asians, 3–5% of Caucasians and Blacks[181]
- Heterozygous extensive metabolizers have twofold higher voriconazole exposure compared to homozygous extensive metabolizers[181]

Table 6.14 Voriconazole dosing[181]

Infection	Loading dose IV	Maintenance dose IV[a]	PO[b]
Invasive aspergillosis, scedosporiosis, and fusariosis	6 mg/kg every 12 h for two doses	4 mg/kg every 12 h	200 mg every 12 h for patients ≥40 kg;
Candidemia in non-neutropenic patients and other deep tissue *Candida* infections	6 mg/kg every 12 h for two doses	3–4 mg/kg every 12 h	100 mg every 12 h for patients <40 kg
Esophageal candidiasis	See recommendations for oral therapy	See recommendations for oral therapy	

Note: When a loading dose is administered, steady state plasma concentrations are achieved within 1 day. If a loading dose is not administered, steady state plasma concentrations are achieved after about 5–6 days of IV therapy

[a]If patients are unable to tolerate 4 mg/kg IV, reduce the IV maintenance dose to 3 mg/kg/dose every 12 h

[b]PO maintenance dose:

- For patients weighing ≥40 kg, may increase the to 300 mg every 12 h if response is inadequate
- For patients weighting <40 kg, may increase the dose to 150 mg every 12 h if response is inadequate
- In patients unable to tolerate 300 mg every 12 h, decrease the dose by 50 mg increments to a minimum of 200 mg every 12 h (or 100 mg every 12 h for patients weighing <40 kg)

Safety Concerns

Safety concern	Rationale	Comments/recommendations
Reversible visual disturbances	About 21% of patients in clinical trials experienced abnormal vision, such as blurry vision, color vision changes and/or photophobia. Optic neuritis and papilledema have also occurred in patients receiving voriconazole. Visual disturbances may be associated with higher voriconazole concentrations and/or doses[181]	Visual disturbances usually disappear over time with continued therapy and/or discontinuation of voriconazole. In one study, vision returned to normal 14 days after discontinuation of therapy[181]

(continued)

Safety concern	Rationale	Comments/recommendations
QTc interval prolongation	Arrhythmias, cardiac arrests, and sudden deaths rarely occur in patients taking voriconazole[181]	Use caution in patients with a history of proarrhythmic conditions, cardiotoxic chemotherapy, hypokalemia, and other agents that prolong the QTc interval. Agents that have the potential to increase the QTc interval such as terfenadine, astemizole, cisapride, pimozide or quinidine, are contraindicated with voriconazole Correct potassium, magnesium, and calcium concentrations before initiating voriconazole[181]
Elevations in liver function tests and clinical signs of liver damage, such as jaundice, hepatitis, and hepatic failure	About 12% of patients in all clinical studies developed clinically significant transaminase abnormalities[181]	Liver function tests (AST, ALT, alkaline phosphatase, total bilirubin) should be monitored at the start of and during therapy. Discontinue voriconazole if liver damage due to voriconazole is suspected[181]
Photosensitivity	Photosensitivity reactions have been reported and squamous cell carcinoma of the skin and melanoma have been reported during long-term therapy[181]	Patients should avoid strong, direct sunlight during therapy[181]
Dermatological reactions	About 7% of patients in clinical trials developed mild to moderate rashes with voriconazole therapy[181]	Monitor for dermatological reactions[181]
Rare serious cutaneous reactions	Stevens-Johnson syndrome, toxic epidermal necrolysis, and erythema muliforme have been reported during therapy[181]	Discontinue voriconazole if an exfoliative cutaneous reaction occurs[181]
Drug–drug interactions	Agents that have increased or expected increased concentrations when used with voriconazole	Alfentanil, fentanyl, oxycodone, methadone, warfarin, statins, benzodiazepines, calcium channel blockers, sulfonylureas, vinca alkaloids, NSAIDS – monitor patients closely for adverse effects of these agents and adjust their doses as needed Cyclosporine – decrease the cyclosporine dose by 50% when initiating voriconazole; monitor cyclosporine concentrations when initiating and discontinuing voriconazole; when discontinuing voriconazole, increase cyclosporine dose as needed

Safety concern	Rationale	Comments/recommendations
		Tacrolimus – decrease the tacrolimus dose by 33% when initiating voriconazole; monitor tacrolimus concentrations when initiating and discontinuing voriconazole; when discontinuing voriconazole, increase tacrolimus dose as needed[181]
Drug–drug interactions	Two-way interactions	
	Voriconazole is a CYP2C19, 2 C9, and 3A4 substrate and inhibitor[181]	
	Efavirenz is a CYP450 inducer and CYP3A4 inhibitor and substrate. With concurrent administration, efavirenz C_{max} and AUC_τ are increased and voriconazole C_{max} and AUC_τ are decreased[181]	For concurrent administration of voriconazole and efavirenz, the voriconazole maintenance dose is increased to 400 mg Q 12 h and the efavirenz dose decreased to 300 mg every 24 h; when voriconazole is discontinued, the efavirenz dose should be increased to 600 mg every 24 h.[181]
	Other non-nucleoside reverse transcriptase inhibitors (NNRTIs) (see above for efavirenz) are CYP450 inducers and CYP3A4 inhibitors and substrates. With concurrent administration, there is a potential for inhibition of the metabolism of the NNRTI or of voriconazole[181,185]	For concurrent administration of delavirdine, nevirapine, and etravirine, monitor for adverse effects of voriconazole and the other agent[181,185]
	Phenytoin is a CYP450 inducer and CYP2C9 substrate. With concurrent administration, phenytoin C_{max} and AUC_τ are increased and voriconazole C_{max} and AUC_τ are decreased[181]	For concurrent administration of voriconazole and phenytoin, increase the voriconazole maintenance dose from 4 to 5 mg/kg IV every 12 h or from 200 to 400 mg PO every 12 h (or 100–200 mg every 12 h in patients <40 kg). Monitor patients closely for phenytoin adverse effects and monitor phenytoin concentrations[181]
	Omeprazole is a CYP2C19 inhibitor and 2C19 and 3A4 substrate. With concurrent administration, omeprazole and voriconazole C_{max} and AUC_τ are increased[181]	For concurrent administration of voriconazole and omeprazole ≥40 mg every 24 h, decrease the omeprazole dose by 50% when initiating voriconazole. No dose adjustments are recommended for voriconazole[181]

(continued)

Safety concern	Rationale	Comments/recommendations
	Oral contraceptives are CYP2C19 inhibitors and 3A4 substrates. With concurrent administration, both the oral contraceptive and voriconazole C_{max} and AUC_τ are increased[181]	For concurrent administration of voriconazole and oral contraceptives, monitor for adverse effects of voriconazole and the oral contraceptives[181]
	Protease inhibitors (except indinavir) are CYP3A4 inhibitors and substrates. With concurrent administration, there is a potential for inhibition of the metabolism of the protease inhibitor or of voriconazole[181]	For concurrent administration of voriconazole and protease inhibitors, monitor for adverse effects of voriconazole and the protease inhibitors[181]
Contraindicated drug	Agents that decrease or are expected to decrease voriconazole concentrations	Rifampin, high-dose ritonavir (400 mg every 12 h), St. John's Wort, carbamazepine, long-acting barbiturates[181]
	Agents that have significantly increased or expected significantly increased concentrations when used with voriconazole	Sirolimus, terfenadine, astemizole, cisapride, pimozide, quinidine, ergot alkaloids[181]
	Two-way interactions	Rifabutin[181]
Infusion rate	Maximum rate of infusion is 3 mg/kg/h[181]	IV voriconazole must not be infused concomitantly with any blood product or short-term infusion of concentrated electrolytes, even if the two infusions are running in separate IV lines.[181]
Pregnancy	Pregnancy category D[181]	Contraception should be used in women of childbearing potential during treatment[181]

References

1. Hernandez JO, Norstrom J, Wysock G. Acyclovir-induced renal failure in an obese patient. *Am J Health Syst Pharm.* 2009;66:1288-1291.
2. Naranjo CA, Busto U, Sellers EM, et al. A method for estimating the probability of adverse drug reactions. *Clin Pharmacol Ther.* 1981;30:239-245.
3. Davis RL, Quenzer RW, Weller S, et al. Acyclovir pharmacokinetics in morbid obesity. In: Programs and abstracts of the 31st Interscience Conference on antimicrobial agents and chemotherapy. American Society for Microbiology; 1991; Washington, DC.
4. Acyclovir for injection (package insert). Bedford, OH: Bedford Laboratories™; June 2005.
5. McEvoy GK, ed. Acyclovir. American hospital formulary service drug information. American Society of Health-System Pharmacists; Bethesda, MD; 2010:812–822.

6. Krasny HC, Liao SH, de Miranda P, Laskin OL, Whelton A, Lietman PS. Influence of hemodialysis on acyclovir pharmacokinetics in patients with chronic renal failure. *Am J Med.* 1982;73:202-204.
7. Heintz BH, Matzke GR, Dager WE. Antimicrobial dosing concepts and recommendations for critically ill adult patients receiving continuous renal replacement therapy or intermittent hemodialysis. *Pharmacotherapy.* 2009;29:562-577.
8. Seth SK, Visconti JA, Hebert LA, Krasny HC. Acyclovir pharmacokinetics in a patient on continuous ambulatory peritoneal dialysis. *Clin Pharm.* 1985;4:320-322.
9. Boelaert J, Schurgers M, Daneels R, Van Landuyt HW, Weatherley BC. Multiple dose pharmacokinetics of intravenous acyclovir in patients on continuous ambulatory peritoneal dialysis. *J Antimicrob Chemother.* 1987;20:69-76.
10. Sigaloff KC, de Fijter CW. Herpes zoster-associated encephalitis in a patient undergoing continuous ambulatory peritoneal dialysis: case report and literature review. *Perit Dial Int.* 2007;27:391-394.
11. Boulieu R, Bastien O, Gaillard S, Flamens C. Pharmacokinetics of acyclovir in patients undergoing continuous venovenous hemodialysis. *Ther Drug Monit.* 1997;19:701-704.
12. Khajehdehi P, Jamal JA, Bastani B. Removal of acyclovir during continuous venovenous hemodialysis and hemodiafiltration with high-efficiency membranes. *Clin Nephrol.* 2000; 54:351-355.
13. Pai MP, Bearden DT. Antimicrobial dosing considerations in obese adult patients. *Pharmacotherapy.* 2007;27:1081-1091.
14. Erstad BL. Dosing of medications in morbidly obese patients in the intensive care unit setting. *Intensive Care Med.* 2004;30:18-32.
15. Nicolau DP, Freeman CD, Belliveau PP, Nightingale CH, Ross JW, Quintiliani R. Experience with a once-daily aminoglycoside program administered to 2,184 adult patients. *Antimicrob Agents Chemother.* 1995;39:650-655.
16. Traynor AM, Nafziger AN, Bertino JS Jr. Aminoglycoside dosing weight correction factors for patients of various body sizes. *Antimicrob Agents Chemother.* 1995;39:545-548.
17. Hull JH, Sarubbi FA Jr. Gentamicin serum concentrations: pharmacokinetic predictions. *Ann Intern Med.* 1976;85:183-189.
18. Lesar TS, Rotschafer JC, Strand LM, et al. Gentamicin dosing errors with four commonly used nomograms. *JAMA.* 1982;248:1190-1193.
19. Fish DN. Extended-interval dosing of aminoglycoside antibiotics in critically ill patients. *J Pharm Pract.* 2002;15:85-95.
20. Teigen MM, Duffull S, Dang L, et al. Dosing of gentamicin in patients with end-stage renal disease receiving hemodialysis. *J Clin Pharmacol.* 2006;46:1259-1267.
21. O'Shea S, Duffull S, Johnson DW. Aminoglycosides in hemodialysis patients: is the current practice of post dialysis dosing appropriate? *Semin Dial.* 2009;22:225-230.
22. Dang L, Duffull S. Development of a semimechanistic model to describe the pharmacokinetics of gentamicin in patients receiving hemodialysis. *J Clin Pharmacol.* 2006;46:662-673.
23. Kamel Mohamed OH, Wahba IM, Watnick S, et al. Administration of tobramycin in the beginning of the hemodialysis session: a novel intradialytic dosing regimen. *Clin J Am Soc Nephrol.* 2007;2:694-699.
24. Sowinski KM, Magner SJ, Lucksiri A, et al. Influence of hemodialysis on gentamicin pharmacokinetics, removal during hemodialysis, and recommended dosing. *Clin J Am Soc Nephrol.* 2008;3:355-361.
25. Sampliner R, Perrier D, Powell R, et al. Influence of ascites on tobramycin pharmacokinetics. *J Clin Pharmacol.* 1984;24:43-46.
26. Hampel H, Bynum GD, Zamora E, et al. Risk factors for the development of renal dysfunction in hospitalized patients with cirrhosis. *Am J Gastroenterol.* 2001;96:2206-2210.
27. McCormick PA, Greenslade L, Kibbler CC, et al. A prospective randomized trial of ceftazidime versus netilmicin plus mezlocillin in the empirical therapy of presumed sepsis in cirrhotic patients. *Hepatology.* 1997;25:833-836.

28. Mercer JM, Neyens RR. Aminoglycoside pharmacokinetic parameters in neurocritical care patients undergoing induced hypothermia. *Pharmacotherapy*. 2010;30:654-660.
29. Moore RD, Lietman PS, Smith CR. Clinical response to aminoglycoside therapy: importance of the ratio of peak concentration to minimal inhibitory concentration. *J Infect Dis*. 1987;155: 93-99.
30. Drusano GL, Ambrose PG, Bhavnani SM, et al. Back to the future: using aminoglycosides again and how to dose them optimally. *Clin Infect Dis*. 2007;45:753-760.
31. Taccone FS, Laterre PF, Spapen H, et al. Revisiting the loading dose of amikacin for patients with severe sepsis and septic shock. *Crit Care*. 2010;14:R53.
32. Bailey JA, Virgo KS, DiPiro JT, Nathens AB, Sawyer RG, Mazuski JE. Aminoglycosides for intra-abdominal infection: equal to the challenge? *Surg Infect (Larchmt)*. 2002;3:315-335.
33. Simmen HP, Battaglia H, Kossmann T, et al. Effect of peritoneal fluid pH on outcome of aminoglycoside treatment of intraabdominal infections. *World J Surg*. 1993;17:393-397.
34. Wong PF, Gilliam AD, Kumar S, et al. Antibiotic regimens for secondary peritonitis of gastro-intestinal origin in adults. Cochrane Database Syst Rev. 2005:CD004539.
35. Mingeot-Leclercq MP, Tulkens PM. Aminoglycosides: nephrotoxicity. *Antimicrob Agents Chemother*. 1999;43:1003-1012.
36. Schentag JJ, Meagher AK, Jelliffe RW. Aminoglycosides. In: Burton ME, Shaw LM, Schentag JJ, Evans WE, eds. *Applied Pharmacokinetics & Pharmacodynamics: Principles of Therapeutic Drug Monitoring*. 4th ed. Baltimore: Lippincott Williams & Wilkins; 2006:286-319.
37. Rybak MJ, Albrecht LM, Boike SC, Chandrasekar PH. Nephrotoxicity of vancomycin, alone and with an aminoglycoside. *J Antimicrob Chemother*. 1990;25:679-687.
38. Cosgrove SE, Vigliani GA, Fowler VG Jr, et al. Initial low-dose gentamicin for Staphylococcus aureus bacteremia and endocarditis is nephrotoxic. *Clin Infect Dis*. 2009;48:713-721.
39. Olsen KM, Rudis MI, Rebuck JA, et al. Effect of once-daily dosing vs. multiple daily dosing of tobramycin on enzyme markers of nephrotoxicity. *Crit Care Med*. 2004;32:1678-1682.
40. ter Braak EW, de Vries PJ, et al. Once-daily dosing regimen for aminoglycoside plus beta-lactam combination therapy of serious bacterial infections: comparative trial with netilmicin plus ceftriaxone. *Am J Med*. 1990;89:58-66.
41. Rybak MJ, Abate BJ, Kang SL, Ruffing MJ, Lerner SA, Drusano GL. Prospective evaluation of the effect of an aminoglycoside dosing regimen on rates of observed nephrotoxicity and ototoxicity. *Antimicrob Agents Chemother*. 1999;43:1549-1555.
42. Selimoglu E. Aminoglycoside-induced ototoxicity. *Curr Pharm Des*. 2007;13:119-126.
43. Tablan OC, Reyes MP, Rintelmann WF, et al. Renal and auditory toxicity of high-dose, pro-longed therapy with gentamicin and tobramycin in pseudomonas endocarditis. *J Infect Dis*. 1984;149:257-263.
44. Pavlidis P, Nikolaidis V, Gouveris H, et al. Ototoxicity caused by once- and twice-daily admin-istration of amikacin in rabbits. *Int J Pediatr Otorhinolaryngol*. 2010;74:361-364.
45. Takumida M, Nishida I, Nikaido M, Hirakawa K, Harada Y, Bagger-Sjöbäck D. Effect of dos-ing schedule on aminoglycoside ototoxicity: comparative cochlear ototoxicity of amikacin and isepamicin. *ORL J Otorhinolaryngol Relat Spec*. 1990;52:341-349.
46. Ali MZ, Goetz MB. A meta-analysis of the relative efficacy and toxicity of single daily dosing versus multiple daily dosing of aminoglycosides. *Clin Infect Dis*. 1997;24:796-809.
47. Bailey TC, Little JR, Littenberg B, Reichley RM, Dunagan WC. A meta-analysis of extended-interval dosing versus multiple daily dosing of aminoglycosides. *Clin Infect Dis*. 1997;24: 786-795.
48. Munckhof WJ, Grayson ML, Turnidge JD. A meta-analysis of studies on the safety and effi-cacy of aminoglycosides given either once daily or as divided doses. *J Antimicrob Chemother*. 1996;37:645-663.
49. Tice AD, Rehm SJ, Dalovisio JR, et al. Practice guidelines for outpatient parenteral antimicro-bial therapy. IDSA guidelines. *Clin Infect Dis*. 2004;38:1651-1672.
50. Sha SH, Qiu JH, Schacht J. Aspirin to prevent gentamicin-induced hearing loss. *N Engl J Med*. 2006;354:1856-1857.

51. Feldman L, Efrati S, Eviatar E, et al. Gentamicin-induced ototoxicity in hemodialysis patients is ameliorated by N-acetylcysteine. *Kidney Int.* 2007;7:359-363.

52. Finnell DL, Davis GA, Cropp CD, et al. Validation of the Hartford nomogram in trauma surgery patients. *Ann Pharmacother.* 1998;32:417-421.

53. Toschlog EA, Blount KP, Rotondo MF, et al. Clinical predictors of subtherapeutic aminoglycoside levels in trauma patients undergoing once-daily dosing. *J Trauma.* 2003;55:255-260.

54. Barletta JF, Johnson SB, Nix DE, Nix LC, Erstad BL. Population pharmacokinetics of aminoglycosides in critically ill trauma patients on once-daily regimens. *J Trauma.* 2000;49: 869-872.

55. Buijk SE, Mouton JW, Gyssens IC, Verbrugh HA, Bruining HA. Experience with a once-daily dosing program of aminoglycosides in critically ill patients. *Intensive Care Med.* 2002;28: 936-942.

56. Bond CA, Raehl CL. Clinical and economic outcomes of pharmacist-managed aminoglycoside or vancomycin therapy. *Am J Health Syst Pharm.* 2005;62:1596-1605.

57. Amphotericin B for injection (package insert). Big Flats, NY: X-GEN Pharmaceuticals, Inc.; April 2010.

58. Amphotericin B cholesteryl sulfate complex (Amphotec®) for injection (package insert). Warrendale, PA: Three Rivers Pharmaceuticals, LLC; January 2009.

59. Amphotericin B lipid complex (Abelcet®) injection (package insert). Bridgewater, NJ: Enzon Pharmaceuticals, Inc.; February 2009.

60. Amphotericin B liposome (Ambisome®) for injection (package insert). Deerfield, IL: Astellas Pharma US, Inc.; October 2008.

61. Morgan DJ, Ching MS, Raymond K, et al. Elimination of amphotericin B in impaired renal function. *Clin Pharmacol Ther.* 1983;34:248-253.

62. Block ER, Bennet JE, Livoti LG, Klein WJ, MacGregor RR, Henderson L. Flucytosine and amphotericin B: hemodialysis effects on the plasma concentration and clearance. Studies in man. *Ann Intern Med.* 1974;80:613-617.

63. Heinemann V, Bosse D, Jehn U, et al. Pharmacokinetics of liposomal amphotericin B (AmBisome®) in critically ill patients. *Antimicrob Agents Chemother.* 1997;41:1275-1280.

64. Wong PN, Lo KY, Tong GM, et al. Treatment of fungal peritonitis with a combination of intravenous amphotericin B and oral flucytosine, and delayed catheter replacement in continuous ambulatory peritoneal dialysis. *Perit Dial Int.* 2008;28:155-162.

65. Muther RS, Bennett WM. Peritoneal clearance of amphotericin B and 5-fluorocytosine. *West J Med.* 1980;133:157-160.

66. Bellmann R, Egger P, Gritsch W, et al. Amphotericin B lipid formulations in critically ill patients on continuous veno-venous haemofiltration. *J Antimicrob Chemother.* 2003;51: 671-681.

67. Humphreys H, Oliver DA, Winter R, Warnock DW. Liposomal amphotericin B and continuous venous-venous haemofiltration. *J Antimicrob Chemother.* 1994;33:1070-1071.

68. McEvoy GK, ed. Amphotericin B. American Hospital Formulary Service Drug Information. American Society of Health-System Pharmacists; Bethesda, MD; 2010:555–566.

69. Rex JH, Steven DA. Systemic antifungal agents: amphotericin B–based preparations. In: Mandell GL, Bennett JE, Dolin R, eds. *Mandell, Douglas, and Bennett's: Principles and Practice of Infectious Diseases*, vol. 1. 7th ed. Philadelphia: Churchill Livingstone Elsevier; 2010:549-553.

70. Laniado-Laborín R, Cabrales-Vargas MN. Amphotericin B: side effects and toxicity. *Rev Iberoam Micol.* 2009;26:223-227.

71. Anidulafungin (Eraxis™) for injection (package insert). New York, NY: Roerig, Division of Pfizer, Inc.; November 2010.

72. Mazzei T, Novelli A. Pharmacological properties of antifungal drugs with a focus on anidulafungin. *Drugs.* 2009;69(Suppl 1):79-90.

73. Sucher AJ, Chahine EB, Balcer HE. Echinocandins: the newest class of antifungals. *Ann Pharmacother.* 2009;43:1647-1657.

74. Menichetti F. Anidulafungin, a new echinocandin: effectiveness and tolerability. *Drugs.* 2009;69(Suppl 1):95-97.

75. McEvoy GK, ed. Anidulafungin. American Hospital Formulary Service Drug Information. American Society of Health-System Pharmacists; Bethesda, MD; 2010:545–547.

76. Caspofungin acetate (Cancidas®) for injection (package insert). Whitehouse Station, NJ: Merck & Co., Inc.; June 2010.

77. Caspofungin summary of product characteristics. Electronic Medicines Compendium (eMC), United Kingdom. http://www.medicines.org.uk/emc/document.aspx?documentId=12843#PRODUCTINFO. July 2009. Accessed June 13, 2010.

78. Nguyen TH, Hoppe-Tichy T, Geiss HK, et al. Factors influencing caspofungin plasma concentrations in patients of a surgical intensive care unit. *J Antimicrob Chemother.* 2007;60:100-106.

79. Kubiak DW, Bryar JM, McDonnell AM, et al. Evaluation of caspofungin or micafungin as empiric antifungal therapy in adult patients with persistent febrile neutropenia: a retrospective, observational, sequential cohort analysis. *Clin Ther.* 2010;32:637-648.

80. Dodds Ashley ES, Lewis R, Lewis JS, Martin C, Andes D. Pharmacology of systemic antifungal agents. *Clin Infect Dis.* 2006;43(Suppl 1):28-39.

81. Lee MC, Ni YW, Wang CH, Lee CH, Wu TW. Caspofungin-induced severe toxic epidermal necrolysis. *Ann Pharmacother.* 2010;44:1116-1118.

82. Lalezari JP, Drew WL, Glutzer E, et al. (S)-1-[3-hydroxy-2-(phosphonylmethoxy)propyl]cytosine (cidofovir): results of a phase I/II study of a novel antiviral nucleotide analogue. *J Infect Dis.* 1995;171:788-796.

83. Cundy KC, Petty BG, Flaherty J, et al. Clinical pharmacokinetics of cidofovir in human immunodeficiency virus-infected patients. *Antimicrob Agents Chemother.* 1995;39:1247-1252.

84. Cidofovir (Vistide®) injection (package insert). Foster City, CA: Gilead Sciences, Inc.; September 2000.

85. Brody SR, Humphreys MH, Gambertoglio JG, Schoenfeld P, Cundy KC, Aweeka FT. Pharmacokinetics of cidofovir in renal insufficiency and in continuous ambulatory peritoneal dialysis or high-flux hemodialysis. *Clin Pharmacol Ther.* 1999;65:21-28.

86. Bernard GR, Vincent JL, Laterre PF, et al. Efficacy and safety of recombinant human activated protein C for severe sepsis. *N Engl J Med.* 2001;344:699-709.

87. Loveland SM, Lewin JJ III, Amabile CM, et al. Obese man treated with drotrecogin alfa (activated). *Ann Pharmacother.* 2003;37:918-919.

88. Levy H, Small D, Heiselman DE, et al. Obesity does not alter the pharmacokinetics of drotrecogin alfa (activated) in severe sepsis. *Ann Pharmacother.* 2005;39:262-267.

89. Macias WL, Dhainaut JF, Yan SC, et al. Pharmacokinetic-pharmacodynamic analysis of drotrecogin alfa (activated) in patients with severe sepsis. *Clin Pharmacol Ther.* 2002;72: 391-402.

90. Xigris® (package insert). Indianapolis, IN: Eli Lilly and Company. October 2008.

91. Böhler J, Donauer J, Keller F. Pharmacokinetic principles during continuous renal replacement therapy: drugs and dosage. *Kidney Int.* 1999;72:S24-S28.

92. Pastores SM. Drotrecogin alfa (activated): a novel therapeutic strategy for severe sepsis. *Postgrad Med J.* 2003;79:5-10.

93. Dhainaut JF, Yan SB, Margolis BD, et al. Drotrecogin alfa (activated) (recombinant human activated protein C) reduces host coagulopathy response in patients with severe sepsis. *Thromb Haemost.* 2003;90:642-653.

94. Martí-Carvajal A, Salanti G, Cardona AF. Human recombinant activated protein C for severe sepsis. *Cochrane Database Syst Rev.* 2008:CD004388.

95. Bernard GR, Macias WL, Joyce DE, et al. Safety assessment of drotrecogin alfa (activated) in the treatment of adult patients with severe sepsis. *Crit Care.* 2003;7:155-163.

96. Camporota L, Wyncoll D. Practical aspects of treatment with drotrecogin alfa (activated). *Crit Care.* 2007;11:S7.

97. Gentry CA, Gross KB, Sud B, et al. Adverse outcomes associated with the use of drotrecogin alfa (activated) in patients with severe sepsis and baseline bleeding precautions. *Crit Care Med.* 2009;37:19-25.

98. Sweeney DA, Natanson C, Eichacker PQ. Recombinant human activated protein C, package labeling, and hemorrhage risks. *Crit Care Med.* 2009;37:327-329.

99. Fry DE, Beilman G, Johnson S, et al. Safety of drotrecogin alfa (activated) in surgical patients with severe sepsis. *Surg Infect (Larchmt).* 2004;5:253-259.

100. Barie PS, Williams MD, McCollam JS, et al. Benefit/risk profile of drotrecogin alfa (activated) in surgical patients with severe sepsis. *Am J Surg.* 2004;188:212-220.

101. Abraham E, Laterre PF, Garg R, et al. Drotrecogin alfa (activated) for adults with severe sepsis and a low risk of death. *N Engl J Med.* 2005;353:1332-1341.

102. Payen D, Sablotzki A, Barie PS, et al. International integrated database for the evaluation of severe sepsis and drotrecogin alfa (activated) therapy: analysis of efficacy and safety data in a large surgical cohort. *Surgery.* 2007;141:548-561.

103. Dellinger RP, Levy MM, Carlet JM, et al. Surviving Sepsis Campaign: international guidelines for management of severe sepsis and septic shock: 2008. *Crit Care Med.* 2008;36: 296-327.

104. Levi M, Levy M, Williams MD, et al. Prophylactic heparin in patients with severe sepsis treated with drotrecogin alfa (activated). *Am J Respir Crit Care Med.* 2007;176:483-490.

105. Bijsterveld NR, Moons AH, Meijers JC, et al. Rebound thrombin generation after heparin therapy in unstable angina: a randomized comparison between unfractionated and low-molecular-weight heparin. *J Am Coll Cardiol.* 2002;39:811-817.

106. Vincent JL, Bernard GR, Beale R, et al. Drotrecogin alfa (activated) treatment in severe sepsis from the global open-label trial ENHANCE: further evidence for survival and safety and implications for early treatment. *Crit Care Med.* 2005;33:2266-2277.

107. Wheeler A, Steingrub J, Schmidt GA, et al. A retrospective observational study of drotrecogin alfa (activated) in adults with severe sepsis: comparison with a controlled clinical trial. *Crit Care Med.* 2008;36:14-23.

108. European Medicines Agency; Xigris (Drotrecogin alfa activated) Prescribing Information; Available from: http://www.ema.europa.eu/docs/en_GB/document_library/EPAR_-_Product_Information/human/000396/WC500058067.pdf. Accessed December 2, 2010.

109. Gillum JG, Johnson M, Lavoie S, Venitz J. Flucytosine dosing in an obese patient with extrameningeal cryptococcal infection. *Pharmacotherapy.* 1995;15(2):251-253.

110. Flucytosine (Ancobon®) (package insert). Aliso Viejo, CA: Valeant™ Pharmaceuticals North America; January 2008.

111. Vermes A, Guchelaar HJ, Dankert J. Flucytosine: a review of its pharmacology, clinical indications, pharmacokinetics, toxicity and drug interactions. *J Antimicrob Chemother.* 2000; 46:171-179.

112. McEvoy GK, ed. Flucytosine. American hospital formulary service drug information. American Society of Health-System Pharmacists; Bethesda, MD; 2010:567–570.

113. Cutler RE, Blair AD, Kelly MR. Flucytosine kinetics in subjects with normal and impaired renal function. *Clin Pharmacol Ther.* 1978;24:333-342.

114. Lau AH, Kronfol NO. Elimination of flucytosine by continuous hemofiltration. *Am J Nephrol.* 1995;15:327-331.

115. Thomson AH, Shankland G, Clareburt C, Binning S. Flucytosine dose requirements in a patient receiving continuous veno-venous haemofiltration. *Intensive Care Med.* 2002;28:999.

116. Block ER. Effect of hepatic insufficiency on 5-fluorocytosine concentrations in serum. *Antimicrob Agents Chemother.* 1973;3:141-142.

117. Foscarnet for injection (package insert). Lake Forest, IL: Hospira, Inc; February 2008.

118. Aweeka FT, Jacobson MA, Martin-Munley S, et al. Effect of renal disease and hemodialysis on foscarnet pharmacokinetics and dosing recommendations. *J Acquir Immune Defic Syndr Hum Retrovirol.* 1999;20:350-357.

119. MacGregor RR, Graziani AL, Weiss R, Grunwald JE, Gambertoglio JG. Successful foscarnet therapy for cytomegalovirus retinitis in an AIDS patient undergoing hemodialysis: rationale for empiric dosing and plasma level monitoring. *J Infect Dis.* 1991;164:785-787.

120. Sam R, Patel SB, Popli A, Leehey DJ, Gambertoglio JG, Ing TS. Removal of foscarnet by hemodialysis using dialysate-side values. *Int J Artif Organs.* 2000;23:165-167.

121. Alexander AC, Akers A, Matzke GR, Aweeka FT, Fraley DS. Disposition of foscarnet during peritoneal dialysis. *Ann Pharmacother*. 1996;30:1106-1109.
122. Deray G, Martinez F, Katlama C, et al. Foscarnet nephrotoxicity; mechanism, incidence, and prevention. *Am J Nephrol*. 1989;9:316-321.
123. Nyberg G, Blohmé I, Persson H, Svalander C. Foscarnet-induced tubulointerstitial nephritis in renal transplant patients. *Transplant Proc*. 1990;22:241.
124. Cacoub P, Deray G, Baumelou A, et al. Acute renal failure induced by foscarnet: 4 cases. *Clin Nephrol*. 1988;29:315-318.
125. Jacobson MA, Crowe S, Levy J, et al. Effect of foscarnet therapy on infection with immuno-deficiency virus in patients with AIDS. *J Infect Dis*. 1988;158:862-865.
126. Wagstaff AJ, Bryson HM. Foscarnet. A reappraisal of its antiviral activity, pharmacokinetic properties and therapeutic use in immunocompromised patients with viral infections. *Drugs*. 1994;48:199-226.
127. Fletcher C, Sawchuk R, Chinnock B, de Miranda P, Balfour HH Jr. Human pharmacokinetics of the antiviral drug DHPG. *Clin Pharmacol Ther*. 1986;40:281-286.
128. Ganciclovir sodium (Cytovene®) for injection (package insert). South San Francisco, CA: Genentech USA, Inc.; February 2010.
129. Czock D, Scholle C, Rasche FM, Schaarschmidt D, Keller F. Pharmacokinetics of valganci-clovir and ganciclovir in renal impairment. *Clin Pharmacol Ther*. 2002;72:142-150.
130. Lake KD, Fletcher CV, Love KR, Brown DC, Joyce LD, Pritzker MR. Ganciclovir pharma-cokinetics during renal impairment. *Antimicrob Agents Chemother*. 1988;32:1899-1900.
131. Sommadossi JP, Bevan R, Ling T, et al. Clinical pharmacokinetics of ganciclovir in patients with normal and impaired renal function. *Rev Infect Dis*. 1988;10(Suppl 3):S507-S514.
132. Swan SK, Munar MY, Wigger MA, Bennett WM. Pharmacokinetics of ganciclovir in a patient undergoing hemodialysis. *Am J Kidney Dis*. 1991;17:69-72.
133. Gando S, Kameue T, Nanzaki S, Hayakawa T, Nakanishi Y. Pharmacokinetics and clearance of ganciclovir during continuous hemodiafiltration. *Crit Care Med*. 1998;26:184-187.
134. Boulieu R, Bastien O, Bleyzac N. Pharmacokinetics of ganciclovir in heart transplant patients undergoing continuous venovenous hemodialysis. *Ther Drug Monit*. 1993;15:105-107.
135. Bastien O, Boulieu R, Bleyzac N, Estanove S. Clinical use of ganciclovir during renal failure and continuous hemodialysis. *Intensive Care Med*. 1994;20:47-48.
136. Gumbo T, Hiemenz J, Ma L, Keirns JJ, Buell DN, Drusano GL. Population pharmacokinetics of micafungin in adult patients. *Diagn Microbiol Infect Dis*. 2008;60:329-331.
137. Micafungin sodium (Mycamine®) for injection (package insert). Deerfield, IL: Astellas Pharma US, Inc.; January 2008.
138. McEvoy GK, ed. Micafungin. American Hospital Formulary Service Drug Information. American Society of Health-System Pharmacists; Bethesda, MD; 2010:552-555.
139. Yoshizawa S, Gotoh M, Kitahara T, et al. Micafungin-induced hemolysis attack due to drug-dependent antibody persisting for more than 6 weeks. *Leuk Res*. 2010;34:e60-e61.
140. Nanri T, Iwanaga E, Fujie S, et al. Micafungin-induced immune hemolysis attacks. *Int J Hematol*. 2009;89:139-141.
141. Kauffman CA, Carver PL. Update on echinocandin antifungals. *Semin Respir Crit Care Med*. 2008;29:211-219.
142. Rybak M, Lomaestro B, Rotschafer JC, et al. Therapeutic monitoring of vancomycin in adult patients: a consensus review of the American Society of Health-System Pharmacists, the Infectious Diseases Society of America, and the Society of Infectious Diseases Pharmacists. *Am J Health Syst Pharm*. 2009;66:82-98.
143. Bauer LA, Black DJ, Lill JS. Vancomycin dosing in morbidly obese patients. *Eur J Clin Pharmacol*. 1998;54:621-625.
144. Blouin RA, Bauer LA, Miller DD, et al. Vancomycin pharmacokinetics in normal and mor-bidly obese subjects. *Antimicrob Agents Chemother*. 1982;21:575-580.
145. Vance-Bryan K, Guay DR, Gilliland SS, et al. Effect of obesity on vancomycin pharmacoki-netic parameters as determined by using a Bayesian forecasting technique. *Antimicrob Agents Chemother*. 1993;37:436-440.

146. Matzke GR, Zhanel GG, Guay DR. Clinical pharmacokinetics of vancomycin. *Clin Pharmacokinet.* 1986;11:257-282.

147. Moellering RC Jr, Krogstad DJ, Greenblatt DJ. Vancomycin therapy in patients with impaired renal function: a nomogram for dosage. *Ann Intern Med.* 1981;94:343-346.

148. Matzke GR, McGory RW, Halstenson CE, et al. Pharmacokinetics of vancomycin in patients with various degrees of renal function. *Antimicrob Agents Chemother.* 1984;25: 433-437.

149. Brown DL, Mauro LS. Vancomycin dosing chart for use in patients with renal impairment. *Am J Kidney Dis.* 1988;11:15-19.

150. Thomson AH, Staatz CE, Tobin CM, et al. Development and evaluation of vancomycin dosage guidelines designed to achieve new target concentrations. *J Antimicrob Chemother.* 2009;63:1050-1057.

151. Pea F, Furlanut M, Negri C, et al. Prospectively validated dosing nomograms for maximizing the pharmacodynamics of vancomycin administered by continuous infusion in critically ill patients. *Antimicrob Agents Chemother.* 2009;53:1863-1867.

152. Polk RE, Espinel-Ingroff A, Lockridge R. In vitro evaluation of a vancomycin radioimmuno-assay and observations on vancomycin pharmacokinetics in dialysis patients. *Drug Intell Clin Pharm.* 1981;15:15-20.

153. Launay-Vacher V, Izzedine H, Mercadal L, et al. Clinical review: use of vancomycin in haemodialysis patients. *Crit Care.* 2002;6:313-316.

154. Pallotta KE, Manley HJ. Vancomycin use in patients requiring hemodialysis: a literature review. *Semin Dial.* 2008;21:63-70.

155. Welage LS, Mason NA, Hoffman EJ, et al. Influence of cellulose triacetate hemodialyzers on vancomycin pharmacokinetics. *J Am Soc Nephrol.* 1995;6:1284-1290.

156. Pai AB, Pai MP. Vancomycin dosing in high flux hemodialysis: a limited-sampling algorithm. *Am J Health Syst Pharm.* 2004;61:1812-1816.

157. Ariano RE, Fine A, Sitar DS, et al. Adequacy of a vancomycin dosing regimen in patients receiving high-flux hemodialysis. *Am J Kidney Dis.* 2005;46:681-687.

158. Brown N, Ho DH, Fong KL, et al. Effects of hepatic function on vancomycin clinical pharmacology. *Antimicrob Agents Chemother.* 1983;23:603-609.

159. Aldaz A, Ortega A, Idoate A, et al. Effects of hepatic function on vancomycin pharmacokinetics in patients with cancer. *Ther Drug Monit.* 2000;22:250-257.

160. Forouzesh A, Moise PA, Sakoulas G. Vancomycin ototoxicity: a reevaluation in an era of increasing doses. *Antimicrob Agents Chemother.* 2009;53:483-486.

161. Brummett RE, Fox KE. Vancomycin- and erythromycin-induced hearing loss in humans. *Antimicrob Agents Chemother.* 1989;33:791-796.

162. Wood CA, Kohlhepp SJ, Kohnen PW, et al. Vancomycin enhancement of experimental tobramycin nephrotoxicity. *Antimicrob Agents Chemother.* 1986;30:20-24.

163. King DW, Smith MA. Proliferative responses observed following vancomycin treatment in renal proximal tubule epithelial cells. *Toxicol In Vitro.* 2004;18:797-803.

164. Nishino Y, Takemura S, Minamiyama Y, et al. Inhibition of vancomycin-induced nephrotoxicity by targeting superoxide dismutase to renal proximal tubule cells in the rat. *Redox Rep.* 2002;7:317-319.

165. Bailie GR, Neal D. Vancomycin ototoxicity and nephrotoxicity. A review. *Med Toxicol Adverse Drug Exp.* 1988;3:376-386.

166. Jeffres MN, Isakow W, Doherty JA, et al. A retrospective analysis of possible renal toxicity associated with vancomycin in patients with health care-associated methicillin-resistant Staphylococcus aureus pneumonia. *Clin Ther.* 2007;29:1107-1115.

167. Hidayat LK, Hsu DI, Quist R, et al. High-dose vancomycin therapy for methicillin-resistant Staphylococcus aureus infections: efficacy and toxicity. *Arch Intern Med.* 2006;166: 2138-2144.

168. Lodise TP, Lomaestro B, Graves J, Drusano GL. Larger vancomycin doses (at least four grams per day) are associated with an increased incidence of nephrotoxicity. *Antimicrob Agents Chemother.* 2008;52:1330-1336.

169. Moise-Broder PA, Forrest A, Birmingham MC, Schentag JJ. Pharmacodynamics of vancomycin and other antimicrobials in patients with Staphylococcus aureus lower respiratory tract infections. *Clin Pharmacokinet*. 2004;43(13):925-942.

170. Haque NZ, Cahuayme Zuniga L, et al. Relationship of vancomycin MIC to mortality in patients with methicillin-resistant Staphylococcus aureus hospital-acquired, ventilator-associated and healthcare-associated pneumonia. *Chest*. 2010;138:1356-1362.

171. Sakoulas G, Moise-Broder PA, Schentag J, et al. Relationship of MIC and bactericidal activity to efficacy of vancomycin for treatment of methicillin-resistant Staphylococcus aureus bacteremia. *J Clin Microbiol*. 2004;42:2398-2402.

172. Soriano A, Marco F, Martínez JA, et al. Influence of vancomycin minimum inhibitory concentration on the treatment of methicillin-resistant Staphylococcus aureus bacteremia. *Clin Infect Dis*. 2008;46:193-200.

173. Wang JL, Wang JT, Sheng WH, et al. Nosocomial methicillin-resistant Staphylococcus aureus (MRSA) bacteremia in Taiwan: mortality analyses and the impact of vancomycin, MIC = 2 mg/L, by the broth microdilution method. *BMC Infect Dis*. 2010;10:159.

174. Lodise TP, Graves J, Evans A, et al. Relationship between vancomycin MIC and failure among patients with methicillin-resistant Staphylococcus aureus bacteremia treated with vancomycin. *Antimicrob Agents Chemother*. 2008;52:3315-3320.

175. Polk RE. Red man syndrome. *Ann Pharmacother*. 1998;32:840.

176. Polk RE, Healy DP, Schwartz LB, et al. Vancomycin and the red-man syndrome: pharmacodynamics of histamine release. *J Infect Dis*. 1988;157:502-507.

177. Sivagnanam S, Deleu D. Red man syndrome. *Crit Care*. 2003;7:119-120.

178. Healy DP, Sahai JV, Fuller SH, et al. Vancomycin-induced histamine release and "red man syndrome": comparison of 1- and 2-hour infusions. *Antimicrob Agents Chemother*. 1990;34:550-554.

179. Von Drygalski A, Curtis BR, Bougie DW, et al. Vancomycin-induced immune thrombocytopenia. *N Engl J Med*. 2007;356:904-910.

180. Pea F, Porreca L, Baraldo M, et al. High vancomycin dosage regimens required by intensive care unit patients cotreated with drugs to improve haemodynamics following cardiac surgical procedures. *J Antimicrob Chemother*. 2000;45:329-335.

181. Voriconazole (Vfend®) (package insert). New York, NY: Roerig, Division of Pfizer, Inc.; June 2010.

182. Luke DR, Tomaszewski K, Damle B, Schlamm HT. Review of the basic and clinical pharmacology of sulfobutylether-beta-cyclodextrin (SBECD). *J Pharm Sci*. 2010;99:3291-3301.

183. Hafner V, Czock D, Burhenne J, et al. Pharmacokinetics of sulfobutylether-beta-cyclodextrin and voriconazole in patients with end-stage renal failure during treatment with two hemodialysis systems and hemodiafiltration. *Antimicrob Agents Chemother*. 2010;54:2596-2602.

184. Robatel C, Rusca M, Padoin C, Marchetti O, Liaudet L, Buclin T. Disposition of voriconazole during continuous veno-venous hemodiafiltration (CVVHDF) in a single patient. *J Antimicrob Chemother*. 2004;54:269-270.

185. Etravirine (Intelence®) (package insert). Raritan, NJ: Tibotec Therapeutics, Division of Centocor Ortho Biotech Products, L.P.; July 2010.

Chapter 7
Antiarrhythmics

Christopher A. Paciullo

Introduction

Antiarrhythmic medications are used in the prevention and treatment of numerous cardiac diseases in the intensive care unit. Additionally, the critical care practitioner is often faced with the dilemma of patients who are admitted to the intensive care unit on antiarrhythmic medications as an outpatient. Due to the tendency of these agents to cause harm when used in error, the Institute for Safe Medication Practices considers intravenous antiarrhythmics to be high-risk medications. Intravenous antiarrhythmics have a propensity for adverse drug events such as causing arrhythmias, organ dysfunction and hypotension. Therapeutic drug monitoring is important for some of the antiarrhythmics, and most are susceptible to multiple drug interactions. This chapter discusses commonly encountered IV antiarrhythmic agents as well as provides practical considerations on dosing, safety and adverse reactions.

Adenosine

Dosing Considerations

Obesity: No dosage adjustment required.
Thinness/emaciation: No dosage adjustment required.
Kidney Injury: Adenosine is rapidly metabolized by red blood cells and vascular endothelium, and no dosage adjustments are required.

C.A. Paciullo
Department of Pharmaceutical Services, Emory University Hospital, Atlanta, GA, USA
e-mail: christopher.paciullo@emoryhealthcare.org

S.L. Kane-Gill and J. Dasta (eds.),
High-Risk IV Medications in Special Patient Populations,
DOI: 10.1007/978-0-85729-606-1_7, © Springer-Verlag London Limited 2011

Hemodialysis/Continuous Renal Replacement Therapy: No dosage adjustment required.

Liver Dysfunction: No dosage adjustment required.

Hypothermia: There are no data on the effects of hypothermia on adenosine administration.

Safety Concerns

Safety concern	Rationale	Comments/recommendations
Asystole	Rarely, prolonged asystole may occur with adenosine	Epinephrine or atropine are first line agents in the treatment of asystole due to adenosine. Aminophylline may be considered for asystole unresponsive to epinephrine or atropine[1]
Proarrhythmia	Adenosine has been known to induce atrial fibrillation as well as bradyarrhythmias, sinus pauses and ventricular tachycardia (VT)[2]	Continuous electrocardio-gram (EKG) monitoring is necessary when administering adenosine. Advanced life support medications and equipment should be readily available
Patients with central venous access	When administered via central venous access, adenosine may produce complete atrioventricular (AV) nodal blockade	A lower starting dose (3 mg) is advised for patients with central venous access[3]
Peripheral vasodilation	Adenosine causes peripheral vasodilation when administered intravenous (IV) push. Due to adenosine's short half-life this effect is short lived and of little clinical concern. However, the vasodilation also causes patients to experience slight discomfort, manifested as brief chest pain, flushing and shortness of breath[4]	Counsel awake patients on the side effects of adenosine
Bronchospasm	Adenosine causes transient bronchospasm	Caution the use of adenosine in patients with reactive airway disease

Safety concern	Rationale	Comments/recommendations
Heart transplant patients	The denervated donor heart of a heart transplant patient has been found to have enhanced sensitivity to the effects of adenosine[5]	Lower starting doses (3 mg) should be used in patients following heart transplantation
Drug interactions	Addition of adenosine to other medications known to slow AV conduction (non-dihydropyridine calcium channel blockers, beta blockers) may lead to prolonged AV block and sustained bradycardia	Lower doses of adenosine should be attempted first when combining adenosine with other medications known to block AV conduction
	Dipyridamole and carbamazepine potentiate the pharmacologic effect of adenosine, leading to profound bradycardia and chest pain[6,7]	Patients taking dipyridamole or carbamazepine should receive lower starting doses of adenosine (3 mg)
	Methylxanthines (theophylline, caffeine) antagonize the effect of adenosine[8]	Larger initial doses of adenosine may be required when administering adenosine to patients taking theophylline or caffeine

Amiodarone

Dosing Considerations

Obesity: Amiodarone is highly lipophilic and distributes extensively into adipose tissue.[9] Theoretically this may affect the pharmacokinetics of amiodarone in obese patients, but the clinical significance is unknown.

Thinness/emaciation: Due to the highly lipophilic properties of amiodarone, alterations in the pharmacokinetics of amiodarone in extremely underweight patients would be expected, but the clinical significance is unknown.

Kidney Injury: Kidney injury has no effect on the clearance of amiodarone.[10]

Hemodialysis/Continuous Renal Replacement Therapy: Amiodarone and its metabolite are not removed by renal replacement therapy.[10]

Liver Dysfunction: Although no published data exist, it has been suggested that liver disease would decrease the clearance of amiodarone due to its extensive liver metabolism.[11]

Hypothermia: Decreased activity of the P450 enzyme system during hypothermia is well described.[12] Therefore, the decreased clearance of amiodarone during hypothermia would be expected.

Safety Concerns

Safety concern	Rationale	Comments/recommendations
Dysrhythmia	Amiodarone will cause a prolongation of QTc due to its ability to block potassium channels. However, the absolute risk of torsades de pointes (TdP) is low due to amiodarone's multiple electrophysiological effects[13]	Do not discontinue amiodarone if the patient displays a prolonged QTc in the absence of any additional medications that are known to prolong QTc[13]
Hypotension	Intravenous amiodarone has been associated with dose related hypotension.[14] The current parenteral formulation is solubilized with polysorbate-80 and benzyl alcohol, which are thought to be responsible for the hypotensive effect seen with IV amiodarone[15]	Hypotension with IV amiodarone does not preclude treatment with oral amiodarone. Patients who display hypotension after initiation of amiodarone may benefit from a slower infusion rate (<0.5 mg/min) or a change to oral therapy[15]
Acute pulmonary toxicity	Pulmonary toxicity due to amiodarone usually presents after years of chronic therapy, however acute pulmonary toxicity presenting as acute respiratory distress syndrome (ARDS) has been reported.[16,17] Patients undergoing cardiac or lung surgery seem to be at higher risk[18,19]	Patients receiving IV amiodarone who subsequently develop ARDS should have their amiodarone discontinued if other causes of ARDS (i.e., sepsis) have been ruled out
Hepatotoxicity	Long term use of amiodarone has been associated with hepatotoxicty.[20] Short term, intravenous bolus doses have also rarely been suspected of causing an acute hepatitis.[21,22] The cause of acute hepatitis from amiodarone is likely due to the solubilizing agent polysorbate-80, which has been implicated in the hepatotoxic effects of other IV medications[23]	Clinicians should examine all other potential causes of hepatotoxicity before discontinuing amiodarone. Hepatotoxicity from IV amiodarone is likely due to polysorbate-80, and does not preclude treatment with oral amiodarone

Safety concern	Rationale	Comments/recommendations
Drug interactions	Amiodarone interacts with several medications. Drug interactions due to amiodarone usually are due to one of two mechanisms, amiodarone's inhibitory effects on the cytochrome P450 enzyme system (specifically 1A2, 2C9, 2D6 and 3A4) or potentiation of cardiac effects such as bradycardia and/or QTc prolongation	Caution is advised whenever medications known to prolong the QTc interval (i.e., macrolide antibiotics, class Ia antiarrhythmics, first-generation antipsychotics, methadone, fluoroquinolones, and tricyclic antidepressants) are used concurrently with amiodarone. A baseline EKG should be compared with EKGs taken after the second drug is initiated. Clinicians should be aware of additional patient specific risk factors for QTc prolongation and TdP such as elderly patients with underlying heart disease, renal or hepatic dysfunction, electrolyte abnormalities, or bradycardia. Discontinue offending drugs if the QTc prolongs >60 ms above baseline or to >500 ms[13]
		Additionally, drugs that cause AV nodal blockade (beta blockers, non-dihydropyridine calcium channel blockers, digoxin, propafenone, and adenosine) should be used cautiously with amiodarone
	Amiodarone decreases renal and non-renal clearance of digoxin[24]	Empirically decrease digoxin dosage by 50% when initiating amiodarone
	Amiodarone decreases the clearance of phenytoin[25]	Monitor phenytoin serum concentrations and adjust dosage as necessary
	Amiodarone decreases the clearance and increases the free fraction of warfarin[26]	Monitor international normalized ratio (INR) daily when initiating amiodarone, empirically decrease warfarin dose by 25%[20]
	Amiodarone decreases clearance of cyclosporine[27]	Monitor cyclosporine concentrations daily when initiating amiodarone and adjust as necessary
Defibrillation threshold (DFT)	Amiodarone may increase the amount of energy needed during a defibrillation for unstable ventricular tachycardia[28]	Patients undergoing internal cardio defibrillator (ICD) implantation on amiodarone should have their DFT evaluated. Patients with an ICD who are initiated on amiodarone after initial DFT placement should have their DFT threshold re-evaluated[29]

Digoxin

Dosing Considerations

Obesity: Digoxin is widely distributed into skeletal muscle with a high degree of tissue binding. Maintenance doses of digoxin should be based on lean body weight.

Thinness/emaciation: Lower starting dosages of digoxin should be used in patients with low lean body mass (0.0625–0.125 mg) assuming normal renal function.

Kidney Injury: 85% of a digoxin dose is excreted unchanged in the urine. Kidney injury is one of the leading causes of digoxin toxicity.

Hemodialysis/Continuous Renal Replacement Therapy: Due to digoxin's large volume of distribution, it is not effectively removed by hemodialysis or CRRT.

Liver Dysfunction: No dosage change is necessary in patients with liver dysfunction.

Hypothermia: Although hypothermia is not expected to change the pharmacokinetics of digoxin, changes in potassium concentrations during the cooling and rewarming phases may impact the pharmacodynamic effect of digoxin. Careful monitoring of serum potassium during these phases is essential. Practitioners should carefully weigh the potential risks and benefits of continuing digoxin in this patient population.

Safety Concerns

Safety concern	Rationale	Comments/recommendations
Pro-arrhythmia	Digoxin commonly induces several arrhythmias via decreasing conduction through the AV node and increasing automaticity. Premature ventricular contractions, heart block, atrial tachycardia, accelerated junctional rhythms and bidirectional VT have been reported.[30] Arrhythmias caused by digoxin are most commonly at higher serum concentrations (>1.2 ng/mL).[31] Patient specific factors such as decreased renal function, hypokalemia, hypomagnesemia, and hypercalcemia increase the risk of digoxin toxicity	Closely monitor serum concentrations and other factors that can influence changes in serum concentrations (changes in renal function, drug interactions, electrolyte abnormalities and altered pharmacokinetics in critically ill patients)

Safety concern	Rationale	Comments/recommendations
Use in conversion of atrial fibrillation	Digoxin has been given a class III recommendation (procedure/treatment should not be performed/administered since it is not helpful and may be harmful) by the American Heart Association for conversion of atrial fibrillation.[32] Trials of intravenous digoxin have failed to show any efficacy in conversion to sinus rhythm[33,34]	Consider alternative agents for conversion of atrial fibrillation. Digoxin remains an effective alternative agent for ventricular rate control in atrial fibrillation, especially in patients with systolic heart failure
Therapeutic drug monitoring	Blood samples taken during digoxin's distribution phase do not correspond to drug concentrations in the heart[35]	Allow at least 4 h between IV administration and the drawing of blood samples
	High serum concentrations of digoxin (>0.8 ng/mL) have been associated with an increased mortality in patients with heart failure with reduced ejection fraction[31]	Serum digoxin concentrations should be maintained at <0.8 ng/mL in patients with an ejection fraction of <45%
Drug interactions[36]	Amiodarone decreases clearance of digoxin and increases digoxin concentrations by 70–100%	Empirically reduce digoxin dose by 50% when initiating amiodarone
	Quinidine decreases both renal and non-renal clearance of digoxin, as well as decreases digoxin's volume of distribution	Empirically reduce digoxin dose by 50% when initiating quinidine
	Azole antifungals decrease clearance of digoxin	Empirically reduce digoxin dose by 50% when initiating azole antifungals.
	Verapamil decreases clearance of digoxin	Empirically reduce digoxin dose by 50% when initiating verapamil, strongly consider the use of alternative calcium channel blockers
	Potassium wasting diuretics and amphotericin B cause lower serum potassium concentrations	Hypokalemia is the leading cause of digoxin toxicity, patient receiving potassium wasting diuretics with digoxin should have their serum potassium checked frequently and corrected to a normal level
	Macrolide antibiotics increase digoxin bioavailability and decrease renal clearance	Alternative antibiotic regimens or careful monitoring of serum digoxin concentrations during macrolide therapy is warranted

Ibutilide

Dosing Considerations

Obesity: No data exist on the effects of obesity on ibutilide pharmacokinetics.

Thinness/emaciation: Patients with smaller body size are at increased risk of ibutilide induced TdP.[37] Patients weighing <60 kg should be administered a weight-based dose of 0.01 mg/kg.[38]

Kidney Injury: No change of dosage is necessary in renal dysfunction.

Hemodialysis/Continuous Renal Replacement Therapy (CRRT): No data exist on the effects of CRRT on ibutilide pharmacokinetics.

Liver Dysfunction: No data exist on the effects of liver dysfunction on ibutilide metabolism. However, because approximately 90% of a dose of ibutilide is metabolized in the liver, extended monitoring of patients (beyond 4 h) with liver disease receiving ibutilide is recommended.[38]

Hypothermia: No data are available regarding the dosing of ibutilide in hypothermia.

Safety Concerns

Safety concern	Rationale	Comments/recommendations
Ventricular arrhythmia	Sustained and nonsustained monomorphic and polymorphic VT have been reported with the use of ibutilide[39–42]	Continuous EKG monitoring and access to advanced life support medications and equipment is required when administering ibutilide
		Do not administer ibutilide to patients with baseline QTc >440 ms[37]
Heart failure	Patients with known chronic heart failure are at greater risk for ibutilide induced proarrhythmia[37]	Caution the use of ibutilide in patients with chronic heart failure
Electrolyte abnormalities	Hypomagnesemia and hypokalemia may increase the risk of ibutilide-induced torsades de pointes (TdP)	Hypomagnesemia and hypokalemia should be corrected prior to the initiation of ibutilide[38]
Drug interactions	Patients receiving medications known to prolong QTc interval (antipsychotics, antidepressants, erythromycin, fluoroquinolones, methadone) may be at higher risk for ibutilide-induced TdP	Monitor QTc interval before, during, and after ibutilide administration

Safety concern	Rationale	Comments/recommendations
	Concurrent use of class Ia and class III antiarrhythmic medications may increase the risk of ibutilide induced TdP	A four–five half-life washout of previously administered class Ia or class III antiarrhythmics is recommended prior to ibutilide administration. Class Ia or class III antiarrhythmics should not be restarted within 4 h of ibutilide administration[38]

Lidocaine

Dosing Considerations

Obesity: No data exist on the effects of obesity on lidocaine pharmacokinetics.

Thinness/emaciation: Elderly, frail patients are at higher risk for central nervous system (CNS) side effects of lidocaine.[43]

Kidney Injury: Although lidocaine pharmacokinetics are not affected by renal disease, glycinexylidide, a metabolite of lidocaine is excreted renally. Accumulation of this metabolite has lead to central nervous system toxicity (seizures, headache) in animals, but no data exist in humans and no dosage adjustment appears necessary.[44]

Hemodialysis/Continuous Renal Replacement Therapy: No adjustment of lidocaine dosage in necessary during HD.[45] No data exist for the removal of lidocaine by continuous renal replacement.

Liver Dysfunction: Lidocaine is extensively metabolized by the liver. Patients with advanced hepatic disease (Child class B or C) will require dose reduction.[11]

Hypothermia: No data exist regarding the effect of hypothermia on lidocaine metabolism. However, due to the extensive liver metabolism by lidocaine, it would be reasonable to expect a decrease in lidocaine metabolism in hypothermic patients.

Safety Concerns

Safety concern	Rationale	Comments/recommendations
Acute myocardial infarction (AMI)	Observational data have shown that prophylactic use of lidocaine after AMI reduces rates of ventricular fibrillation. However, randomized controlled trials have shown increases in mortality in patients receiving lidocaine after AMI[46,47]	Lidocaine should not be administered after acute myocardial infarction

(continued)

Safety concern	Rationale	Comments/recommendations
Drug interactions	Medications that inhibit cytochrome P450 2D6 (paroxetine, quinidine) and 3A4 (protease inhibitors, azole antifungals, clarithromycin, amiodarone) may increase serum lidocaine concentrations	A decreased dosage of lidocaine may be required when therapy with a P450 2D6 or 3A4 inducer is initiated
	Medications that induce cytochrome P450 2D6 (rifampin) and 3A4 (barbiturates, phenytoin, carbam-azepime) increase the clearance of lidocaine	Increases in dosage may be required when P450 2D6 or 3A4 inducers are added to lidocaine
	Lidocaine potentiates the action of neuromuscular blocking agents and delays recovery from neuromuscular blockade to a varying degree	Practitioners should be aware of the risk of prolonged paralysis when neuromuscular blockers are adminis-tered to patients receiving lidocaine. Additionally, these patients may require lower doses of neuromuscular blocking agents, but no precise dose adjustment has been recommended
	Drugs that reduce hepatic blood flow (i.e., Beta blockers, cimetidine, vasopressors)[48]	Due to the extensive liver metabolism and high hepatic extraction (0.83) of lidocaine, any decrease in hepatic blood flow will cause a decrease in lidocaine clearance. Agents that decrease hepatic blood flow should be avoided or initiated under careful monitoring
CNS toxicity	CNS toxicity is the most common side effect of intravenous lidocaine, which may progress to seizures in severe cases[43]	Monitoring for early signs of central nervous system toxicity (restlessness, anxiety, tinnitus, dizziness, blurred vision, tremors, depression, or drowsi-ness) should be performed routinely while patients are receiving lidocaine infusions

Safety concern	Rationale	Comments/recommendations
Heart failure	Hepatic clearance of lidocaine is dependent on liver blood flow (extraction ratio 0.83). Therefore patients with heart failure have an expected 50% decrease in lidocaine clearance[49]	Reduce maintenance dosage of lidocaine in patients with low cardiac output
Defibrillation threshold	Conflicting data exists regarding the effect of lidocaine on DFT. High doses or prolonged infusions may cause ICD failure[28]	Patients with an ICD on high dose or prolonged lidocaine infusions should have alternative methods for defibrillation readily available

Procainamide

Dosing Considerations

Obesity: The pharmacokinetics of procainamide are similar in obese and normal weight individuals. Ideal body weight should be used for the initial bolus dose as well as the maintenance infusion for procainamide in obese patients.[50]

Thinness/emaciation: There are no reports of dosing considerations in underweight or nutritionally depleted patients.

Kidney Injury: 40–70% of procainamide as well as a significant amount of its active metabolite (N-acetylprocainamide, NAPA) are cleared by the kidneys. A lower initial infusion rate (1–2 mg/min) and more careful monitoring of procainamide and NAPA concentrations are recommended for patients with kidney injury.[51]

Hemodialysis/Continuous Renal Replacement Therapy: Both procainamide and NAPA are significantly removed by conventional hemodialysis. Patients receiving procainamide while on hemodialysis (HD) or continuous renal replacement therapy (CRRT) should have both procainamide and NAPA concentrations measured routinely.[52] Supplemental doses of procainamide after HD should be based on serum concentrations of procainamide and NAPA.

Liver Dysfunction: Studies evaluating the effect of liver dysfunction on clearance of procainamide have yielded conflicting results. Careful monitoring of procainamide and NAPA concentrations is recommended.[11]

Hypothermia: There are no data on the pharmacokinetics of procainamide during hypothermia.

Safety Concerns

Safety concern	Rationale	Comments/recommendations
Administration rate	Fast administration rates (>50 mg/min) lead to peripheral vasodilation and hypotension[53]	Limit administration rates to <50 mg/min
Ester anesthetic allergy	Patients with an ester anesthetic allergy may have cross sensitivity to procainamide	Procainamide is contraindicated in patients with a known allergy to ester anesthetics
Systemic lupus erythematosus (SLE)	Procainamide is known to cause SLE.[54] Patients with SLE would be expected to have an aggravation of their disease	Procainamide is contraindicated in patients with SLE. Patients experiencing signs or symptoms of SLE should have procainamide discontinued immediately
Arrhythmia	QRS prolongation is the most common electrophysiologic adverse effect of procainamide administration. QRS prolongation may lead to VT or TdP[55]	Carefully monitor QRS and QTc interval while patients are on procainamide. Discontinue infusion if QRS becomes >50% of baseline
Agranulocytosis	Agranulocytosis, although rare, it is the most severe reaction to procainamide, with mortality rates of about 20–25%[55]	Patients initiated on procainamide should have routine monitoring of their complete blood counts for the first 12 weeks of therapy. For patients with pre-existing cytopenia, procainamide should not be used
Heart failure	Procainamide is a negative inotrope	Extreme caution should be used if initiating procainamide in patients with left ventricular dysfunction or in combination with other negative inotropic medications (non-dihydropyridine calcium channel blockers, beta blockers)
Therapeutic drug monitoring	Serum concentrations of procainamide and NAPA are available. The therapeutic range of procainamide is 4–10 mcg/mL. The therapeutic range of NAPA is 5–20 mcg/mL[56]	NAPA concentrations can be used to monitor for toxicity more than efficacy. Fast acetylators will have higher concentrations of NAPA than slow acetylators. NAPA concentrations, as compared to procainamide concentrations may be disproportionally increased in patients with renal failure
Drug interactions	Combination therapy with other medications known to prolong QTc may lead to TdP	Monitor QTc closely when initiating additional agents known to prolong QTc (antipsychotics, antidepressants, erythromycin, flouroquinolones, class III antiarrythmics)

Safety concern	Rationale	Comments/recommendations
	Amiodarone decreases procainamide clearance and increases procainamide concentrations by 23–57%[57]	Empirically reduce procainamide dose by 20–30% when initiating amiodarone[57]
	Trimethoprim decreases renal clearance of procainamide and NAPA and increases procainamide concentrations by 37–63%[48,58]	Empirically reduce procainamide dose by 50% when initiating trimethoprim
	Cimetidine decreases renal clearance of procainamide and increases serum concentrations by 30–35%[59]	Measure serum procainamide and NAPA concentrations when initiating cimetidine and adjust infusion accordingly

References

1. Mader TJ, Smithline HA, Durkin L, Scriver G. A randomized controlled trial of intravenous aminophylline for atropine-resistant out-of-hospital asystolic cardiac arrest. *Acad Emerg Med*. 2003;10:192-197.
2. Tisdale JE. Supraventricular arrhythmias. In: Tisdale JE, Miller DA, eds. *Drug Induced Diseases: Prevention, Detection and Management*. 2nd ed. Bethesda: American Society of Health-System Pharmacists; 2010:445-884.
3. Chang M, Wrenn K. Adenosine dose should be less when administered through a central line. *J Emerg Med*. 2002;22:195-198.
4. diMarco JP, Sellers TD, Lerman BB, Greenberg ML, Berne RM, Belardinelli L. Diagnostic and therapeutic use of adenosine in patients with supraventricular tachyarrhythmias. *J Am Coll Cardiol*. 1985;6:417-425.
5. Ellenbogen KA, Thames MD, DiMarco JP, Sheehan H, Lerman BB. Electrophysiological effects of adenosine in the transplanted human heart. Evidence of supersensitivity. *Circulation*. 1990;81:821-828.
6. Emergency Cardiovascular Care Committee, Subcommittees and Task Forces of the American Heart Association guidelines for cardiopulmonary resuscitation and emergency cardiovascular care. *Circulation*. 2005;112:IV1-IV203.
7. German DC, Kredich NM, Bjornsson TD. Oral dipyridamole increases plasma adenosine levels in human beings. *Clin Pharmacol Ther*. 1989;45:80-84.
8. Evoniuk G, von Borstel RW, Wurtman RJ. Antagonism of the cardiovascular effects of adenosine by caffeine or 8-(p-sulfophenyl)theophylline. *J Pharmacol Exp Ther*. 1987;240:428-432.
9. Roden DM. Pharmacokinetics of amiodarone: implications for drug therapy. *Am J Cardiol*. 1993;72:45F-50F.
10. Ujhelyi MR, Klamerus KJ, Vadiei K, et al. Disposition of intravenous amiodarone in subjects with normal and impaired renal function. *J Clin Pharmacol*. 1996;36:122-130.

11. Klotz U. Antiarrhythmics: elimination and dosage considerations in hepatic impairment. *Clin Pharmacokinet*. 2007;46:985-996.
12. Tortorici MA, Kochanek PM, Poloyac SM. Effects of hypothermia on drug disposition, metabolism, and response: a focus of hypothermia-mediated alterations on the cytochrome P450 enzyme system. *Crit Care Med*. 2007;35:2196-2204.
13. Drew BJ, Ackerman MJ, Funk M, et al. Prevention of Torsade de Pointes in hospital settings: a scientific statement from the American Heart Association and the American College of Cardiology Foundation endorsed by the American Association of Critical-Care Nurses and the International Society for Computerized Electrocardiology. *J Am Coll Cardiol*. 2010;55:934-947.
14. Scheinman MM, Levine JH, Cannom DS, et al. Dose-ranging study of intravenous amiodarone in patients with life-threatening ventricular tachyarrhythmias. The intravenous amiodarone Multicenter Investigators Group. *Circulation*. 1995;92:3264-3272.
15. Munoz A, Karila P, Gallay P, et al. A randomized hemodynamic comparison of intravenous amiodarone with and without Tween 80. *Eur Heart J*. 1988;9:142-148.
16. Kaushik S, Hussain A, Clarke P, Lazar HL. Acute pulmonary toxicity after low-dose amiodarone therapy. *Ann Thorac Surg*. 2001;72:1760-1761.
17. Skroubis G, Galiatsou E, Metafratzi Z, Karahaliou A, Kitsakos A, Nakos G. Amiodarone-induced acute lung toxicity in an ICU setting. *Acta Anaesthesiol Scand*. 2005;49:569-571.
18. Ashrafian H, Davey P. Is amiodarone an underrecognized cause of acute respiratory failure in the ICU? *Chest*. 2001;120:275-282.
19. Van Mieghem W, Coolen L, Malysse I, Lacquet LM, Deneffe GJ, Demedts MG. Amiodarone and the development of ARDS after lung surgery. *Chest*. 1994;105:1642-1645.
20. Loke YK, Derry S, Aronson JK. A comparison of three different sources of data in assessing the frequencies of adverse reactions to amiodarone. *Br J Clin Pharmacol*. 2004;57:616-621.
21. Giannattasio F, Salvio A, Varriale M, Picciotto FP, Di Costanzo GG, Visconti M. Three cases of severe acute hepatitis after parenteral administration of amiodarone: the active ingredient is not the only agent responsible for hepatotoxicity. *Ann Ital Med Int*. 2002;17:180-184.
22. Ratz Bravo AE, Drewe J, Schlienger RG, Krahenbuhl S, Pargger H, Ummenhofer W. Hepatotoxicity during rapid intravenous loading with amiodarone: description of three cases and review of the literature. *Crit Care Med*. 2005;33:128-134; discussion 245–246.
23. Rhodes A, Eastwood JB, Smith SA. Early acute hepatitis with parenteral amiodarone: a toxic effect of the vehicle? *Gut*. 1993;34:565-566.
24. Fenster PE, White NW Jr, Hanson CD. Pharmacokinetic evaluation of the digoxin-amiodarone interaction. *J Am Coll Cardiol*. 1985;5:108-112.
25. Nolan PE Jr, Erstad BL, Hoyer GL, Bliss M, Gear K, Marcus FI. Steady-state interaction between amiodarone and phenytoin in normal subjects. *Am J Cardiol*. 1990;65:1252-1257.
26. Martinowitz U, Rabinovich J, Goldfarb D, Many A, Bank H. Interaction between warfarin sodium and amiodarone. *N Engl J Med*. 1981;304:671-672.
27. Nicolau DP, Uber WE, Crumbley AJ III, Strange C. Amiodarone-cyclosporine interaction in a heart transplant patient. *J Heart Lung Transplant*. 1992;11:564-568.
28. Dopp AL, Miller JM, Tisdale JE. Effect of drugs on defibrillation capacity. *Drugs*. 2008;68:607-630.
29. Leong-Sit P, Gula LJ, Diamantouros P, et al. Effect of defibrillation testing on management during implantable cardioverter-defibrillator implantation. *Am Heart J*. 2006;152:1104-1108.
30. Ma G, Brady WJ, Pollack M, Chan TC. Electrocardiographic manifestations: digitalis toxicity. *J Emerg Med*. 2001;20:145-152.
31. Rathore SS, Curtis JP, Wang Y, Bristow MR, Krumholz HM. Association of serum digoxin concentration and outcomes in patients with heart failure. *JAMA*. 2003;289:871-878.
32. Fuster V, Ryden LE, Cannom DS, et al. ACC/AHA/ESC 2006 guidelines for the management of patients with atrial fibrillation: a report of the American College of Cardiology/American Heart Association Task Force on practice guidelines and the European Society of Cardiology Committee for practice guidelines (Writing Committee to revise the 2001 guidelines for the management of patients with atrial fibrillation): developed in collaboration with the European Heart Rhythm Association and the Heart Rhythm Society. *Circulation*. 2006;114:e257-e354.

33. The Digitalis in Acute Atrial Fibrillation (DAAF) Trial Group. Intravenous digoxin in acute atrial fibrillation. Results of a randomized, placebo-controlled multicentre trial in 239 patients. *Eur Heart J.* 1997;18:649-54.
34. Falk RH, Knowlton AA, Bernard SA, Gotlieb NE, Battinelli NJ. Digoxin for converting recent-onset atrial fibrillation to sinus rhythm. A randomized, double-blinded trial. *Ann Intern Med.* 1987;106:503-506.
35. Valdes R Jr, Jortani SA, Gheorghiade M. Standards of laboratory practice: cardiac drug monitoring. National Academy of Clinical Biochemistry. *Clin Chem.* 1998;44:1096-1109.
36. Tamargo J, Delpon E, Caballero R. The safety of digoxin as a pharmacological treatment of atrial fibrillation. *Expert Opin Drug Saf.* 2006;5:453-467.
37. Kowey PR, VanderLugt JT, Luderer JR. Safety and risk/benefit analysis of ibutilide for acute conversion of atrial fibrillation/flutter. *Am J Cardiol.* 1996;78:46-52.
38. Product Information: Corvert (ibutilide). New York, NY: Pharmacia & Upjohn Company; 2006.
39. Stambler BS, Wood MA, Ellenbogen KA. Antiarrhythmic actions of intravenous ibutilide compared with procainamide during human atrial flutter and fibrillation: electrophysiological determinants of enhanced conversion efficacy. *Circulation.* 1997;96:4298-4306.
40. Stambler BS, Wood MA, Ellenbogen KA, Perry KT, Wakefield LK, VanderLugt JT. Efficacy and safety of repeated intravenous doses of ibutilide for rapid conversion of atrial flutter or fibrillation. Ibutilide Repeat Dose Study Investigators. *Circulation.* 1996;94:1613-1621.
41. Volgman AS, Carberry PA, Stambler B, et al. Conversion efficacy and safety of intravenous ibutilide compared with intravenous procainamide in patients with atrial flutter or fibrillation. *J Am Coll Cardiol.* 1998;31:1414-1419.
42. Vos MA, Golitsyn SR, Stangl K, et al. Superiority of ibutilide (a new class III agent) over DL-sotalol in converting atrial flutter and atrial fibrillation. The Ibutilide/Sotalol Comparator Study Group. *Heart.* 1998;79:568-575.
43. DeToledo JC. Lidocaine and seizures. *Ther Drug Monit.* 2000;22:320-322.
44. Waller ES. Pharmacokinetic principles of lidocaine dosing in relation to disease state. *J Clin Pharmacol.* 1981;21:181-194.
45. Jacobi J, McGory RW, McCoy H, Matzke GR. Hemodialysis clearance of total and unbound lidocaine. *Clin Pharm.* 1983;2:54-57.
46. Hine LK, Laird N, Hewitt P, Chalmers TC. Meta-analytic evidence against prophylactic use of lidocaine in acute myocardial infarction. *Arch Intern Med.* 1989;149:2694-2698.
47. MacMahon S, Collins R, Peto R, Koster RW, Yusuf S. Effects of prophylactic lidocaine in suspected acute myocardial infarction. An overview of results from the randomized, controlled trials. *JAMA.* 1988;260:1910-1916.
48. Trujillo TC, Nolan PE. Antiarrhythmic agents: drug interactions of clinical significance. *Drug Saf.* 2000;23:509-532.
49. Rodighiero V. Effects of cardiovascular disease on pharmacokinetics. *Cardiovasc Drugs Ther.* 1989;3:711-730.
50. Christoff PB, Conti DR, Naylor C, Jusko WJ. Procainamide disposition in obesity. *Drug Intell Clin Pharm.* 1983;17:516-522.
51. Bauer LA, Black D, Gensler A, Sprinkle J. Influence of age, renal function and heart failure on procainamide clearance and n-acetylprocainamide serum concentrations. *Int J Clin Pharmacol Ther Toxicol.* 1989;27:213-216.
52. Gibson TP, Lowenthal DT, Nelson HA, Briggs WA. Elimination of procainamide in end stage renal failure. *Clin Pharmacol Ther.* 1975;17:321-329.
53. Gonzalez ER, Ornato JP. Procainamide-induced hypotension during CPR. *Clin Pharm.* 1985;4:504-505.
54. Tan EM, Rubin RL. Autoallergic reactions induced by procainamide. *J Allergy Clin Immunol.* 1984;74:631-634.
55. Kim SY, Benowitz NL. Poisoning due to class IA antiarrhythmic drugs. Quinidine, procainamide and disopyramide. *Drug Saf.* 1990;5:393-420.
56. Giardina EG. Procainamide: clinical pharmacology and efficacy against ventricular arrhythmias. *Ann NY Acad Sci.* 1984;432:177-188.

57. Windle J, Prystowsky EN, Miles WM, Heger JJ. Pharmacokinetic and electrophysiologic interactions of amiodarone and procainamide. *Clin Pharmacol Ther*. 1987;41:603-610.
58. Kosoglou T, Rocci ML Jr, Vlasses PH. Trimethoprim alters the disposition of procainamide and N-acetylprocainamide. *Clin Pharmacol Ther*. 1988;44:467-477.
59. Christian CD Jr, Meredith CG, Speeg KV Jr. Cimetidine inhibits renal procainamide clearance. *Clin Pharmacol Ther*. 1984;36:221-227.

Chapter 8
Antihypertensives and Prostanoids

Pamela L. Smithburger and Sandra L. Kane-Gill

Introduction

Acute hypertension managed with intravenous antihypertensives has an all-cause in-hospital mortality rate of nearly 7%; with 59% of patients developing worsening organ dysfunction.[1] The cost of hypertension associated with a secondary diagnosis in hospitalized patients is $2,734.[2] Currently, national treatment guidelines for acute hypertension are not available for adult intensive care unit (ICU) patients. Recently, a survey was conducted to evaluate the management of acute hypertension.[3] This survey discovered that only 8.2% of responders had a guideline in place to treat acute hypertension in non-stroke patients. There is also substantial variability in the intravenous agents selected to treat acute hypertension.[1,3] In regards to the number of patients admitted to the ICU with acute hypertension, physicians surveyed reported that approximately five patients are admitted with a hypertensive emergency to their ICU each month and approximately the same number develop a hypertensive emergency during their ICU stay.[3] With the frequency of acute hypertension and the safety concerns associated with intravenous antihypertensive agents, a review of the medications commonly used in the ICU to treat acute hypertension in special populations was conducted.

Pulmonary arterial hypertension, a debilitating disease of the lung vasculature, is associated with a poor prognosis if left untreated.[4] Although no curative drug therapy has been developed, recent advancements have been shown to improve survival and quality of life.[5,6] One class of medications that has impacted quality of life and

P.L. Smithburger (✉)
Department of Pharmacy and Therapeutics, University of Pittsburgh,
Pittsburgh, PA, USA
e-mail: smithburgerpl@upmc.edu

S.L. Kane-Gill and J. Dasta (eds.),
High-Risk IV Medications in Special Patient Populations,
DOI:10.1007/978-0-85729-606-1_8, © Springer-Verlag London Limited 2011

survival is the prostanoids. This medication class contains potent vasodilators that posses antithrombotic, antiproliferative, and anti-inflammatory properties.[7] Three prostacyclin analogues are available in the United States. They include epoprostenol, treprosinil, and iloprost. Complex dosing regimens, detailed patient administration instructions, coupled with complex pharmacokinetics and possible life threatening adverse effects necessitate a closer review of these agents.[8]

Esmolol

Dosing Considerations

Obesity: Esmolol requires weight-based dosing; however, studies have not examined dosing changes in obese patients. It is recommended to not exceed a maintenance dose of 200 mcg/kg/min as a precaution to avoid hypotension. Bolus doses range from 50 to 500 mcg/kg administered over 1-min.[7]

Thinness/emaciation: Esmolol requires weight-based dosing; however, studies have not examined dosing changes in nutritionally depleted patients.

Kidney Injury: Only 2% of the dose administered of the parent drug is excreted unchanged in the urine. The free acid metabolite, ASL-8123, is excreted in the urine. The elimination half-life of 3.7 h is increased about ten-fold. ASL-8123 has 1500-fold less beta-blocking activity than the parent compound and has not resulted in significant toxicity in humans.[9,10] There are no specific dosing changes recommended for patients with kidney injury.[11] It is reasonable to increase monitoring in patients with substantial renal dysfunction receiving high doses for a long duration of time due to the accumulation of the acid metabolite.

Hemodialysis: The elimination half-life of the parent compound remains unchanged in patients receiving hemodialysis or peritoneal dialysis. The elimination half-life of the metabolite ASL-8123 is ten-fold greater in patients receiving hemodialysis or peritoneal dialysis.[9,10] ASL-8123 has not resulted in significant toxicity in humans. Dosing alterations are not likely necessary in patients receiving either hemodialysis or peritoneal dialysis.

Liver Failure: Esmolol is primarily metabolized by nonspecific blood esterases. Pharmacokinetic parameters (total body clearance, elimination half-life and volume of distribution) for esmolol and its metabolite were not significantly different in a small sample of patients with liver disease (Laennec's cirrhosis) compared to controls.[12] Dosing changes do not appear to be required for patients with liver disease.

Safety Concerns

Safety concern	Rationale	Comments/recommendations
Contraindications	Esmolol is a beta-1 selective adrenergic receptor blocking agent	Esmolol is contraindicated in patients with sinus bradycardia, heart block greater than first degree, cardiogenic shock or overt heart failure[13]
Heart failure	Esmolol has negative inotropic effects, slows AV conduction, and could potentiate hypotension and bradycardia in heart failure patients[13]	Esmolol should be used with caution in patients with congestive heart failure. If beta-blockade therapy is necessary, begin at low dosages. If signs or symptoms of heart failure develop, esmolol should be discontinued[13-17]
Hypotension	20–50% of patients experience hypotension in clinical trials.[16] This effect can be exacerbated when administered with other antihypertensive and vasodilatory agents	Esmolol has a short half-life of 9 min. Discontinuation of the drug should result in return to baseline hemodynamic parameters within 30-min[18,19]
Drug interactions (this is not an all inclusive list of potential drug interactions)	Digoxin concomitant administration results in a 10–20% increase in digoxin concentrations in healthy volunteers; however no changes in blood pressure or heart rate occurred. Esmolol pharmacokinetics were not altered[20]	Esmolol and digoxin have been used for purposes of rate control in atrial fibrillation and atrial flutter safely.[21] Monitor digoxin concentrations during prolonged administration of esmolol
	Drugs with negative inotropic effects such as diltiazem and verapamil could potentiate the negative intotropic effects of esmolol[22]	Monitor blood pressure and heart rate
	Drugs with beta-blocking activity such as metoprolol and amiodarone could result in additive effects on hemodynamics[23]	Monitor blood pressure and heart rate
	Morphine can increase the steady state concentrations of esmolol by 46%[20]	Monitor blood pressure and heart rate

Labetalol

Dosing Considerations

Obesity: Labetalol pharmacokinetics have been evaluated in a small sample of obese patients. There was a trend toward a larger volume of distribution compared to normal volunteers; however, this did not appear to be due to a greater distribution in adipose tissue, so other factors contribute to this pharmacokinetic difference.[24] The area under the curve, clearance and half-life did not differ between the obese patients and normal volunteers. Dosing adjustments are not recommended in this population. Labetalol dosing is not typically weight based.

Thinness/emaciation: Labetalol studies have not examined dosing changes in nutritionally depleted patients

Kidney Injury: In patients with chronic renal dysfunction, the half-life and volume of distribution are similar to controls.[25-27] Also, clinical experience in several patients with varying degrees of renal dysfunction revealed labetalol dosing does not require adjustments.[26] Labetalol has no active metabolites.[28,29]

Dialysis: A minimal amount of labetalol is removed by hemodialysis and peritoneal dialysis so supplemental dosing should be unnecessary.[30]

Liver Dysfunction: The pharmacokinetic parameters of oral and intravenous labetalol were studied in patients with chronic liver failure. Oral administration is not the focus of this book, but dosing adjustment is required. In contrast, intravenous administration of labetalol does not require dosing adjustment. The area under the plasma concentration time curve and half-life were not significantly different between patients with chronic liver failure and healthy controls.[31]

Safety Concerns

Safety concern	Rationale	Comments/recommendations
Contraindications	Non-selective beta-blocker with alpha-1 activity	Labetalol is contraindicated in patients with bronchial asthma, overt cardiac failure, greater than first-degree heart block, cardiogenic shock, severe bradycardia, other conditions associated with severe and prolonged hypotension[29]
Maximum intravenous dose		300 mg/day[32]
Hypotension	Higher doses associated with substantial drop in blood pressure	Avoid bolus doses > 1 mg/kg[33,34]

Safety concern	Rationale	Comments/recommendations
Postural hypotension and dizziness[35,36]	Non-selective beta-blocker with alpha-1 activity	Most common (up to 58%) adverse effect of labetalol. When initiating labetalol therapy be sure that changes between sitting to standing or standing to lying are done slowly[28,29]
Congestive heart failure/ acute left ventricular failure	Negative inotropic effect limiting applicability in this patient population[35]	Use with caution in patients with a history of congestive heart failure
Hepatic injury	Unclear	Hepatic injury is not common and is typically reversible[37,38]
Drug interactions (this is not an all inclusive list of potential drug interactions)	Drugs with negative inotropic effects (diltiazem, verapamil)[22]	Monitor blood pressure and heart rate
	Drugs with beta-blocking activity (metoprolol, amiodarone)[23]	Monitor blood pressure and heart rate
	Labetalol blunts the reflex tachycardia associated with nitroglycerin[29]	Monitor blood pressure and heart rate
	Effect of bronchodilator can be blunted by non-selective beta-blockers	Monitor need for bronchodilator. Additional doses may be necessary

Metoprolol

Dosing Considerations

Obesity: The volume of distribution of metoprolol is increased in patients with obesity because metoprolol is a lipid soluble drug. However, the increased volume of distribution has not shown to impact the antihypertensive effects of the drug.[29] It is also reported that beta blockers, in general, can cause weight gain due to a reduction in basal metabolic rate and energy expenditure and an impairment of glucose tolerance.[39,40]

Kidney Injury: No dose adjustment is needed in patients with acute or chronic renal dysfunction.[41-43]

Hemodialysis/CRRT: No dose adjustment is needed in patients receiving dialytic therapies.[41-43] It is recommended that patients should receive their maintenance dose after the dialysis session.[44]

Liver Dysfunction: Metoprolol is metabolized by the liver; however, there is a lack of clinical information to recommend dosage adjustments.[41,45]

Safety Concerns

Safety concern	Rationale	Comments/recommendations
Bronchospasm/wheezing	Caution should be used in patients with a history of bronchospastic diseases[41]	Metoprolol is a beta-1 selective beta-blocker; however, caution should still be used due to the possibility to of beta-2 blockade. The lowest effective dose should be used
History of heart block	Metoprolol is contraindicated in patients with second and third degree heart block and in patients with significant first degree heart block (PR interval ≥ 0.24 s). Metoprolol slows AV conduction, and may produce first, second or third degree heart block[41]	If heart block occurs, metoprolol should be discontinued and atropine should be administered to the patient if necessary[41]
Acute heart failure and history of heart failure	Metoprolol is contraindicated in patients with overt cardiac failure. Metoprolol has the potential to further depress myocardial contractility in patients with a history of heart failure and may lead to additional cardiac failure	Careful monitoring is needed when initiating therapy or increasing doses in patients with a history of heart failure. If heart failure occurs or persists despite treatment, therapy should be discontinued[41]
Withdrawal	Abrupt withdrawal from metoprolol therapy causes rebound hypertension and in patients with angina pectoris, myocardial infarction, serious arrhythmias, and sudden death has occurred[41,46-48]	A gradual tapering of the beta blocker may help avoid these reactions. Tapering should occur over 1–2 weeks to avoid tachycardia, hypertension and/or ischemia. If angina worsens or coronary insufficiency worsens, metoprolol should be restarted[41,46-48]

Clevidipine

Dosing Considerations

Obesity: There are no reports of dosing considerations in obese patients. Individualized dosing should be based upon the blood pressure response.[49]

Thinness/emaciation: There are no reports of dosing considerations in under-weight/nutritionally deplete patients. Individualized dosing should be based upon the blood pressure response.[49]

Kidney Injury: Patients with kidney injury were not specifically studied in clinical trials. However, the manufacturer reports that 121 patients with moderate to severe renal failure did receive clevidipine in various clinical trials, and a dose of 1–2 mg/h was appropriate in these patients.[49] Clevidipine is metabolized by esterases in the blood to inactive metabolites which are eliminated in the urine and feces. Therefore, clevidipine clearance is unlikely affected by renal dysfunction.[50,51]

Hemodialysis/CRRT: There is no information available for clevidipine administration in patients receiving hemodialysis or continuous renal replacement therapy.

Liver Dysfunction: Patients with liver dysfunction were not specifically studied in clinical trials. However, the package insert reports that 78 patients with abnormal hepatic function (with the presence of one or more of the following: elevated serum bilirubin, AST/SGOT, ALT/SGPT) did receive clevidipine in clinical trials, and a dose of 1–2 mg/h has been found to be appropriate in these patients.[49] Clevidipine is metabolized by esterases in the blood to inactive metabolites which are eliminated in the urine and feces. Therefore clevidipine metabolism should not be affected by liver dysfunction.[50,51]

Patients with Disorders of Lipid Metabolism: Clevidipine contains approximately 0.2 g of lipid per mL (2.0 kcal). Therefore, additional lipid intake may need to be reduced while receiving clevidipine.

Hypothermia: The clearance of clevidipine is lower and its terminal elimination half-life is prolonged during hypothermic cardiopulmonary bypass.[52,53]

Safety Concerns

Safety concern	Rationale	Comments/recommendations
Increased triglycerides	Clevidipine contains phospholipids, consisting of approximately 0.2 g of lipid per mL. Clevidipine is contraindicated in patients with defective lipid metabolism.[49] Due to the lipid emulsion, clevidipine may increase triglyceride concentrations.[54] However, in the VELOCITY trial, long term infusion of clevidipine did not alter the median percentage of change in triglyceride concentrations. In the ECLIPSE trials, no specific data on the effect of clevidipine on triglycerides were provided. The investigators did state that the changes in triglycerides were similar between the clevidipine and comparator groups[55]	Patients with disorders of lipid metabolism may need to have a reduction of their lipid intake while receiving clevidipine. Clevidipine is also contraindicated in patients with pathologic hyperlipidemia, lipoid nephrosis, or acute pancreatitis if it is accompanied with hyperlipidemia.[49] The total lipid load should be assessed in patients also receiving Intralipid or propofol

(continued)

Safety concern	Rationale	Comments/recommendations
Rebound hypertension	Patients receiving clevidipine for a prolonged time and are not transitioned to other antihypertensive agents may develop rebound hypertension up to 8 h after the clevidipine infusion has been stopped[49]	Patients not transitioned to oral antihypertensive therapy should be monitored for at least 8 h after the clevidipine infusion has stopped[49]
Reflex tachycardia	An increase in mean heart rate has been observed in both healthy adult males (from 53 to 72 beats per minute) and patients in clinical trials. Patients treated with clevidipine in the ESCAPE-1 trial had a 18% vs. 10% occurrence of tachycardia compared to the placebo group[56-58]	If reflex tachycardia occurs, it is recommended to decrease the dose of clevidipine. Beta blockers are not recommended to be used to correct the reflex tachycardia[49]
Oral conversion	The short elimination half-life of clevidipine requires starting an oral antihypertensive before the antihypertensive effect of clevidipine has ended	The oral antihypertensive agent can be administered 1–2 h before stopping clevidipine, depending on the pharmacokinetics of the oral antihypertensive[59]
Need for aseptic technique	Clevidipine is a single use parenteral product that may support bacterial growth due to its formulation of phospholipids and the lack of a microbial retardant.[49] However, clinical trials have not reported infections in the patients using this product[54,55,57]	The package insert recommends that once the stopper is punctured, unused product, including what is being infused, be discarded after 4 h[49]
Drug-compatibility data	Clevidipine should not be administered in the same line as other medications[49]	Currently, compatibility data are not available for clevidipine and precipitation would be difficult to detect due to clevidipine's milky white appearance[49,50]
Drug interactions	Because of its pharmacokinetic properties, clevidipine has a low potential to interact with drugs that are metabolized through cytochrome P450.[49,60] Pharmacodynamic interactions could be a concern with compounded or additive effects with the administration of drugs known to reduce blood pressure	An in-vitro study suggests that it is not likely that cytochrome p450 enzymes would be induced or inhibited by clevidipine or its metabolite at therapeutic concentrations.[49,60] In-vivo drug interaction data are currently unavailable.[51] Care should be taken if it is necessary to administer clevidipine with another drug that may result in additional blood pressure lowering effects
Contraindications	Several contraindications exist	Allergy to eggs or soy; Defective lipid metabolism; severe aortic stenosis[49]

Enalaprilat

Dosing Considerations

Obesity: There are no reports of dosing considerations in obese patients. It is recommended that continuous monitoring of the blood pressure and heart rate be conducted during use of enalaprilat. Individualized dosing should be based upon the resulting blood pressure.[61]

Thinness/emaciation: There are no reports of dosing considerations in underweight or nutritionally depleted patients. It is recommended that continuous monitoring of the blood pressure and heart rate be conducted during use of enalaprilat. Individualized dosing should be based upon the blood pressure obtained.[61]

Kidney Injury: Most angiotensin-converting enzyme (ACE) inhibitors and their metabolites are excreted by the kidney, and usually require reduction in dosage when administered to patients with renal dysfunction. When the patient's creatinine clearance is ≤ 30 mL/min the peak and trough concentrations of enalaprilat concentrations increase, as does the time to achieve steady state. The elimination half-life of enalaprilat is also increased when creatinine clearance is ≤ 30 mL/min.[61-64] Case reports reveal profound, refractory hypotension when enalaprilat is given to a patient with renal artery stenosis.[65]

Hemodialysis/CRRT: Enalaprilat is removed by hemodialysis. In one study, plasma concentrations fell by an average of $45.7 \pm 11.5\%$ over a 4 h hemodialysis session.[64] Enalaprilat is dialyzable at a rate of 62 mL/min.[61] It is recommended to administer the dose after hemodialysis.

Pregnancy: Enalaprilat is a rated pregnancy category C during the 1st trimester and a pregnancy category D during the 2nd and 3rd trimester.

African Americans: Controlled clinical trials have demonstrated that ACE inhibitors, in general, have less effect on blood pressure as monotherapy in African American patients than non-African Americans.[66,67] It is also thought that the adverse effects of cough and angioedema are more prevalent in African Americans treated with ACE inhibitors compared to other populations.[68,69]

Safety Concerns

Safety concern	Rationale	Comments/recommendations
Angioedema	Angioedema associated with laryngeal edema may be fatal and has been associated with enalaprilat use.[61] This is seen more commonly in African American patients[68,69]	If angioedema of the face, tongue, lips, glottis, and/or larynx occurs, enalaprilat should be discontinued immediately and appropriate therapy should be initiated[61]

(continued)

Safety concern	Rationale	Comments/recommendations
		This medication is contraindicated in patients that have previously experienced angioedema with an ACE inhibitor or have hereditary or idiopathic angioedema
Hepatic failure	Cholestatic jaundice, which may progress to Fulminant hepatic necrosis has been reported with ACE inhibitor therapy[61,70,71]	If a patient receiving an ACE inhibitor develops jaundice or elevations in hepatic enzymes, the ACE inhibitor should be discontinued[61,70]
Hypotension associated with concurrent diuretic use	There is a pharmacodynamic drug interaction with patients concurrently taking diuretic therapy with enalaprilat. These patients may experience a greater reduction in blood pressure than those receiving enalaprilat monotherapy[61]	Consideration should be given to discontinuing the diuretic therapy, increasing salt intake prior to enalaprilat administration or administering an intravenous infusion of normal saline[61]
Increased serum potassium	ACE inhibitors increase serum potassium concentrations. When used in combination with a potassium sparing diuretic, such as spironolactone, or potassium supplementation, markedly elevated serum potassium concentrations may result[61]	Use caution when concurrently administrating potassium-sparing diuretics, potassium supplements, or potassium containing salt substitutes. Frequent monitoring of serum potassium concentrations may be indicated if concurrent use of the above agents is necessary[61]
Compatibility and stability	Concern for incompatibility	Enalaprilat is compatible and stable for 24 h when mixed with the following solutions: 5% Dextrose; 0.9% Sodium Chloride; 0.9% Sodium Chloride in 5% Dextrose; 5% Dextrose in Lactated ringers[61]

Hydralazine

Dosing Considerations

Obesity: There are no reports of dosing considerations in obese patients.

Thinness/emaciation: There are no reports of dosing considerations in underweight or nutritionally depleted patients

Kidney Injury: A prolongation of the dosing interval or a lower dose may be necessary in patients with a creatinine clearance < 50 mL/min. Blood pressure should also be checked more frequently in these patients.[72,73]

Hemodialysis/CRRT: For patients receiving intermittent hemodialysis, doses should be given after the dialysis session. In patients receiving continuous renal replacement therapy, patients should be dosed as if they had a creatinine clearance of 10–50 mL/min and titrate based upon blood pressure.[72,73]

Liver dysfunction: No recommendations are made regarding dosing in liver dysfunction.

Pregnancy: Hydralazine is rated Pregnancy category C. This medication should be used during pregnancy if the benefits outweigh the risks to the fetus.[72]

Elderly: Lower starting doses are recommended in the elderly because they may experience more orthostatic hypotension and impairment of motor function than younger individuals.[74]

Safety Concerns

Safety concern	Rationale	Comments/recommendations
Drug-induced lupus erythematosus	Case reports have described the development of drug-induced lupus with the use of hydralazine. Risk factors include: female gender; slow acetylator; high daily doses; therapy longer than 3 months; family history of autoimmune diseases[72,75]	Patients should be closely monitored when initiating therapy, especially during chronic therapy. Skeletal muscle symptoms are the most common manifestation of hydralazine-induced systemic lupus[75]
Reflex tachycardia	Tachycardia is reflexively induced and the magnitude is related to the sensitivity of baroreceptors[72,76]	Reflex tachycardia can be minimized by administering hydralazine with a beta blocker, such as propranolol[72]
Contraindications	Hypersensitivity to hydralazine; coronary artery disease; mitral valvular rheumatic heart disease[72]	Hydralazine has been implicated in myocardial ischemia and infarction in patients with known coronary artery disease[72,77,78]
Administration	After the vial of hydralazine is opened it should be used immediately and it should not be added to infusion solutions. Hydralazine hydrochloride may become discolored when it comes into contact with metal. Discolored solutions should be discarded[72]	

Nicardipine

Dosing Considerations

Obesity: No dosing recommendations in obese patients are available. It has been shown that nicardipine has no effect on glucose tolerance, and release of insulin and glucagon in obese patients.[79,80]

Thinness/Emaciation: No dosing recommendations in thin/emaciated patients have been made.[79,80]

Kidney Injury (acute, chronic): The plasma clearance of nicardipine is slower and the area under the curve and maximum concentration are greater in patients with renal dysfunction. Caution should be used when initiating or increasing doses in this patient population.[81]

Hemodialysis: Dialysis does not affect nicardipine pharmacokinetics and additional doses following dialysis sessions are not necessary.[81]

Liver dysfunction: Due to the extensive hepatic metabolism of nicardipine, higher peak blood pressure decreases and serum concentrations are found in patients with hepatic dysfunction.[81,82] Clinicians should consider slow titration of dosing and use lower doses when initiating therapy. Nicardipine has also been reported to increase hepatic venous pressure in patients with cirrhosis. Caution should be used in patients with portal hypertension.[81]

Neurovascular conditions: Nicardipine has been recommended as the first-line agent to treat hypertension in patient with ischemic stroke, intracerebral hemorrhage, craniotomy, and spinal surgery. It appears that this recommendation is based on clinical opinion and there are limited randomized controlled data to support its use. Selection of a first-line antihypertensive agent remains controversial.[83]

Pregnancy/breast feeding: Pregnancy category C. Significant concentrations of nicardipine have been ofund in maternal mile. Therefore, it is recommended to not use nicardipine if breast feeding.[81]

Safety Concerns

Safety concern	Rationale	Comments/recommendations
Headache	Headache is the most commonly reported adverse reaction and occurs in 14.6% of patients[81]	Decrease rate if possible and treat symptoms
Hypotension	Hypotension occurs in 5.6% of patients[81]	Closely monitor blood pressure during therapy. Reduce the rate of infusion and administer intravenous fluids as appropriate

Safety concern	Rationale	Comments/recommendations
Tachyarrhythmia	Tachyarrhythmias have been reported to occur in up to 3.5% of patients. In one report, severe maternal tachycardia occurred in 2 out of 20 patients receiving nicardipine for pre-eclampsia[81,84]	It is recommended to reduce the infusion rate if tachyarrhythmias occur. The use of beta-blockers to control heart rate has also been shown to be effective.[84] Tachycardia may result in angina and or a myocardial infarction in patients with coronary artery disease, Additional care should be used in this patient population
Nausea/Vomiting	Nausea/vomiting is reported to occur in 4.9% of patients[81]	Decrease rate if possible and treat symptoms
Contraindication	Hypersensitivity to the drug; Advanced aortic stenosis[81]	Reduced diastolic pressure may worsen myocardial oxygen balance[81]
Peripheral vein irritation	Phlebitis at the injection site is reported to occur with IV administration[81]	Vein irritation can be minimized if the nicardipine infusion site is changed every 12 h. The pH of the Cardene™ premixed injection is between 3.7 and 4.7[81]

Nitroglycerin

Dosing Considerations

Obesity: A study was conducted that compared the effectiveness of nitroglycerin in obese and lean rats. It was found that the pharmacodynamics of nitroglycerin are not affected by adipose tissue, therefore dose adjustments should not be necessary.[85] Currently there are no human data.

Elderly: The elderly are more susceptible to adverse effects, including hypotension and bradycardia. Therefore, it is recommended that lower doses should be used initially to minimize the development of adverse effects.[86,87]

Hemodialysis/CRRT: There is no information available for nitroglycerin administration in patients receiving hemodialysis or continuous renal replacement therapy.[88]

Safety Concerns

Safety concern	Rationale	Comments/recommendations
Methemoglobinemia	Nitrate ions that are liberated during metabolism of nitroglycerin can oxidize hemoglobin into methemoglobin[88]	This diagnosis should be suspected in patients that exhibit signs of impaired oxygen delivery and have adequate cardiac output and arterial PO_2.[88]
Hypotension	In an evaluation of antihypertensive use in clincial practice, 5% of patients had subsequent hypotension and nitroglycerin was the most common cause[89] Even at low doses, severe hypotension can occur Elderly patients are at an increased risk for hypotension	Severe hypotension may be treated by the administration of IV fluids. Due to the short duration of hemodynamic effects of nitroglycerin, additional measures may not be necessary. However, if additional therapy is indicated, administration of an IV adrenergic agonist should be considered
Headache	Most common side effect which occurs between 50% and 63% of the time.[88] About 10–20% of patients are unable to tolerate the nausea and prostration from the nitrate-induced headaches.[90] Nitroglycerin may also provoke a migraine headache in patients with a personal or family history of migraine attacks[91]	If headaches occur, dose reduction should be attempted. Headaches usually disappear within several days of continued treatment[92]
Administration: adsorption of nitroglycerin into plastics, particularly polyvinyl chloride (PVC)	Increased adsorption of nitroglycerin by PVC tubing occurs when the tubing is long, the flow rates are low, and the nitroglycerin concentration of the solution is high. The delivered percentage of drug has been reported to be as low as 20% when PVC tubing has been used. Some in-line intravenous filters also have been shown to adsorb nitroglycerin[88]	Due to these issues of adsorption, nitroglycerin injection administration should monitored when PVC tubing is used, as drug delivery will increase over time as tubing becomes saturated[88] The nitroglycerin concentration should not exceed 400 mcg/mL
Development of tolerance	Blood pressure lowering effects of a continuous infusion of nitroglycerin have been lost after 24 h.[93] To avoid the development of tolerance to nitroglycerin, it is recommended that drug free intervals occur[88]	Studies have shown that nitrates need to absent from the body for several hours for their anti-anginal effects to become restored after tolerance develops
Drug-compatibility data	Concern for diluent incompatibilities	Dilute in Dextrose 5% or Normal Saline 0.9%

Safety concern	Rationale	Comments/recommendations
Drug interactions	Amplification of vasodilatory effects and the possibility of resulting in severe hypotension when administered with a phosphodiesterase five inhibitor (i.e., sildenafil)[88,94]	Confirm the patient has not taken a phosphodiesterase inhibitor in the past 24 h before administering nitroglycerin
	Concurrent use of nitroglycerin with heparin has lead to a decrease in the partial thromboplastin time (PTT). A rebound effect in the PTT has also been observed upon discontinuation of the nitroglycerin[88]	It is recommended to closely monitor the PTT and the heparin dose while nitroglycerin is co-administered with heparin
Contraindications	Pericardial tamponade, restrictive cardiomyopathy, or constrictive pericarditis, conditions whereby cardiac output is dependent upon venous return[88]	Avoid use of nitroglycerin
Storage/Stability	Concern for drug degradation	Nitroglycerin should be protected from light and kept in its carton until use[88]

Nitroprusside

Dosing Considerations

Obesity: Data are not available for dosing in obese patients.

Thinness/Emaciation: Data are not available for dosing in underweight patients.

Kidney Injury (acute, chronic): Approximately 44% of nitroprusside consists of cyanide which becomes free cyanide upon administration. Cyanide is then converted to cyanocobalamin or thiocyanate. Thiocyanate is excreted via the kidneys and can accumulate in patients with renal injury.[95,96] Caution should be used when administering nitroprusside to patients with kidney injury and should probably be avoided in patients with a glomerular filtration rate of less than 10 mL/min.[97]

Hemodialysis/CRRT: Data evaluating the removal of nitroprusside via hemodialysis are not available but should probably be avoided due to the concern for cyanide toxicity.[97] Cyanide is not removed via dialysis. The removal of thiocyanate is approximately the blood flow rate of the dialyzer.[98] Thiocyanate is rapidly removed by continuous venovenous hemodialfiltration.[99]

Liver Dysfunction: The free cyanide (cyanogens) is converted to thiocyanate by thiosulfate sulfurtransferase, an enzyme in the liver. This conversion is dependent on the availability of sulfur donors such as thiosulfate, cystine or cysteine. Patients with hepatic injury can accumulate cyanide. Caution should be used when administering nitroprusside to patients with hepatic injury.[96] Specific dosing recommendations are not available.

Hypothermia: Cyanide to thiocyanate conversion could be slowed during hypothermia increasing the risk for cyanide toxicity.[100,101]

Safety Concerns

Safety concern	Rationale	Comments/recommendations
Contraindications	Increases intracranial pressure by dilating cerebral vessels Significant reduction in regional blood flow (coronary steal) can occur in patients with coronary artery disease[34,103]	Avoid in patients with hypertensive encephalopathy and cerebrovascular accident and coronary artery disease[34,102]
Hypotension	Potent peripheral (arterial and venous) vasodilator	Use intra-arterial monitoring of blood pressure
Maximum dose	10 mcg/kg/min results in significant concerns of cyanide toxicity since the human body cannot convert and remove cyanide as quickly as administered	Monitor for cyanide toxicity in doses above 4 mcg/kg/min for greater than 2–3 h.[104] Use nitroprusside for as minimal time as possible and in doses not greater then 2 mcg/kg/min when possible. An infusion of thiosulfate should be considered in patients receiving doses between 4 and 10 mcg/kg/min[34]
Patients who smoke	Tobacco contains cyanide and theoretically the combination can increase cyanide concentrations[95]	Monitor signs of cyanide toxicity including confusion, dyspnea, headache, hyperreflexia, tinnitus, seizures and metabolic acidosis
Hypoalbuminemia	Impairs cyanide detoxification[95]	Monitor signs of cyanide toxicity including confusion, dyspnea, headache, hyperreflexia, tinnitus, seizures and metabolic acidosis
Hypertensive emergency in the presence of acute myocardial infarction	Nitroprusside administration within 9 h of the onset of chest pain in patients with acute myocardial ischemia and elevated left ventricular filling pressure is associated with an increased mortality[105,106]	Avoid nitroprusside administration within close proximity to the occurrence of a myocardial infarction

Safety concern	Rationale	Comments/recommendations
Cardiopulmonary bypass	Cyanide detoxification is slowed since plasma thiosulfate concentrations are decreased in patients during and immediately after cardiopulmonary bypass surgery.[95,107] Another proposed mechanism is that the hemolysis occurring during cardiopulmonary surgery catalyzes the release of free cyanide[108]	Use with caution during cardiopulmonary bypass. Monitor signs of cyanide toxicity including confusion, dyspnea hyperreflexia, headache, tinnitus, seizures and metabolic acidosis

Epoprostenol

Dosing Considerations

Obesity: Thinness/emaciation: There are no reports of dosing considerations in the obese or underweight patient. However, the short half-life of the drug would most likely not allow for much distribution and therefore would not be expected to distribute in adipose tissue.[109]

Kidney Injury: There are no reports of dosing considerations in patients with kidney dysfunction

Hemodialysis/CRRT: Dosing considerations of epoprostenol during dialysis are not available. Prostacyclin analogs inhibit platelet aggregation which may lasts up to 2 h after epoprostenol administration. Studies have been conducted that evaluate the prostacylcin analog as the sole anti-hemostatic agent during continuous and intermittent hemodialysis.[109-114]

Liver Dysfunction: Dosing considerations are not available for patients with liver dysfunction, however, there are reports detailing the use of epoprostenol in patients with porto-pulmonary hypertension waiting for liver transplantation.[115,116]

Pregnancy: Epoprostenol is rated pregnancy category B for all trimesters, however, there have been no well-controlled studies in humans. It is recommended that epoprostenol only be used during pregnancy if needed.[109]

Elderly: During clinical trials epoprostenol, there were not enough patients >65 years of age to determine if they react differently to drug therapy than younger patients. However, it is recommended that older patients should be started on therapy at the lower end of the dosing range (package insert).[109]

Safety Concerns

Safety concern	Rationale	Comments/recommendations
Most common dose-limiting adverse effects	Flushing (58%) ; headache (49%); Nausea/vomiting (32%); hypotension (16%); Chest pain (11%); Anxiety, nervousness, agitation (11%)[109]	Some adverse effects may be attributable to the underlying disease state. However during chronic therapy, the occurrence of dose-limited adverse drug events may require a decrease in the infusion rate. However, some adverse events may occasionally resolve without dose adjustment. Dose reductions should be made in increments of 2 ng/kg/min every 15 min until the adverse effect resolves. Do not abruptly discontinue epoprostenol[109]
Avoid abrupt disruptions or large dose reductions	An abrupt withdrawal of drug delivery, such as in a ambulatory pump malfunction, or large reduction in infusion rate may result in rebound pulmonary hypertension[109]	Symptoms of rebound pulmonary hypertension include; dyspnea, dizziness, and asthenia. In one clinical trial, the death of one patient was attributed to an abrupt withdrawal of therapy[5,109,117]
Local infection attributable to drug delivery system	Upon evaluating 7 centers, individual center blood stream infection rates ranged from 0.23 to 1.02 per 1,000 medicine days[118] Another investigation reported rates of 0.24 per person-year for local infections and 70 episodes or 0.14 per person-year incidence of sepsis[5]	Sterile preparation of the reconstituted medication as well as infection control of the central venous catheter are important in the prevention of sepsis and blood stream infections[109,118,119]
Drug delivery system for chronic infusions	Due to its short half-life, epoprostenol must be administered as a continuous infusion. Chronic infusions of epoprostenol should be administered through a central venous catheter by an ambulatory infusion pump. However, a temporary peripheral intravenous infusion may be used until central venous access can be established[109]	It is recommended that the patient have access to a back-up infusion device to avoid potential interruptions in of drug delivery.[109]

Safety concern	Rationale	Comments/recommendations
Storage/Stability	Flolan® is supplied as a freeze-dried powder which must be diluted with "sterile diluent for Flolan®" It must not be mixed with any other parenteral medications or solutions. The reconstituted solutions must be protected from light and stored in a cold pouch at temperatures between 2 and 8 C for 12 h. Reconstituted solutions should be discarded if not used 48 h after reconstitution[109]	During use, a reconstituted solution can be used at room temperature for up to 8 h. If used with a cold pack, the drug can be administered up to 24 h[109]

Iloprost

Dosing Considerations

Obesity: Thinness/ Emaciation: There are no reports of dosing considerations in the obese or underweight patient.

Kidney Injury: Iloprost is metabolized to an inactive metabolite that is found in the urine. Iloprost has not been evaluated in patients with renal disease. Therefore no dosing recommendations are available.

Hemodialysis/CRRT: The effect of dialysis on iloprost exposure has not been evaluated, therefore no dosing recommendations are available.

Liver Dysfunction: Iloprost is primarily metabolized by Beta-oxidation. The cytochrome P450 enzyme system only has a minor role in its metabolism. The metabolism of iloprost is thought to be reduced in patients with Child Pugh Class B or C hepatic impairment, therefore it is recommended that the dosing interval be increased depending upon the patient's response at the end of the dosing interval.

Pregnancy: Iloprost has been shown to be teratogenic in rats, and therefore is a given a Pregnancy category C rating. This medication should only be used during pregnancy if the benefit of therapy outweighs the risk.[120]

Elderly: During clinical trials, there were insufficient numbers of subjects ≥65 years old to see if there is difference in response. However, based upon the greater frequency of hepatic, renal, and/or cardiac dysfunction associated with this age group, it is recommended to start at the lower end of the dosing range and titrate slowly.[120]

Pulmonary Disease: Iloprost induces bronchospasm. Although iloprost has not been evaluated in patients with hyperactive airway diseases, such as asthma, chronic obstructive pulmonary disease, or acute pulmonary infections, it is thought that bronchospasm may be more severe or occur more frequently in these patient populations.[120]

Safety Concerns

Safety concern	Rationale	Comments/recommendations
Most common Dose-limiting Adverse Effects	Flushing (18%); cough (13%); headache (10%); trismus (9%); insomnia (6%); nausea (5%); hypotension (5%)[120]	Several adverse reactions are the result of irritation to the respiratory tract including, cough, bronchospasm, and wheezing. Epistaxis and gingival bleeding have been reported with use of inhaled iloprost[120]
Administration	Iloprost can be administered by inhalation through 2 pulmonary drug devices: the I-neb® ADD® System or the Prodose® ADD® system. Iloprost is supplied as 1 mL glass ampules that either contain 10 mcg/mL or 20 mcg/mL. Iloprost should be inhaled in dosing intervals not less than 2 h. Patients may adjust intervals to cover planned activities. In patients that experience extended treatment time, the 20 mcg/mL concentration should be considered because this will decrease treatment times	The ampules should be broken with a rubber pad or an ampule breaker to avoid injury. Dispose of the top of the ampule in a sharps container. After the solution is drawn-up from the ampule, the open ampule should be disposed of in a sharps container. After each inhalation session, the remaining solution in the ampule should be discarded. Patients should clean the inhalation device according to the manufacturer's instructions. Patients should have access to a back-up inhalation device to avoid interruption in therapy if there is equipment malfunction[120]
Storage/Stability	Do not mix other medications with inhaled iloprost in the inhalation device. Ampules and the remaining solution should be discarded after each inhalation session. should be discarded after each	Ventavis® is supplied as cartons of 30 × 1 mL clear single-use ampules. They should be stored at room temperature

Treprostinil -Injection

Dosing Considerations

Obesity; Thinness/emaciation: There are no reports of dosing considerations in the obese or underweight patient. However, the short half-life of the drug would most likely not allow for much distribution and therefore would not be expected to distribute in adipose tissue.[121]

Kidney Injury: No studies have been conducted in patients with renal insufficiency, however, it is recommended to titrate the dose slower in this patient population.[121]

Hemodialysis/CRRT: Dosing information in this patient population is not available.

Liver dysfunction: Treprostinil is metabolized primarily in the liver by CYP2C8 to four inactive metabolites, hence the clearance of treprostinil is reduced in patients with hepatic insufficiency. The initial dose should be decreased in patients with mild or moderate hepatic insufficiency. It is also recommended to titrate the dose slower in this patient population.[121] One case series describes the safe and effective use of intravenous treprostinil therapy in three patients with end-stage liver disease.[122]

Subcutaneous vs. intravenous injection: Subcutaneous infusion is the preferred mode of administration, however, intravenous administration should be used if the subcutaneous infusion is not tolerated.[121] The subcutaneous mode of administration of treprostinil was completely absorbed and results in a slightly longer half-life than the intravenous route. (subcutaneous half-life = 1.38 h vs. 0.87 h for intravenous injection).[123] Based upon pharmacokinetic assessments, the two routes of administration are considered bioequivalent at steady state.[124]

Pregnancy: Pregnancy category B.[121]

Safety Concerns

Safety concern	Rationale	Comments/recommendations
Most common dose-limiting adverse effects	Infusion site pain (85%); infusion site reaction (83%); headache (27%); diarrhea (25%); nausea (22%); rash (14%); jaw pain (13%); edema (9%)[121]	Infusion site reactions were sometimes severe and may lead to discontinuation of the drug. Pain at the infusion site has been a major drawback of subcutaneous administration, which has lead to impaired dose titration resulting in a 10% discontinuation rate.[125] Other adverse reactions (diarrhea, jaw pain, edema) are generally considered related to the pharmacologic effects of the drug.[121] Each side effect should be evaluated for frequency, duration, intensity, location and correlation with the increased dose of treprostinil

(continued)

Safety concern	Rationale	Comments/recommendations
Local infection attributable to Drug delivery system	The administration of treprostinil with a chronic indwelling catheter is associated with an increased risk of bloodstream infections and sepsis. Subcutaneous administration of treprostinil is the preferred route of administration[126]	Sterile preparation of the reconstituted medication as well as infection control of the central venous catheter is important in the prevention of sepsis and bloodstream infections.[121] A recent report by the Centers for Disease Control and Prevention raised the concern for an increase in bloodstream infections, specifically with gram-negative organisms in patients receiving intravenous treprostinil. The overall infection rate was higher in patients treated with treprostinil than epoprostenol[118,119]
Drug-drug interactions	Treprostinil does not induce or inhibit the metabolism of cytochrome P450 enzymes. However, it is a substrate of the CYP2C8 isoenzyme. When treprostinil is co-administered with a CYP 2C8 inhibitor (i.e., gemfibrozil) the metabolism of treprostinil is reduced, and when it administered with a CYP 2C8 inducer (rifampin), the metabolism of treprostinil is increased[121]	Clinicians should be aware when concomitant administration of a CYP 2C8 enzyme inhibitor or inducer is given with treprostinil therapy. The addition of a CYP 2C8 inhibitor may result in increased treprostinil concentrations and may increase the adverse effects associated with treprostinil administration. When treprostinil is co-administered with a CYP 2C8 inducer, the result may be a decreased concentration of treprostinil, leading to a reduction in clinical efficacy[121]
	Pharmacodynamic interactions include the concomitant use of diuretics, antihypertensives or vasodilators, which may result in symptomatic hypotension	Pharmacodynamic interactions are also possible. The clinician should monitor for the development of symptomatic hypotension when diuretics, antihypertensive agents or vasodilators are given in combination with treprostinil
	Treprostinil inhibits platelet aggregation, therefore there is an increased risk of bleeding when anticoagulants or anti-platelet agents are given with treprostinil	Patients taking anticoagulants and antiplatelet agents should also be monitored for signs and symptoms of bleeding when theses agents are taken with treprostinil due to the platelet inhibitory properties of treprostinil

Safety concern	Rationale	Comments/recommendations
Drug delivery system for chronic infusions: subcutaneous administration	Due to the properties of treprostinil, including a neutral pH, being stable at room temperature, and possessing a longer half-life when administered chronically, this prostanoid is administered as a subcutaneous infusion. Treprostinil can be administered subcutaneously by a self-inserted subcutaneous catheter and using an infusion pump designed for subcutaneous drug delivery. For subcutaneous administration, no further dilution of the treprostinil is needed	Avoid abrupt disruptions or large dose reductions to prevent rebound pulmonary hypertension. It is recommended that the patient have access to a back-up infusion device to avoid potential interruptions in of drug delivery. However, the 4 h half-life imparts greater safety than the shorter half-life of epoprostenol[121]
Drug delivery system for chronic infusions: intravenous administration	Treprostinil may also be administered intravenously. A surgically implanted indwelling catheter is necessary, however, a peripheral intravenous cannula may be used for short-term administration. Treprostinil must be diluted with either sterile water for injection or 0.9% normal saline or Flolan® sterile diluent for injection when used intravenously[121]	Although treprostinil has a longer half-life than epoprostenol, patients should avoid abrupt disruptions or large dose reductions. It is recommended that the patient have access to a back-up infusion device to avoid potential interruptions of drug delivery[121]
Storage/Stability	Treprostinil has greater chemical stability than epoprostenol, which allows for subcutaneous administration	For intravenous administration, treprostinil must be diluted before being administered, however, the diluted treprostinil is stable at room temperature for up to 48 h, which negates the need for ice packs and daily reconstitution. Subcutaneously administered treprostinil is administered without further dilution and can be administered up to 72 h at 37°C[121,127]

Treprostinil-Inhalation

Additional Dosing Considerations for Inhalation Administration

Pulmonary Disease or Pulmonary Infections: It is recommended that patients with acute pulmonary infections be monitored closely to identify any decline in lung function or the loss of drug effect. Safety and efficacy of inhaled treprostinil has not been established in patients with underlying lung disease. (package insert)

Safety Concerns

Safety concern	Rationale	Comments/recommendations
Most common dose-limiting adverse effects	Cough (54%); headache (41%); throat irritation (25%); nausea (19%); flushing (17%) syncope (6%)[128]	Several adverse reactions are the result of irritation to the respiratory tract. In the open-label study section, serious adverse reactions included eight cases of pneumonia, and three episodes of hemoptysis[128]
Administration	Inhaled treprostinil (Tyvaso®) should only be administered with the Tyvaso® Inhalation System. Treprostinil should be administered 4 times daily during waking hours, and can be adjusted for planned activities. Patients will use 1 ampule per day Each session will take 2–3 min and consist of 1–9 breaths of treprostinil per session depending upon patient dose. Patients should clean the inhalation system once daily after the last use[128,129]	Tyvaso® ampules are a sterile formulation that are supplied in a foil pouch. One ampule should be used daily, and at the conclusion of the day, the remaining solution should be discarded If treatment is missed or interrupted, therapy should be resumed as soon as possible Patients should have access to a back-up inhalation device to avoid interruption in therapy if there is an equipment malfunction[128]
Storage/Stability	Do not mix other medications with inhaled treprostinil in the inhalation device. Compatibility studies have not been completed[128]	The Tyvaso® ampules are stored in a foil pack. Once the foil pack is opened, the ampules should be used within 7 days. Tyvaso® is light sensitive, therefore unopened ampules should be protected from light and remain in the foil pouch[128]

References

1. Katz JN, Gore JM, Amin A, et al. on behalf of the STAT Investigators. Practice patterns, outcomes, and end-organ dysfunction for patients with acute severe hypertension: results from the Studying the Treatment of Acute hyper Tension Registry. *Am Heart J.* 2009;158:599-606.

2. Wang G, Zhang Z, Ayala C. Hospitalization costs associated with hypertension as a secondary diagnosis among insured patients aged 18–64 years. *Am J Hypertens.* 2010;23:275-281.

3. Benson J, Gerlach A, Dasta J. National survey of acute hypertension management. *Crit Care Shock.* 2008;11:154-166.

4. Humbert M, Sitbon O, Simonneau G. Treatment of pulmonary arterial hypertension. *N Engl J Med.* 2004;351(14):1425-1436.

5. McLaughlin VV, Shillington A, Rich S. Survival in primary pulmonary hypertension: the impact of epoprostenol therapy. *Circulation.* 2002;106(12):1477-1482.

6. Barst RJ, Rubin LJ, Long WA, McGoon MD, et al. A comparison of continuous intravenous epoprostenol (prostacyclin) with conventional therapy for primary pulmonary hypertension. The Primary Pulmonary Hypertension Study Group. *N Engl J Med.* 1996;334(5):296-302.

7. Gokhman R, Smithburger PL, Seybert AL, Kane-Gill SL. Pharmacokinetic Rationale for Combination Therapy in Pulmonary Arterial Hypertension. *J Cardiovasc Pharmacol* 2010;56(6):686-695.

8. Gessler T, Seeger W, Schmehl T. Inhaled prostainaoids in the therapy of pulmonary hypertension. *J Aerosol Med Pulm Drug Deliv.* 2008;21(1):1-12.

9. Flaherty JF, Wong B, LaFollette G, Warnock DG, Julse JD, Gambertoglio JG. Pharmacokinetics of esmolol and ASL-8123 in renal failure. *Clin Pharmacol Ther.* 1989;45:321-327.

10. Turlapaty P, Laddu A, Murthy VS, Singh B, Lee R. Esmolol: a titratable short-acting intravenous beta blocker for acute critical care settings. *Am Heart J.* 1987;114:866-885.

11. Lowenthal DT, Porter S, Saris SD, et al. Clinical pharmacology, pharmacodynamics and interactions with esmolol. *Am J Cardiol.* 1985;56:14F-18F.

12. Buchi KN, Rollins DE, Tolman KG, et al. Pharmacokinetics of esmolol in hepatic disease. *J Clin Pharmacol.* 1987;27:880-884.

13. Esmolol hydrochloride injection (package insert). Bedford, OH: Bedford Laboratories, Inc.; August 2008.

14. Hunt SA, Abraham WT, Chin MH, et al. ACC/AHA 2005 guideline update for the diagnosis and management of chronic heart failure in the adult: a report of the American College of Cardiology/American Heart Association Task Force on Practice Guidelines. *Circulation.* 2005;112(12):e154-e235.

15. Felix SB, Stangl V, Kieback A, et al. Acute hemodynamic effects of beta-blockers in patients with severe congestive heart failure: comparison of celiprolol and esmolol. *J Cardiovasc Pharmacol.* 2001;38:666-671.

16. Barbier GH, Shettigar UR, Appunn DO. Clinical rationale for the use of an ultra-short acting beta-blocker: esmolol. *Int J Clin Pharmacol Ther.* 1995;33:212-218.

17. Anonymous. Intravenous esmolol for the treatment of supraventricular tachyarrhytmia: results of a multicenter, baseline-controlled safety and efficacy study in 160 patients. *Am Heart J.* 1986;112:498-505.

18. Askenazi J, MacCosbe PE, Hoff J, Turlapaty P, Hua TA, Laddu A. Hemodynamic effects of esmolol, an ultra-short acting beta blocker. *J Clin Pharmacol.* 1987;27:567-573.

19. Angaran DM, Schultz NJ, Tschida VH. Esmolol hydrochloride: an ultrashort-acting, β-adrenergic blocking agent. *Clin Pharm.* 1986;5:288-303.

20. Lowenthal DT, Porter RS, Schari R, Turapaty P, Laddu AR, Matier WL. Esmolol-digoxin drug interaction. *J Clin Pharmacol.* 1987;27:561-566.

21. Shettigar UR, Toole JG, Appunn DO. Combined use of esmolol and digoxin in the acute treatment of atrial fibrillation and flutter. *Am Heart J.* 1993;126:368-374.

22. Sagie A, Strasberg B, Kusnieck J, Sclarovsky S. Symptomatic bradycardia induced by the combination of oral diltiazem and beta blockers. *Clin Cardiol.* 1991;14:314-316.

23. Leor J, Levartowsky D, Sharon C, Farfel Z. Amiodarone and B-adrenergic blockers: An interaction with metoprolol but not with atenolol. *Am Heart J*. 1988;116:206-207.

24. Cheymol G, Poirier JM, Carrupt PA, Testa B, et al. Pharmacokinetics of β-adrenoceptor blockers in obese and normal volunteers. *Br J Clin Pharmacol*. 1997;43:563-570.

25. Walstad RA, Berg Kj, Wessel-Aas T, Nilsen OG. Labetalol in the treatment of hypertension in patients with normal and impaired renal function. *Acta Med Scand Suppl*. 1982;665: 135-141.

26. Wood AJ, Ferry DG, Bailey RR. Elimination kinetics of labetalol in severe renal failure. *Br J Clin Pharmacol*. 1982;13(suppl 1):81S-86S.

27. Thompson FD, Joekes AM, Hussein MM. Monotherapy with labetalol for hypertensive patients with normal and impaired renal function. *Br J Clin Pharmacol*. 1979;8(suppl 2):129S-133s.

28. MacCarthy EP, Bloomfield SS. Labetalol: a review of its pharmacology, pharmacokinetics, clinical uses and adverse effects. *Pharmacotherapy*. 1983;3:193-219.

29. Labetalol hydrochloride injection (package insert). Bedford, OH: Bedford Laboratories, Inc.; June 2000.

30. Halstenson Ce, Opsahl JA, Pence TV, et al. The disposition and dynamics of labetalol in patients on dialysis. *Clin Pharmacol Ther*. 1986;40:462-468.

31. Homeida M, Jackson L, Roberts CJ. Decreased first-pass metabolism of labetalol in chronic liver disease. *Br Med J*. 1978;2:1048-1050.

32. Wilson DJ, Wallin JD, Vlachakis ND, et al. Intravenous labetalol in the treatment of severe hypertension and hypertensive emergencies. *Am J Med*. 1983;75:95-102.

33. Rosei EA, Trust PM, Brown JJ. Intravenous labetalol in severe hypertension. *Lancet*. 1975;2:1093-1094.

34. Marik PE, Varon J. Hypertensive crises challenges and management. *Chest*. 2007;131:1949-1962.

35. Bailey RR. Labetalol in the treatment of patients with hypertension and renal function impairment. *Br J Clin Pharmacol*. 1979;8(suppl 2):135S-140S.

36. Williams JG, DeVoos K, Craswell PW. Labetalol in the treatment of hypertensive renal patients. *Med J Aust*. 1978;25:225-228.

37. Clark JA, Zimmerman HJ, Tanner LA. Labetalol hepatotoxicity. *Ann Intern Med*. 1990;113:210-213.

38. Douglas DD, Yang Rd, Jensen P, Thiele DL. Fatal labetalol-induced injury. *Am J Med*. 1989;87:235-236.

39. Mason JM, Dickinson HO, Nicolson DJ, Campbell F, et al. The diabetogenic potential of thiazide-type diuretic and beta-blocker combinations in patients with hypertension. *J Hypertens*. 2005;23:1777-1781.

40. Kunz I, Schorr U, Klaus S, Sharma AM. Resting metabolic rate and substrate use in obesity hypertension. *Hypertension*. 2000;36:26-32.

41. Lopressor (metoprolol tartrate). Suffern, NY: Novartis Pharmaceuticals Corporation; 2009.

42. Lloyd P, John VA, Signy M, Smith SE. The effect of impaired renal function on the pharmacokinetics of metoprolol after single administration of a 14/190 metoprolol OROS system. *Am Heart J*. 1990;20(2):478-482.

43. Seiler KU, Schuster KJ, Meyer GJ, et al. The pharmacokinetics of metoprolol and its metabolites in dialysis patients. *Clin Pharmacokinet*. 1980;5(2):192-198.

44. Bennett WM, Aronoff GR, Morrison G, et al. Drug prescribing in renal failure: dosing guidelines for adults. *Am J Kidney Dis*. 1983;3:155-193.

45. Bortolotti A, Castelli D, Verotta D, Bonati M. Pharmacokinetic and pharmacodynamic modeling of metoprolol in rabbits with liver failure. *Eur J Drug Metab Pharmacokinet*. 1989;14(2):145-151.

46. Ross PJ, Lewis MJ, Sheridan DJ, et al. Adrenergic hypersensitivity after beta-blocker withdrawal. *Br Heart J*. 1981;45:637-642.

47. Fishman WH. Bea-adrenergic blocker withdrawal. *Am J Cardiol*. 1987;59(13):26f-32f.

48. Walden RJ, Tomlinson B, Bhattacharjee P, Prichard BN. The beta-adrenergic blockade phenomenon. *J Pharmacol*. 1983;14(2):35-48.
49. Cleviprex (package insert). Parsippany, NJ: The Medicines Company; 2008.
50. Phung OJ, Baker WL, White CM, Coleman CI. Focus on clevidipine. *Formulary*. 2009;44(4):102-107.
51. Deeks ED, Keating GM, Keam SJ. Clevidipine: a review of its use in the management of acute hypertension. *Am J Cardiovasc Drugs*. 2009;9(2):117-134.
52. Vuylsteke A, Milner Q, Ericsson H, et al. Pharmacokinetics and pulmonary extraction of clevidipine, a new vasodilating ultrashort-acting dihydropyridine, during cardiopulmonary bypass. *Br J Anaesth*. 2000;85(5):683-689.
53. Ericsson H, Tholander B, Regardh CG. In vitro hydrolysis rate and protein-binding of clevidipine, a new ultrashort-acting calcium antagonist metabolized by esterases, in different animal species and man. *Eur J Pharm Sci*. 1999;8(1):29-37.
54. Pollack CV, Varon J, Garrison NA, et al. Clevidipine, and intravenous dihydropyridine calcium channel blocker, is safe and effective for the treatment of patients with acute severe hypertension. *Ann Emerg Med*. 2009;53:329-338.
55. Aronson S, Dyke CM, Stierer KA, et al. The ECLIPSE trials: comparative studies of clevidipine to nitroglycerin, sodium nitroprusside, and nicardipine for acute hypertension treatment in cardiac surgery patients. *Anesth Analg*. 2008;107:1110-1121.
56. Ericsson H, Bredburg U, Eriksson U, et al. Pharmacokinetics and arteriovenous differences in clevidipine concentration following a short- and a long-term intravenous infusion in healthy volunteers. *Anesthesiology*. 2000;92:993-1001.
57. Levy JH, Mancoa MY, Gitter R, et al. Clevidipine effectively and rapidly controls blood pressure preoperatively in cardiac surgery patients" The results of the randomized, placebo-controlled efficacy study of clevidipine assessing its preoperative antihypertensive effect in cardiac surgery-1. *Anesth Analg*. 2007;105:918-925.
58. Erickson AL, DeGrado JR, Fanikos JR. Clevidipine: a short acting intravenous dihydropyridine calcium channel blocker for the management of hypertension. *Pharmacotherapy*. 2010;30(5):515-528.
59. Dasta J, Boucher B, Brophy G, et al. Intravenous to oral conversion of antihypertensives: a toolkit for guideline development. *Ann Pharmacother*. 2010;44:1430-1447.
60. Zhang JG, Dehal SS, Ho T, et al. Human Cytochrome P450 induction and inhibition potential of clevidipine and its primary metabolite H152/81. *Drug Metab Dispos*. 2006;34(5):734-737.
61. Enalaprilat (package insert). Bedford, OH: Bedford Laboratories; June 2005.
62. Elung-Jensen T, Heisterberg J, Kamoer AL, et al. High serum enalaprilat in chronic renal failure. *J Renin Angiotensin Aldosterone Syst*. 2001;2(4):240-245.
63. Greenbaum R, Zucchelli P, Caspi A, et al. Comparison of the pharmacokinetics of fosinoprilat with enalaprilat and lisinopril in patients with congestive heart failure and chronic renal insufficiency. *Br J Clin Pharmacol*. 2001;49:23-31.
64. Kelly JG, Doyle GD, Carmody M, et al. Pharmacokinetics of lisinopril, enalapril and enalaprilat in renal failure: effects of hemodialysis. *Br J Clin Pharmacol*. 1988;26:781-786.
65. Mirenda J, Edwards C. Prolonged hypotension by enalaprilat in a case of renal artery stenosis. *Anesth Analg*. 1992;75:1017-1020.
66. Flack JM, Mensah GA, Ferrario CM. Using angiotensin converting enzyme inhibitors in African-American hypertensives: a new approach to treating hypertension and preventing target-organ damage. *Curr Med Res Opin*. 2000;16:66-79.
67. Exner DV, Dries DL, Domanski MJ, et al. Lesser response to angiotensin- converting-enzyme inhibitor therapy in black as compared with white patients with left ventricular dysfunction. *N Engl J Med*. 2001;344:1351-1357.
68. Brown NJ, Ray WA, Snowden M, et al. Black Americans have an increased rate of angiotensin converting enzyme inhibitor-associated angioedema. *Clin Pharmacol Ther*. 1996;60:8-13.
69. Elliott WJ. Higher incidence of discontinuation of angiotensin converting enzyme inhibitors due to cough in black subjects. *Clin Pharmacol Ther*. 1996;60:582-588.

70. Schattner A, Kozak N, Friedman J. Captopril-induced jaundice: report of 2 cases and a review of 13 additional reports in the literature. *Am J Med Sci.* 2001;322(4):236-240.

71. Chou JW, Yu CJ, Chuang PH, et al. Successful treatment of fosinopril-induced severe cholestatic jaundice with plasma exchange. *Ann Pharmacother.* 2008;42(12):1887-1892.

72. Hydralazine hydrochloride injection (package insert). Shirley, NY: American Regent; January 2009.

73. Bennett WM, Aronoff GR, Golper TA, et al. *Drug Prescribing in Renal Failure.* Philadelphia: American College of Physicians; 1994.

74. Jackson G, Pierscianowski TA, Mahon W, et al. Inappropriate antihypertensive therapy in the elderly. *Lancet.* 1976;2:1317-1318.

75. Finks SW, Finks AL, Self TH. Hydralazine-induced lupus: maintaining vigilance with increased use in patients with heart failure. *South Med J.* 2006;99(1):18-22.

76. Vidrio H, Tena I. Hydralazine tachycardia and sympathetic cardiovascular reactivity in normal subjects. *Clin Pharmacol Ther.* 1980;28:587-591.

77. Gould L, Reddy CVR, Zen B, et al. Electrophysiologic properties of hydralazine in man. *Pace Clin Electrophysiol.* 1980;3:548-554.

78. Haitas B, Meyer TE, Angel ME, Reef E. Comparative haemodynamic effects of intravenous nisoldipine and hydralazine in congestive heart failure. *Br J Clin Pharmacol.* 1990;29(3): 366-368.

79. Pezzarossa A, Cimicchi MC, Orlandi N, et al. Lack of effect of nicardipine and diltiazem on glucose- and arginine-induced insulin release in obese subjects. *Cardiovasc Drugs Ther.* 1988;2(5):669-672.

80. Raccah D, Pettenuzzo-Mollo M, Provendier O, et al. Comparison of the effects of captopril and nicardipine on insulin sensitivity and thrombotic profile in patients with hypertension and android obesity CaptISM Study Group. Captopril Insulin Sensitivity Multicenter Study Group. *Am J Hypertens.* 1994;7(8):731-738.

81. Cardene premixed intravenous injection (nicardipine hydrochloride premixed intravenous injection) package insert. Bedminster, NJ: EKR Therapeutics, Inc.; 2009.

82. Razak TA, McNeil JJ, Sewell BB, et al. The effect of hepatic cirrhosis on the pharmacokinetics and blood pressure response to nicardipine. *Clin Pharmacol Ther.* 1990;47(4):463-469.

83. Reddy P, Yeh YC. Use of injectable nicardipine for neurovascular indications. *Pharmacotherapy.* 2009;29(4):398-409.

84. Aya AGM, Mangin R, Hoffet M, et al. Intravenous nicardipine for severe hypertension in preeclampsia – effects of an acute treatment on mother and fetus. *Intensive Care Med.* 1999;25:1277-1281.

85. Wang EQ, Fung HL. Effects of obesity on the pharmacodynamics of nitroglycerin in conscious rats. *AAPS PharmSci.* 2002;4(4):E28.

86. Alpert JS. Nitrate therapy in the elderly. *Am J Cardiol.* 1990;65:23J-27J.

87. Cahalan MK, Hashimoto Y, Aizawa K, et al. Elderly, conscious patients have an accentuated hypotensive response to nitroglycerin. *Anesthesiology.* 1992;77:646-655.

88. Nitroglycerin injection (package insert). Shirley, NY: American Regent, Inc.; 2005.

89. Devlin J, Dasta JF, Kleinschmidt K, Varon J. Patterns of antihypertensive use in patients with acute severe hypertension from a non-neurological cause: The STAT Registry. *Pharmacotherapy.* 2010;30:1087-1096.

90. Wainwright RJ, Foran JPM, Padaria SF, et al. The long-term safety and tolerability of transdermal glyceryl trinitrate, when used with a patch-free interval in patients with stable angina. *Br J Clin Pharmacol.* 1993;47:178-182.

91. Bank J. Migraine with aura after administration of sublingual nitroglycerin tablets. *Headache.* 2001;41:84-87.

92. Olsson G, Allgen J. Is there an optimal prophylactic nitrate therapy? *Eur Heart J.* 1991;12(suppl A):21-23.

93. GISSI-3 investigators. GISSI-3: Effects of lisinopril and transdermal glyceryl trinitrate singly and together on 6-week mortality and ventricular function after acute myocardial infarction. *Lancet.* 1994;343(8906):1115-1122.

94. Webb DJ, Freestone S, Allen MJ, et al. Sildenafil citrate and blood-pressure-lowering drugs: results of drug interaction studies with an organic nitrate and a calcium antagonist. *Am J Cardiol*. 1999;83:21C-28C.

95. Rindone JP, Sloane EP. Cyanide toxicity from sodium nitroprusside: risks and management. *Ann Pharmacother*. 1992;26:515-519.

96. American Heart Association. Guidelines 2005 Cardiopulmonary resuscitation and emergency cardiovascular care. Part 7.4 Monitoring Medications. Circulation 2005; 112;Iv-78-IV-83.

97. Aronoff GR, Bennett WM, Berns JS, et al. *Drug Prescribing in Renal Failure: Dosing Guidelines for adults and Children*. 5th ed. Philadelphia: American College of Physicians; 2007.

98. Nitropress (sodium nitroprusside) Injection Solution (package insert). Lake Forest, IL: Hospira, Inc.; October 2006.

99. Nessim SL, Richardson RM. Dialysis for thiocyanate intoxication: a case report and review of the literature. *ASAIO J*. 2006;52:749-781.

100. Lindquist P, Rosling H, Tydent H. Cyanide release from sodium nitroprusside drug in bypass in hypothermia. *Acta Anaesthesiol Scand*. 1989;33:686-688.

101. Moore RA, Geller EA, Gallagher JD, Clark DL. Effect of hypothermic cardiopulmonary bypass on nitroprusside metabolism. *Clin Pharmacol Ther*. 1995;37:680-683.

102. Varon J. Treatment of acute severe hypertension. *Drugs*. 2008;68:283-297.

103. Mann T, Cohn PF, Holman LB, et al. Effect of nitroprusside on regional myocardial blood flow in coronary artery disease. Results in 25 patients and comparison with nitroglycerin. *Circulation*. 1978;57:732-738.

104. Pasch T, Schulz V, Hoppenshauser G. Nitroprusside-induced formation of cyanide and its detoxification with thiosulphate during deliberate hypotension. *J Cardiovasc Pharmacol*. 1983;5:77-85.

105. Cohn JN, Franciosa JA, Francis GS, et al. Effect of short-term infusion of sodium nitroprusside on mortality rate in acute myocardial infarction complicated by left ventricular failure: results of a Veterans Administration cooperative study. *N Engl J Med*. 1982;306:1129-1135.

106. Rhoney D, Peacock WF. Intravenous therapies for hypertensive emergencies, part 1. *Am J Health Syst Pharm*. 2009;66:1343-1352.

107. Ivankovich AD, Braverman B, Stephens TS, Shulman M, Heyman HJ. Sodium thiosulfate disposition in humans: relation to sodium nitroprusside toxicity. *Anesthesiology*. 1983;58: 11-17.

108. Cheung AT, Cruz-Shiavone GE, Meng QC, et al. Cardiopulmonary bypass, hemolysis and nitroprusside induced cyanide toxicity. *Anesth Analg*. 2007;105:29-33.

109. Flolan® (package insert). Research Triangle Park, NC: GlaxoSmithKline; January 2008.

110. Moncada S, Vane JR. Prostacyclin and blood coagulation. *Drugs*. 1981;21:430-437.

111. Zussman RM, Rubin RH, Cato AE, et al. Hemodialysis using prostacyclin instead of heparin as the sole antithrombin agent. *N Engl J Med*. 1981;304:934-939.

112. Addonizio VP, Fisher CA, Bowen JC, et al. Prostacyclin in lieu of anticoagulation with heparin for extracorporeal circulation. *Trans Am Soc Artif Intern Organs*. 1981;27:304-307.

113. Hory B, Saint-Miller Y, Perol JC. Prostacyclin as the sole antithrombic agent for acute renal failure hemodialysis. *Nephron*. 1983;73:669-678.

114. Fiaccadori E, Maggiore U, Rotelli C, et al. Continuous haemofiltration in acute renal failure with prostacyclin as the sole anti-haemostatic agent. *Intensive Care Med*. 2002;82:586-593.

115. Sulica R, Emre S, Poon M. Medical management of porto-pulmonary hypertension and right heart failure prior to living-related liver transplantation. *Congest Heart Fail*. 2004;10(4): 192-194.

116. Swanson KL, Wiesner RH, Nyberg SL, et al. Survival in portopulmonary hypertension: Mayo Clinic experience categorized by treatment subgroups. *Am J Transplant*. 2008;8(11):2445-2453.

117. Jones K. Prostacyclin. In: Peacock AJ, ed. *Pulmonary Circulation. A Handbook for Clinicians*. London: Chapman & Hall; 1996:115-122.

118. Centers for Disease Control. Bloodstream infections among patients treated with intravenous epoprostenol or intravenous treprostinil for pulmonary arterial hypertension–seven sites, United States, 2003–2006. *MMWR Morb Mortal Wkly Rep.* 2007;56(8):170-172.

119. Yap RL, Mermel LA. Micrococcus infection in patients receiving epoprostenol by continuous infusion. *Eur J Clin Microbiol Infect Dis.* 2003;22:704-705.

120. Ventavis® (Iloprost inhalation solution) package insert. South San Francisco, CA: Actelion Pharmaceuticals US; April 2010.

121. Remodulin® (Treprostinil injection) package insert. Research Triangle Park, NC: United Therapeutics Corporation; January 2010.

122. Sakai T, Planinsic EM, Mathier MA, et al. Initial experience using continuous intravenous treprostinil to manage pulmonary arterial hypertension in patients with end-stage liver disease. *Eur Soc Organ Transplant.* 2009;22:554-561.

123. Wade MF, Baker FJ, Roscigno R, et al. Absolute bioavailability and pharmacokinetics of treprostinil sodium administered by acute subcutaneous infusion. *J Clin Pharmacol.* 2004;44:83.

124. Laliberte K, Arneson C, Jeffs R, et al. Pharmacokinetics and steady-state bioequivalence of treprostinil sodium (Remoduln) administered by the intravenous and subcutaneous route to normal volunteers. *J Cardiovasc Pharmacol.* 2004;44(2):209-214.

125. Skoro-Sajer N, Lang IM, Harja E, et al. A clinical comparison of slow-and rapid escalation treprostinil (Remodulin) dosing regimens in patients with pulmonary hypertension. *Clin Pharmacokinet.* 2008;47(9):611-618.

126. McLaughlin VV, Gaine SP, Barst RJ, et al. Efficacy and safety of treprostinil: an Epoprostenol analog for primary pulmonary hypertension. *J Cardiovasc Pharmacol.* 2003;41:293-299.

127. Oudiz RJ, Farber HW. Dosing considerations in the use of intravenous prostanoids in pulmonary arterial hypertension: an evidence-based review. *Am Heart J.* 2009;157:625-635.

128. Tyvaso® (Treprostinil inhalation solution) package insert. Research Triangle Park, NC: United Therapeutics Corporation; July 2009.

129. Tyvaso® inhalation system: care and replacement of the system. http://www.tyvaso.com/care_of_the_system.aspx. Accessed June 14, 2010.

Index

S.L. Kane-Gill and J. Dasta (eds.),
High-Risk IV Medications in Special Patient Populations,
DOI: 10.1007/978-0-85729-606-1, © Springer-Verlag London Limited 2011